War and Public Health

War and Public Health

Second Edition

Edited by

Barry S. Levy, MD, MPH
Adjunct Professor of Public Health
Tufts University School of Medicine
Sherborn, Massachusetts

Victor W. Sidel, MD
Distinguished University Professor of Social Medicine
Montefiore Medical Center
Albert Einstein Medical College
Bronx, New York

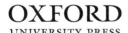

OXFORD
UNIVERSITY PRESS

Published in collaboration with
the American Public Health Association

2008

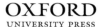

OXFORD
UNIVERSITY PRESS

Oxford University Press, Inc., publishes works that further
Oxford University's objective of excellence
in research, scholarship, and education.

Oxford   New York
Auckland   Cape Town   Dar es Salaam   Hong Kong   Karachi
Kuala Lumpur   Madrid   Melbourne   Mexico City   Nairobi
New Delhi   Shanghai   Taipei   Toronto

With offices in
Argentina   Austria   Brazil   Chile   Czech Republic   France   Greece
Guatemala   Hungary   Italy   Japan   Poland   Portugal   Singapore
South Korea   Switzerland   Thailand   Turkey   Ukraine   Vietnam

Copyright © 2008 by Oxford University Press, Inc.

Published by Oxford University Press, Inc.
198 Madison Avenue, New York, New York 10016

www.oup.com

Oxford is a registered trademark of Oxford University Press

Library of Congress Cataloging-in-Publication Data
War and public health / edited by Barry S. Levy, Victor W. Sidel.—2nd ed.
   p. ; cm.
Includes bibliographical references and index.
ISBN 978-0-19-531118-1
ISBN 978-0-19-531127-3 (pbk.)   1. War—Medical aspects.   2. War and society.
[DNLM: 1. Public Health.   2. War. WA 30 W253 2007]
I. Levy, Barry S.   II. Sidel, Victor W.
RA646.W37 2007
362.109—dc22   2007018265

Printed in the United States of America
on acid-free paper

We dedicate this book to Bernard Lown, M.D.,
and William H. Foege, M.D., M.P.H., for
their outstanding contributions to preventing war
and promoting peace and public health.

Foreword

War and militarism have catastrophic effects on human health and well-being. These effects include casualties during war, long-lasting physical and psychological effects on noncombatant adults and children, the reduction of human and financial resources available to meet social needs, and the creation of a climate in which violence is a primary mode of dealing with conflict.

War and Public Health is a milestone in documenting the impact of war and militarism on human health. It also demonstrates how health professionals, working through organizations like the American Public Health Association, the Centers for Disease Control and Prevention, the International Rescue Committee, and the International Physicians for the Prevention of Nuclear War, can reduce the impact of war and contribute to its prevention.

The participation of respected and trustworthy intermediaries and the willingness of parties to communicate with each other are two key elements in preventing war and resolving conflicts through nonviolent means. Through our work at The Carter Center, I have personally seen the importance of these and other factors in preventing or resolving conflicts in Africa and Latin America, as well as here in the United States.

Reprinted, with permission, from the first edition of *War and Public Health*.

Because they promote healing, most health professionals are respected and trusted. They should be leaders in constantly working to prevent the pain and suffering that result from war, which has an unconscionable impact on human health. It is commendable that the editors and contributing authors of this book have addressed issues of war and militarism in a public health context. But, as the editors state, we, as a global society, need to devote considerably more resources to improving our ability to prevent war. We need to gather and analyze information systematically, and then we need to ensure that this information is used to educate national leaders and others.

Public health workers led the fight to eradicate smallpox. They are now working to eliminate other diseases. We should all strive for a time when, through the efforts of public health workers and others, war too will be eliminated.

Jimmy Carter

Preface

War has an enormous and tragic impact—both directly and indirectly—on public health. Yet, despite all of the effects of war on human health and well-being, war and the prevention of war have generally not been seen as integral parts of the work of public health professionals and have not been adequately covered in their professional education.

Many public health workers provide services in war-torn areas, on either a short-term or a long-term basis; they would benefit from more systematically organized background information on war and its consequences and on the prevention of war. Other public health workers are involved in the prevention of domestic and street violence in their communities and would benefit from systematically organized background information on the attempts to prevent international violence and its consequences. Many public health workers help to set political agendas in their communities; they too would benefit from information on how military budgets divert resources from health and other human services, how arms sales contribute to violence and war in other nations, and how expanded economic development aid could lead to prevention of international violence and war.

This book has two main purposes. The first is to provide a systematic survey of information on the direct and indirect consequences of war on public health and the roles that public health professionals and their organizations can play in preventing war and its consequences. A wide spectrum of other individuals and their organizations, including economists, sociologists, and policy makers, also play roles in the prevention of war and its consequences, and can benefit from this information.

The second purpose of this book is to help make war and its prevention an integral part of public health education, research, and practice. Like other public health problems, war is preventable. The same, or similar, approaches that have been used successfully to prevent or totally eliminate other public health problems can be used to prevent war and its consequences.

The prevention of war needs to be integrated into the curricula of schools of public health, other schools for health workers, and other academic institutions. It needs to become a focus for research into how war and its effects on public health can be prevented. And it needs to become a greater part of public health practice. National associations of health professionals should have peace sections, just as they have sections on health administration, maternal and child health, and early detection of disease.

The first edition of this book, which was published in hard cover by Oxford University Press in 1997 and in an updated paperback edition by the American Public Health Association (APHA) in 2000, arose from a session that we organized at the 1991 APHA Annual Meeting. That session focused primarily on the multiple impacts on public health of the then-recent Persian Gulf War. The strong support of many participants during and after that session, the encouragement of our colleagues, and the leadership of APHA and its Publications Board and staff led us to pursue the development of the first edition of this book.

More than 10 years have passed since then. And, unfortunately, the world is more violent in many ways than it was in 1997.

The book is divided into six parts. Part I places war in the context of public health. Part II addresses the epidemiology of war and the impact of war on health, human rights, and the environment. Part III focuses on major categories of weapons and their adverse health effects. Part IV addresses the adverse effects of war on children, women, refugees and internally displaced persons, and prisoners of war. Part V addresses the health impact of five specific wars of varied type and magnitude. And Part VI discusses the roles of public health professionals and organizations during war and the roles they can play in preventing war and reducing its public health consequences.

The views expressed in this book are those of the contributors and editors and are not necessarily those of the organizations with which they are affiliated.

We would like this book to be used not only to provide necessary information about war and its consequences but also to motivate and inspire public health professionals, students, and others to work for sustainable peace throughout the world, for nonviolent approaches to conflict resolution, and for the freeing of resources and energies that have been used for war and the preparation for war to address the other serious public health issues that threaten humankind.

B.S.L. and V.W.S.
Sherborn, Massachusetts
Bronx, New York
July 2007

Acknowledgments

Developing and producing the second edition of *War and Public Health* has taken the combined skills, resources, and dedication of many people to whom we are profoundly grateful.

We thank all of the contributors to this book, who worked diligently in writing and revising their chapters and in identifying references and illustrative materials.

We express our appreciation to Heather Merrell for her excellent administrative assistance in the development of this book, and to Deyanira Suarez for her excellent help in the preparation of several chapters.

We deeply appreciate the assistance and support of William Lamsback, medical editor of Oxford University Press, and the excellent work of production editor Keith Faivre, assistant editor Ciara Vincent, copyeditor Beverly Braunlich, and indexer Michael Ferreira. We acknowledge the guidance of Jeffrey House, former medical editor of Oxford University Press, in the development of the first edition of this book.

Finally, we express our deep gratitude and appreciation to Nancy Levy and Ruth Sidel for their continuing encouragement and support.

Contents

Foreword by Jimmy Carter, vii

Contributors, xix

Part I Introduction

1. War and Public Health: An Overview, 3
   Barry S. Levy and Victor W. Sidel

     Box 1-1. The Brutality of War (Jennifer Leaning), 6
     Box 1-2. Terrorism and the "War on Terror"
              (Barry S. Levy and Victor W. Sidel), 13

Part II Consequences of War

2. The Epidemiology of War, 23
   Richard Garfield

     Box 2-1. Armed Conflict and Human Development (Richard Garfield), 30

3. War and Human Rights, 37
   George J. Annas and H. Jack Geiger

4. The Impact of War on Mental Health, 51
Evan D. Kanter

5. The Impact of War on the Environment, 69
Arthur H. Westing

>   Box 5-1. Malignancies Associated with Radioactive
>   Fallout (Barry S. Levy and Victor W. Sidel), 78

Part III Types of Weapons

6. Conventional Weapons, 87
Wendy Cukier

>   Box 6-1. Protecting Civilians (Geneva Convention IV), 90

7. Landmines, 102
Susannah Sirkin, James C. Cobey, and Eric Stover

>   Box 7-1. Mine Risk Education (Avid Reza,
>   Reuben Nogueira-McCarthy, and Mark Anderson), 112

8. Chemical Weapons, 117
Ernest C. Lee and Stefanos N. Kales

9. Biological Weapons, 135
Barry S. Levy and Victor W. Sidel

>   Box 9-1. The Case Against Plans for a Biodefense
>   Research Laboratory (David Ozonoff), 139

10. Nuclear Weapons, 152
Patrice M. Sutton and Robert M. Gould

>   Box 10-1. Human Health Effects of Weapons Production
>   (Tim K. Takaro and Laurence J. Fuortes), 163

Part IV Vulnerable Populations

11. The Impact of War on Children, 179
Joanna Santa Barbara

12. The Impact of War on Women, 193
Mary-Wynne Ashford

13. Displaced Persons and War, 207
Michael J. Toole

>   Box 13-1. Darfur (Susannah Sirkin), 210

14. Detainees and the New Face of Torture, 227
Leonard S. Rubenstein and Stephen N. Xenakis

Part V Specific Wars

15. The Iraq War, 243
Barry S. Levy and Victor W. Sidel

   Box 15-1. The New American Militarism
              (Andrew J. Bacevich), 245
   Box 15-2. A Soldier's View (Garett Reppenhagen), 253
   Box 15-3. A Perspective from Military Families
              (Elizabeth Frederick), 254

16. The War in Chechnya, 264
Khassan Baiev

17. War in the Democratic Republic of Congo, 279
Les Roberts and Charles Lubula Muganda

18. Wars in Latin America, 288
Charlie Clements and Tim K. Takaro

19. The Vietnam War, 313
Myron Allukian, Jr., and Paul L. Atwood

Part VI Prevention of War and Its Health Consequences

20. A Public Health Approach to Preventing the Health
Consequences of Armed Conflict, 339
Avid Reza, Mark Anderson, and James A. Mercy

21. International Law, 357
Peter Weiss

22. The Roles of Humanitarian Assistance Organizations, 369
Ronald J. Waldman

23. The Roles of Nongovernmental Organizations, 381
John Loretz

24. The Roles and Ethical Dilemmas for Military
Medical Care Workers, 393
Victor W. Sidel and Barry S. Levy

25. The Roles of Health Professionals in Postconflict Situations, 409
Susannah Sirkin, Susanna Facci Calì, and Mary Ellen Keough

   Box 25-1. The Impact of Postconflict Situations on
              Health Workers (Susannah Sirkin, Susanna Facci Calì,
              and Mary Ellen Keough), 412

26. Peacemaking in the Aftermath of Disasters, 424
Michael Renner

27. Educating Health Professionals on Peace and Human Rights, 440
    Neil Arya, Caecilie Böck Buhmann, and Klaus Melf

      Box 27-1. Potential of Health and Development Work to
                Worsen Health and Safety (Neil Arya,
                Caecilie Böck Buhmann, and Klaus Melf), 443

28. Toward a Culture of Peace, 452
    Mary-Wynne Ashford

    Appendix: A List of Some Organizations That
              Promote Peace, 463

    Index, 469

Contributors

Myron Allukian, Jr, DDS, MPH
Oral Health Consultant
Massachusetts League of Community
  Health Centers and Lutheran
  Medical Center
46 Louders Lane
Boston, MA 02130
617-654-8920
617-426-0097 (fax)
MyAlluk@aol.com

Mark Anderson, MD, MPH
International Emergency and Refugee
  Health Branch
Centers for Disease Control and Prevention
1600 Clifton Road, MS E-97
Atlanta, GA 30333
404-498-0821
404-638-5524 (fax)
manderson@cdc.gov

George J. Annas, JD, MPH
Edward Utley Professor and Chair
Department of Health Law, Bioethics
  & Human Rights
Boston University School of Public Health
715 Albany Street
Boston, Massachusetts 02118
617-638-4626
617-414-1464 (fax)
annasgj@bu.edu

Neil Arya, BASc, MD, CCFP, FCFP
Assistant Clinical Professor of
  Family Medicine, McMaster University
Adjunct Professor of Family Medicine,
  University of Western Ontario
Adjunct Professor of Environment and
  Resource Studies, University of Waterloo
99 Northfield Dr. E. #202
Waterloo, Ontario N2K 3P9
Canada
519-886-2643
519-886-7090 (fax)
narya@admmail.uwaterloo.ca

Mary-Wynne Ashford, MD, PhD
International Physicians for the
   Prevention of Nuclear War
4915 Prospect Lake Road
Victoria, BC V9E 1J5
Canada
250-479-9189
250-479-9309 (fax)
mashford@uvic.ca

Paul L. Atwood, PhD
American Studies Department
Research Associate, The William Joiner
   Center for the Study of War and
   Social Consequences
University of Massachusetts Boston
100 Morrissey Boulevard
Boston, MA 02125
617-287-5850
617-287-5855 (fax)
Paul.Atwood@umb.edu

Andrew J. Bacevich, PhD
Department of International
   Relations
Boston University
154 Bay State Road, Room 201
Boston, MA 02215
617-358-0194
617-358-0190 (fax)
bacevich@bu.edu

Khassan Baiev, MD
Chairman
International Committee for the
   Children of Chechnya
P.O. Box 381305
Cambridge, MA 02238
617-319-6489
drbaiev@hotmail.com

Caecilie Böck Buhmann, MD, BSc
International Physicians for the
   Prevention of Nuclear War
Refnaesgade 53 3 tv
DK-2200 Copenhagen N
Denmark
cbuhmann2002@yahoo.com

Charlie Clements, MD, MPH, MSc
President and Chief Executive
   Officer
Unitarian Universalist Service
   Committee (UUSC)
689 Massachusetts Avenue
Cambridge, MA 02139
617-301-4315
617-868-7102 (fax)
cclements@uusc.org

James C. Cobey, MD, MPH
Orthopedic Surgeon
106 Irving Street, NW, Suite 420
Washington, DC 20010
202-877-7111
202-877-7554 (fax)
cobey@worldnet.att.net

Wendy L. Cukier, MA, MBA, PhD,
   DU (hon), LLD (hon), MSc
Associate Dean, Ryerson University
President, Coalition for Gun Control
575 Bay Street
Toronto, Ontario M5G 2C5
Canada
416-979-5000 x 6740
416-979-5294 (fax)
wcukier@compuserve.com

Susanna Facci Calì
Research Consultant
Physicians for Human Rights
2 Arrow Street
Cambridge, MA 02138
617-301-4200
617-301-4250 (fax)
s_faccicali@yahoo.com

Laurence J. Fortes, MD
Professor, Department of Occupational &
   Environmental Health
University of Iowa School of Public Health
2941 Steindler Building
Iowa City, IA 52242
319-335-9819
319-335-4225 (fax)
laurence-fortes@uiowa.edu

Elizabeth Frederick
Military Families Speak Out
mfsodc@gmail.com

Richard Garfield, RN, DrPH
Henrik H. Bendixen Professor of Clinical
  International Nursing
Columbia University School of Nursing
Advisor to the Assistant Director-General
Health Action in Crises, World Health
  Organization
Box 6
630 West 168th Street
New York, NY 10032
212-305-3248
212-305-6937 (fax)
rmg3@columbia.edu

H. Jack Geiger, MD, MSciHyg
Logan Professor Emeritus of Community
  Health and Social Medicine
Past President, Physicians for Human
  Rights
CUNY Medical School
City College of New York, H-405A
138th Street at Convent Avenue
New York, NY 10031
212-650-6860
718-802-9141 (fax)
jgeiger@igc.org

Robert M. Gould, MD
Associate Pathologist, Kaiser Hospital
San Jose, California
Past-President, Physicians for
  Social Responsibility
311 Douglass Street
San Francisco, CA 94114
408-972-7299
408-972-6429 (fax)
rmgould1@yahoo.com

Stefanos N. Kales, MD, MPH, FACP,
  FACOEM
Director, Employee and Industrial
  Medicine, Cambridge Health
  Alliance
Assistant Professor of Medicine,
  Harvard Medical School
Assistant Professor of Occupational
  Medicine, Harvard School of Public
  Health
1493 Cambridge Street
Cambridge, MA 02139
617-665-1580
617-665-1672 (fax)
skales@challiance.org

Evan D. Kanter, MD, PhD
Staff Psychiatrist
VA Puget Sound Health Care System
Clinical Assistant Professor
Department of Psychiatry and
  Behavioral Sciences
University of Washington School
  of Medicine
Box 358280
Seattle, WA 98195-8280
206-764-2925
206-764-2572 (fax)
ekanter@u.washington.edu

Mary Ellen Keough, MPH
Director for Educational Programs,
  Meyers Primary Care Institute
Instructor, Department of Family
  Medicine and Community Health
University of Massachusetts Medical
  School
630 Plantation Street
Worcester, MA 01605
508-791-7392
508-595-2200 (fax)
meksk@aol.com

Jennifer Leaning, MD
Professor of the Practice of International
   Health, Harvard School of Public Health
Associate Professor of Medicine,
   Harvard Medical School
Co-Director, Harvard Humanitarian
   Initiative
8 Story Street, 2nd Floor
Cambridge, MA 02138
617-384-5661
617-384-5988 (fax)
jleaning@hsph.harvard.edu

Ernest C. Lee, MD, MPH, FAAFP,
   FACOEM
Lieutenant Colonel, United States Air
   Force, Medical Corps
Air Force Institute for Operational Health
2513 Kennedy Circle
Brooks City-Base, TX 78235
ernest.lee.007@post.harvard.edu

Barry S. Levy, MD, MPH
Adjunct Professor of Public Health
Department of Public Health and Family
   Medicine
Tufts University School of Medicine
P.O. Box 1230
20 North Main Street, Suite 200
Sherborn, MA 01770
508-650-1039
508-655-4811 (fax)
blevy@igc.org

John Loretz
Program Director
International Physicians for the
   Prevention of Nuclear War (IPPNW)
727 Massachusetts Avenue, 2nd floor
Cambridge, MA 02139
(617) 868-5050, ext. 280
(617) 868-2560 (fax)
jloretz@ippnw.org

Charles Lubula Muganda
Public Health Nurse
International Rescue Committee
New York, NY
646-479-6576
charlesm@theirc.org

Klaus Melf, MD, MPhil
Peace-Health Project Manager
Centre for International Health (SIH)
Faculty of Medicine & University
   Hospital of North Norway
University of Tromsoe
N-9037 Tromsoe
Norway
47 77 64 92 56
47 77 64 59 90 (fax)
klaus.melf@sih.uit.no

James A. Mercy, PhD
Special Advisor for Strategic Directions
Division of Violence Prevention
National Center for Injury Prevention
   and Control
Centers for Disease Control
   and Prevention
4770 Buford Highway, NE
Mailstop K-68
Atlanta, GA 30341
770-488-4723
770-488-4221 (fax)
jam2@cdc.gov

Reuben Nogueira-McCarthy
Conflict Prevention & Recovery Specialist
UNDP Regional Service Centre
7 Naivasha Road, Private Bag X46
Sunninghill, 2157 Johannesburg
South Africa
27 11 603 5109
reuben.mccarthy@undp.org

David Ozonoff, MD, MPH
Professor of Environmental Health
Chairman Emeritus, Department of
   Environmental Health
Boston University School of
   Public Health
715 Albany Street, T2E
Boston, MA 02118
617-638-4620
617-638-4857 (fax)
dozonoff@bu.edu

Michael Renner
Senior Researcher
Worldwatch Institute
1776 Massachusetts Avenue, NW
Washington, DC 20036
631-369-6896
626-608-3189 (fax)
mrenner@optonline.net

Garett Reppenhagen
Chair of the Board
Iraq Veterans Against the War
P.O. Box 476
Green Mountain Falls, CO 80819
719-235-7030
reppenhagen@gmail.com

Avid Reza, MD, MPH
International Emergency and Refugee
    Health Branch
Centers for Disease Control
    and Prevention
1600 Clifton Road NE, Mailstop E-97
Atlanta GA 30333
404-498-0355
404-498-0064 (fax)
afr6@cdc.gov

Les Roberts, MSPH, PhD
Associate Clinical Professor
Program on Forced Migration and Health
Mailman School of Public Health
Columbia University
60 Haven Street, B4, Suite 432
New York, NY 10032
212-324-5215
les@a-znet.com

Leonard S. Rubenstein, JD
President
Physicians for Human Rights
1156 15th Street, NW
Washington, DC 20005
202-728-5335
lrubenstein@phrusa.org

Joanna Santa Barbara, MB, BS, FRCP(C)
Associate Clinical Professor
Department of Psychiatry and
    Behavioral Neurosciences
McMaster University
1280 Main Street West
Hamilton, Ontario L8S 4L8
Canada
905-648-1520
joanna@web.ca

Victor W. Sidel, MD
Distinguished University Professor
    of Social Medicine
Montefiore Medical Center
Albert Einstein College of Medicine
Adjunct Professor of Public Health
Weill Medical College of
    Cornell University
111 East 210th Street
Bronx, NY 10467
718-920-6586
718-654-7305 (fax)
vsidel@igc.org

Susannah Sirkin
Deputy Director for International Policy
    and Advocacy
Physicians for Human Rights
2 Arrow Street
Cambridge, MA 02138
617-301-4204
617-301-4250 (fax)
ssirkin@phrusa.org

Eric Stover
Faculty Director, Human Rights
    Center
Adjunct Professor, School of Public
    Health
Adjunct Professor, Boalt Hall School
    of Law
University of California, Berkeley
460 Stephens Hall #2300
Berkeley, CA 94720-2300
510-642-0965
510-643-3830 (fax)
stovere@berkeley.edu

Patrice M. Sutton, MPH
Consultant
Occupational and Environmental Health
311 Douglass Street
San Francisco, CA 94114
415-864-6758
psutton2000@yahoo.com

Tim K. Takaro, MD, MPH, MS
Associate Professor
Faculty of Health Sciences
Simon Fraser University
8888 University Drive
Burnaby, BC V5A 1S6
Canada
778-782-7186
778-782-8097 (fax)
ttakaro@sfu.ca

Michael J. Toole, MBBS, BMedSc,
   DTM&H
Center for International Health
The Macfarlane Burnet Institute
   for Medical Research and Public
   Health
85 Commercial Road
Melbourne 3004
Australia
61 3 9282 2216
61 3 9282 2144 (fax)
toole@burnet.edu.au

Ronald J. Waldman, MD, MPH
Mailman School of Public Health
Columbia University
5435 32ⁿᵈ Street NW
Washington, DC 20015
202-460-2341
rw178@columbia.edu

Peter Weiss, JD
President, Lawyers Committee on
   Nuclear Policy
Vice President, Center for
   Constitutional Rights
185 West End Avenue
New York, NY 10023
212-877-0522
petweiss@igc.org

Arthur H. Westing, MF, PhD
Westing Associates in Environment,
   Security, & Education
134 Fred Houghton Road
Putney, VT 05346
802-387-2152
westing@sover.net

Stephen N. Xenakis, MD
Brigadier General (Retired),
   United States Army
Advisor to Physicians for
   Human Rights
2235 Military Road
Arlington, VA 22207-3959
703-527-9393
703-527-2448 (fax)
snxenakis@hotmail.com

I

INTRODUCTION

1

War and Public Health:
An Overview

Barry S. Levy and Victor W. Sidel

War accounts for more death and disability than many major diseases combined. It destroys families, communities, and sometimes whole cultures. It directs scarce resources away from protection and promotion of health, medical care, and other human services. It destroys the infrastructure that supports health. It limits human rights and contributes to social injustice. It leads many people to think that violence is the only way to resolve conflicts—a mindset that contributes to domestic violence, street crime, and other kinds of violence. And it contributes to the destruction of the environment and overuse of nonrenewable resources. In sum, war threatens much of the fabric of our civilization.

War has been conventionally defined as armed conflict conducted by nation-states. The term is also used to describe an armed conflict within a nation (a "civil war" or a "war of liberation") and armed action by a clandestine group against a government or an occupying force (a "guerrilla war" or "intifada"). *Public health* has been defined as "what we, as a society, do collectively to assure the conditions in which people can be healthy."[1] War is generally anathema to public health.

Some of the impacts of war on public health are obvious, but others are not. The direct impact of war on mortality and morbidity is apparent. An increasing percentage of those killed or injured during war have been civilians. An estimated 191 million people died directly or indirectly as a result of conflict during the 20th century, more than half of whom were civilians[2] (see Figure 1-1). The exact figures are unknowable because of poor recordkeeping in many countries and its disruption in times of conflict.[3]

Civilians are increasingly affected by war. There is evidence that in some wars 90 percent or more of the people killed were noncombatants.[4] Many of them were innocent bystanders, caught in the crossfire of opposing armies; others were civilians who were specifically targeted during wars. During each year of the past decade, there have been approximately 20 wars, mainly civil wars that are infrequently reported by the news media in the United States. For example, almost 4 million people died during the civil war in the Democratic Republic of Congo, and 1 million people, about half of whom were civilians, died in the 30-year civil war in Ethiopia.[5]

Since 1999, the number of major armed conflicts has steadily decreased. There were 17 major armed conflicts in 16 locations worldwide during 2005— the lowest number since the end of the Cold War in 1990. Most conflicts in recent years have been civil wars within nations. For example, in the 1990– 2005 period, only 4 of 57 active conflicts were armed conflicts between na-

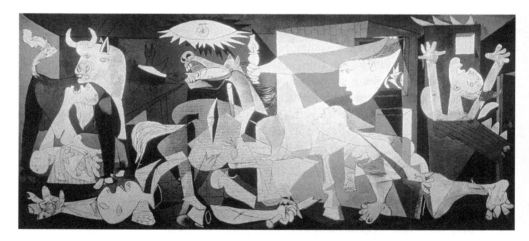

Figure 1-1. *Guernica* (Pablo Picasso, 1937). On April, 26, 1937, German planes bombed the Basque city of Guernica in northern Spain, killing hundreds of civilians. The attack marked the beginning of terror bombing of civilian targets in the Spanish Civil War, which continued through the bombing in World War II of Warsaw, Rotterdam, London, Coventry, Hamburg, Dresden, Osaka, Tokyo, Hiroshima, and Nagasaki, among many other cities. *Guernica* was commissioned by the Spanish Republic, which asked Picasso to prepare it for exhibition at the Spanish pavilion at the 1937 Paris World's Fair. (Image © Archivo Iconografico, S.A./CORBIS, reproduced with permission.)

tions: between Eritrea and Ethiopia in 1998–2000; between India and Pakistan in 1990–1992 and again in 1996–2003; between Iraq and Kuwait (and a large coalition of nations) in 1991; and the Iraq War starting in 2003. (The last of these wars has evolved into sectarian conflict; see Chapter 15.) Of the remaining 53 conflicts within nations during this period, 30 were fought for control over government and 23 were fought for control over territory.[6] Some enduring conflicts have taken place in recent years in the same locations as they did in the 1960s, such as the conflicts between Israel and the Palestinians, between India and Pakistan for control over the territory of Kashmir, in the Democratic Republic of Congo, and in Colombia.[7]

There have been some encouraging developments in recent years. Despite continuing violence in Iraq and Darfur, during the 2002–2005 period the number of wars being fought worldwide decreased from 66 to 56, with the greatest reduction in sub-Saharan Africa. Battle-related deaths during the same period are estimated to have declined by almost 40 percent. More wars are ending in negotiated settlements instead of being fought to the bitter end—a trend that reflects increased commitment of the international community to peacemaking.[8]

There have also been some discouraging developments, however. In four regions of the world, the number of armed conflicts increased between 2002 and 2005. International "terrorist" incidents tripled between 2000 and 2005, with an even greater relative increase in the number of deaths. And the number of organized violence campaigns against civilians annually rose by 56 percent between 1989 and 2005.[8]

Given the brutality of war, many people survive wars only to be physically or mentally scarred for life (see Box 1-1). Millions of survivors are chronically disabled from injuries sustained during war or the immediate aftermath of war. Approximately one-third of the soldiers who survived the civil war in Ethiopia, for example, were injured or disabled, and at least 40,000 individuals lost one or more limbs during the war.[5] Antipersonnel landmines represent a serious threat to many people[9] (see Chapter 7). For example, in Cambodia, 1 in 236 people is an amputee as a result of a landmine explosion.[10]

Millions more people are psychologically impaired from wars, during which they have been physically or sexually assaulted or have physically or sexually assaulted others; have been tortured or have participated in the torture of others; have been forced to serve as soldiers against their will; have witnessed the death of family members; or have experienced the destruction of their communities or entire nations (see Chapter 4). Psychological trauma may be demonstrated in disturbed and antisocial behaviors, such as aggression toward family members and others. Many soldiers, on returning from military action, suffer from posttraumatic stress disorder (PTSD), which also affects many civilian survivors of war.

Box 1-1 The Brutality of War
Jennifer Leaning

All wars impose grave consequences but those with pronounced features of brutality can be seen to exact the most enduring psychosocial impact. Brutality is most prevalent in conflicts characterized by the willful or indiscriminate infliction of death, pain, and suffering on combatants and civilians in violation of the Geneva Conventions.

Aspects of observed brutality during war include mass killing and rape of civilians, torture and other atrocities, and concentration camps. Such brutality may arise in desperate phases of a conflict, especially when local leaders or commanders, attempting to galvanize last-ditch action, incite troops or other fighters. Brutality is also a recurrent feature of communal war, ethnic cleansing, and genocide, in all of which the targets of armed groups are not other soldiers but stigmatized civilians.

Documented instances of brutality in major international wars include grievous instances of gender-based violence—such as the 1937 "Rape of Nanking" during the Japanese invasion of China, the abuse of Korean comfort women by the Japanese military during its Asian campaigns in the 1930s and 1940s, and the rape of German women during the fall of Berlin in 1945; massacres of civilians, such as in the 1941 German sweep across Ukraine; and gross maltreatment of prisoners of war, especially by the Japanese, German, and the Soviet forces throughout World War II. The Holocaust stands out not only as part of the international war waged by the Third Reich, but also as the most extensive genocide in recorded history—implemented independent of any specific war campaign or strategic aim. In the past 20 years, internal and civil wars characterized by high levels of brutality against opponent forces or civilians have included the conflicts in the former Yugoslavia, Liberia, Sierra Leone, the Democratic Republic of Congo, Uganda, Afghanistan, and Iraq. At the extreme, brutality in these wars has extended to ethnic cleansing or outright genocide, as in the former Yugoslavia, Rwanda, and, most recently, Darfur (see Box 13-1 in Chapter 13).

Brutality has long-term psychological consequences (see Chapters 4, 12, and 14). Survivors of rape and torture, depending on the kind of assault they experienced, must deal with their own feelings of fear, shame, and humiliation as well as the physical consequences of these events, which may be severe and long-lasting. They also face harsh social stigma, which may, for example, lead to rape victims' being ejected from their families and isolated from their communities. Often, both the experiences themselves and the reactions from families and communities are so traumatizing that survivors retreat into zones of relative silence—if not denial—about their past.

In wars fought along communal lines of race, religion, language, and ethnicity, individuals and groups targeted on the basis of their communal char-

(continued)

6

acteristics are forced to undergo a profound disorientation in their sense of social stability, trust, and personal identity.[1] Neighbors become killers and rapists. Members of mixed families tear each other apart. What had not previously been perceived as difference, such as dialect, color, or surname, appears suddenly to be the most crucial characteristic of the feared and hated other. For victims of grave abuse in war and for those targeted on the basis of group characteristics, the cognitive and emotional framework that they constructed to make sense of their world proves inadequate to withstand the withering assault that this world has delivered against their own person and consciousness. What was once trusted proves dangerous. Attachments turn lethal.[2]

The perpetrators of these atrocities and wars are also consumed by rage, fear, and humiliation.[3,4] Societies are usually forced to work out their own modes of re-entry and accommodation for the many people known to have committed awful acts during wartime. Punishment may be meted out, but often impunity characterizes the postwar context. There is little truth-telling, no explanation, scant forgiveness. The perpetrators suffer in their own mix of silence, rejection, and denial, blocked from the processes of explanation and expiation that might lead to their reintegration into society.

Societies emerging from brutal wars include tens of thousands, if not hundreds of thousands, of such people, both victims and perpetrators, shackled by their own pain and fear and unable to participate fully in life or in postwar reconstruction, which requires the energy and talent of all survivors.[5] The victims are both men and women, but the perpetrators are usually men. These men cannot retain jobs, become indifferent or absent as parents, have difficulty concentrating, and remain irritable and depressed for years—locked in a past they cannot escape and sleepwalking in a present that holds no future.

These thousands of people, however, constitute only a small fraction of people in the entire community who are burdened by memories of what they did—or did not do—during the brutal aspects of the war. Especially in communities afflicted with communal conflict, the great majority of people are guilty of acts of omission and commission, acquiescence and witnessing, silence and suppression.[6] This guilt contributes to a complicity of silence that already enshrouds victims and perpetrators. What happened is best left unspoken. People are never sure of the mindset of those to whom they are talking. People are never sure what they need to conceal. And people are never sure what they need to conceal from themselves.

Yet, in this silence, stories are constructed and relayed. They serve the interests of the victims or perpetrators, or they serve the needs of those who watched and did nothing or not enough. These stories provide meaning and explanatory frameworks in a postwar context in which people no longer trust in what they used to believe. Often, these stories harken back to old myths derived from epochs that predated the nation-state—the mixed societies of

(continued)

7

Box 1-1 (*continued*)

modernity. Embellished now with the latest tales of treachery and atrocity, these stories provide protective guidance about what to think and what to do in the ravaged and unsettled circumstances wrought by war.

These war stories also serve two other functions that maintain the ugly dynamic of communal conflict. First, they drive and secure a wedge between groups. The stories of one community demonize the other, even as they appear to be mirror images in terms of details, facts, sequence of events, heroes and villains, and key motifs. Occasionally, in somewhat mixed gatherings, often with expatriates providing some political protection, the stories are shared and become the material of bitter jokes. Second, these stories travel across generations. They sustain the trauma narrative by providing encapsulated messages as to why one group must always be perceived as cruel, dominating, racist, or evil and the other group must always stay on guard. There are many informal ways in which this transmission of trauma occurs,[7] including intrafamilial processes, in which powerful injectors of toxic material are provided in admonitions before bedtime from grandmothers to grandchildren and in tales told around the fire with children in earshot.

If subsequent generations receive nothing but these stories, in an overall context of silence and denial about what actually occurred, in all its complexities and contradictions, communal divides are magnified. An example is the U.S. Civil War: Despite more than a century of laws, judicial decisions, and social actions at all levels and despite libraries of analysis and commentary on virtually every aspect of what could conceivably be historically related to the war, disputes over who was right and who was wrong, who was injured and why, and what was gained and what was lost continue to mark the great schism in American consciousness. The failure of ongoing efforts by the Korean comfort women to secure a comprehensive apology from the Japanese government for its activities more than 60 years ago inflames underlying (anticolonial) Korean hostility towards Japan. Similarly, refusals on the part of Japan to undertake a comprehensive accounting of its actions during its military campaigns in China in the 1930s and 1940s continue to fuel latent, but strong, anti-Japanese sentiment in China.

It is difficult to reconcile communities torn apart by war, especially very brutal wars. Social psychologists, lawyers, and other groups of experts believe that layers of grievance, buttressed by trauma stories, prepare societies for nothing more than sectarian conflict or further war.[8] Despite disagreement on methods and approaches, such as truth commissions, international tribunals, and national judicial processes, some type of effort to construct a full accounting must occur in the first or second postwar generation, or there will likely be recurrent conflict. The massive documentation of Germany's actions during the Third Reich, as uncovered in the hundreds of trials under the Nuremberg court system, has been considered pivotal to the ability of Germany and the rest of the world to successfully move on from the grotesque events of the 1933–1945 war period.[9] In stark contrast, the relative incon-

8

clusiveness of the Tokyo War Crimes Trials has been considered pivotal to people in Japan and elsewhere in Asia in continuing to harbor defiantly different and antagonistic perspectives of what happened and who is to blame for the terrible events of the same war period.[10]

The path toward recovery from the profoundly disruptive consequences of brutal war is very long, difficult, and ultimately uncertain—for individuals and society alike. This understanding should weigh heavily in decisions to go to war, in decisions about the conduct of war, and in decisions to intervene to stop wars from spiraling into terrible violations of our most hard-won legal and humanitarian norms.

References

1. Babbitt E. Ethnic conflict and the pivotal states. In Chase R, Hill E, Kennedy P (eds.). The Pivotal States: A New Framework for U.S. Policy in the Developing World. New York: WW Norton, 1999, pp. 338–359.
2. Gjelten T. Sarajevo Daily: A City and Its Newspaper Under Siege. New York: Harper Collins, 1995, pp. 131–167.
3. Gilligan J. Violence: A National Epidemic. New York: Random House, 1996.
4. Mitscherlich A, Mitscherlich M. The Inability to Mourn: Principles of Collective Behavior. New York: Grove Press, 1985.
5. Desjarlais R, Eisenberg L, Good B, Kleinman A. World Mental Health: Problems and Priorities in Low-Income Countries. New York: Oxford University Press, 1995, pp. 116–135.
6. Glover J. Humanity: A Moral History of the Twentieth Century. New Haven, CT: Yale University Press, 1999, pp. 405–410.
7. Volkan VD, Itzkowitz N. Turks and Greeks: Neighbours in Conflict. Cambridge-shire, England: Eothen Press, 1994, pp. 7–10.
8. Minow M. Between Vengeance and Forgiveness. Boston: Beacon Press, 1998.
9. Persico JE. Nuremberg: Infamy on Trial. New York: Penguin, 1994, pp. 438–443.
10. Minear R. The individual, the state, and the Tokyo Trial. In Hosoya C, Ando N, Onuma Y, Minear R (eds.). The Tokyo War Crimes Trial. Tokyo: Kodansha Ltd., 1986, pp. 159–165.

Women are especially vulnerable during war (see Chapter 12). Rape has been used as a weapon in many wars—in Korea, Bangladesh, Algeria, India, Indonesia, Liberia, Rwanda, Uganda, the former Yugoslavia, and elsewhere. As acts of humiliation and revenge, soldiers have raped the female family members of their enemies. For example, at least 10,000 women were raped by military personnel during the war in Bosnia and Herzegovina.[11] The social chaos brought about by war also creates situations and conditions conducive to sexual violence.

Children also are especially vulnerable during and after wars (see Chapter 11). Many die as a result of malnutrition, disease, or military attack. Many are physically or psychologically injured. Many are forced to become soldiers or sexual slaves to military officers. The health of children suffers in numerous other ways, as reflected by increased mortality rates among infants and young children and decreased rates of immunization coverage.[12,13]

The infrastructure that supports social well-being and health—including medical care facilities, electricity-generating plants, food supply systems, water treatment and sanitation facilities, and transportation and communication systems—has been destroyed during many wars, so that many people have inadequate access to food, clean water, medical care, or other conditions necessary for public health. Economic sanctions can have a similar effect. For example, the United Nations Children's Fund (UNICEF) has estimated that between 350,000 and 500,000 excess child deaths occurred in Iraq between 1991 and 1998, many due to inadequate nutrition, contaminated water, and shortages of essential medicines, all of which were worsened by international economic sanctions imposed on Iraq.

Many people during wartime flee to other countries as refugees or become internally displaced persons within their own countries, where it may be difficult for them to maintain their health and safety (see Chapter 13). Refugees and internally displaced persons are vulnerable to malnutrition, infectious diseases, injuries, and criminal and military attacks. A substantial number of the approximately 12 million refugees and 20 to 25 million internally displaced persons in the world today were forced to leave their homes because of war or the threat of war.[14,15]

In addition to the direct effects of war, there are three categories of indirect and less obvious impacts on health of war and preparation for war: diversion of resources, domestic and community violence, and damage to the environment.

Many countries spend large amounts of money per capita for military purposes. The countries with the highest military expenditures are shown in Table 1-1. War and the preparation for war divert huge amounts of resources from health and human services and other productive societal endeavors.[16–18] This diversion of resources occurs in many countries. In some less developed countries, national governments spend $10 to $20 per capita on military expenditures but only $1 per capita on all health-related expenditures. The same type of distorted priorities also exist in more developed countries. For example, the United States ranks first among nations in military expenditures and arms exports, but 38th among nations in infant mortality rate and 45th in life expectancy at birth. Since 2003, during a period when federal, state, and local governments in the United States have been experiencing budgetary shortfalls and finding it difficult to maintain adequate health and human services, the U.S. government has spent almost $500 billion for the Iraq War, and is spending (in 2007) more than $2 billion a week on the war.

Weapons represent a large portion of expenditures for military purposes. Availability of weapons, especially small arms and light weapons, often in-

Table 1-1. The 15 Countries with the Highest Military Expenditures in 2005

Country	Spending (in Billions of Dollars)	Spending per Capita (in Dollars)	World Share of Spending (Percent)
United States	478	1,604	48
United Kingdom	48	809	5
France	46	763	5
Japan	42	329	4
China	41	31	4
Germany	33	401	3
Italy	27	468	3
Saudi Arabia	25	1,025	3
Russia	21	147	2
India	20	19	2
South Korea	16	344	2
Canada	11	327	1
Australia	11	522	1
Spain	10	230	1
Israel	10	1,430	1
Total of top 15	840*	—	84*
All countries	1,001	155	100

*Because of rounding, this total is not the sum of above numbers.

Source: Omitoogun W, Sköns E. Military expenditure data: a 40-year overview. In Stockholm International Peace Research Institute. SIPRI Yearbook 2006: Armaments, Disarmament and International Security. Oxford, UK: Oxford University Press, 2006, p. 302.

creases the likelihood of armed conflict (see Chapter 6). Between 2003 and 2004, there was a substantial increase in international arms sales worldwide, from $233 to $268 billion (not including China). The United States accounted for approximately 63 percent of these international arms sales, the United Kingdom about 19 percent, and France about 12 percent.[19]

War often creates a cycle of violence, increasing domestic and community violence in the countries engaged in war. War teaches people that violence is an acceptable method for settling conflicts. Children growing up in environments in which violence is an established way of settling conflicts may choose violence to settle conflicts in their own lives. Teenage gangs may mirror the activity of military forces. Men, sometimes former military servicemen who have been trained to use violence, commit acts of violence against women; there have been instances of men murdering their wives on return from the battlefield.

Finally, war and the preparation for war have profound impacts on the physical environment (see Chapter 5). The disastrous consequences of war for the environment are often clear. Examples include bomb craters in Vietnam that have filled with water and provide breeding sites for mosquitoes that spread malaria and other diseases; destruction of urban environments by aerial carpet bombing of major cities in Europe and Japan during World

War II; and the more than 600 oil-well fires in Kuwait that were ignited by retreating Iraqi troops in 1991, which had a devastating effect on the ecology of the affected areas and caused acute respiratory symptoms among those exposed. Less obvious are the environmental impacts of the preparation for war, such as the huge amounts of nonrenewable fossil fuels used by the military before (and during and after) wars and the environmental hazards of toxic and radioactive wastes, which can contaminate air, soil, and both surface water and groundwater. For example, much of the area in and around Chelyabinsk, Russia, site of a major nuclear weapons production facility, has been determined to be highly radioactive, leading to evacuation of local residents (see Chapter 10).[20]

In the early 21st century, new geopolitical, tactical, and technological issues concerning war have continued to arise. These issues include the use of new weapons, such as drone (unmanned) aircraft[21] and high-altitude bombers as well as the possible future development and use of space-based weapons[22] ; continuing proliferation of nuclear weapons; an increasing number of suicide (or "homicide") bomber attacks; newly adopted U.S. policies on "preemptive" war and on "usable" nuclear weapons; and the "war on terror" in response to the September 11, 2001, attacks on the World Trade Center and the Pentagon (see Box 1-2). In addition, there has been violent involvement of armed individuals and groups—including rebel opposition groups and other groups not under state control, such as militias, warlords, and vigilantes—that use armed force for a number of purposes, often "shadowing" similar functions of the state. (This description of armed non-state actors does not consider "terrorist groups" as distinct organizations, because armed non-state actors have used terrorist actions for centuries.) Among the issues posed by the involvement of armed non-state actors are (1) the challenges they pose for the management and resolution of conflicts; (2) the denial by state actors of the presence of "conflict" when opposed by non-state actors; and (3) the blurring among conflict, postconflict, and peace periods that occurs when non-state actors are involved in violent activities.[7]

New weaponry has led to new problems. For example, depleted uranium (DU), a toxic and radioactive material, has been used in shells and shell casings because of its density and pyrophoric qualities. It has been used by the United States in the Persian Gulf War, in the Balkans, and in Afghanistan, and by both the United States and the United Kingdom in the Iraq War. An estimated 320 to 1,000 metric tons of DU remain in Iraq, Kuwait, and Saudi Arabia from the Persian Gulf War. Some critics argue that the use of DU constitutes a violation of the Hague Convention (which bans use of "poison or poisoned weapons"), the Geneva Conventions, and the United Nations Charter.[23] In addition to DU, incendiary weapons similar to napalm have been reportedly used against Iraqi troops[24] (see Chapter 15).

Box 1-2 Terrorism and the "War on Terror"
Barry S. Levy and Victor W. Sidel

We define *terrorism* as "politically motivated violence or the threat of violence, especially against civilians, with the intent to instill fear."[1] Terrorism is intended to have psychological effects that go beyond the immediate victims to intimidate a wider population, such as a rival ethnic or religious group, a national government or political party, or an entire country.[2] It is often intended to establish power where there is none or to consolidate power where there is little. Although many nations, including the United States, differentiate terrorism from war, especially a war formally declared by a nation, we perceive little difference between terrorism and a war directed largely against civilian populations.

The term *terrorist* is "generally applied to one's enemies and opponents, or to those with whom one disagrees and would otherwise prefer to ignore."[2] The use of the term, therefore, depends on one's point of view. The term *terrorist* implies a moral judgment; if one group can attach the term to its opponent, then it may persuade others to adopt its moral perspective.[3] In civil wars, revolutions, and other conflicts, those considered "terrorists" by one side are often considered "freedom fighters" by the other. In these situations, groups that have been relatively powerless, in contrast to very powerful foes, have often used terrorist tactics, believing that these tactics represented effective weapons against superior forces.

Some people construe "terrorism" to encompass the use by countries of weapons designed to cause mass casualties among civilian populations, sometimes termed "state terrorism." Examples include the bombing of Guernica, Spain, by Nazi forces in 1937 and the carpet bombing of urban centers during World War II.

The bombings of the World Trade Center in 1993, the Alfred P. Murrah Federal Building in Oklahoma City in 1995, and U.S. military and diplomatic facilities abroad in the late 1990s awakened Americans to the reality of terrorism directed at U.S. targets at home and abroad. Americans' concerns about terrorism on U.S. soil were tragically confirmed by the September 11, 2001, attacks on the World Trade Center and the Pentagon, followed soon afterward by letters contaminated with anthrax spores that were mailed to two U.S. senators and several news organizations. These events highlighted the importance of public health professionals and their agencies and organizations, both in responding to these events and in helping to prepare for and prevent future terrorist attacks and threats.

U.S. law defines *terrorism* as "premeditated, politically motivated violence perpetrated against non-combatant targets by subnational groups or clandestine agents."[5] Based on this definition, the National Counterterrorism Center reported that, during 2006, there were 14,352 terrorist attacks

(continued)

Box 1-2 (*continued*)

worldwide that resulted in 20,573 deaths (13,340 in Iraq), with an additio-nal 36,214 people wounded. There were nearly 300 incidents that resulted in 10 or more deaths, 90 percent of which were in the Near East and South Asia. Armed attacks and bombings led to 77 percent of the fatalities during 2006.[6]

Current Challenges

Since the September 11, 2001, attacks, billions of dollars have been spent by federal, state, and local governments in the United States on emergency pre-paredness and response capabilities for potential terrorist attacks. Although some of this money has been used to improve public health capabilities, work to prepare for low-probability events has diverted much attention and many resources from widespread existing public health problems.[7]

Public health workers need to support measures to ensure emergency preparedness, not only for potential terrorist attacks but also for chemical emergencies, radiation emergencies, natural disasters, severe weather events, and large outbreaks of disease. The Centers for Disease Control and Pre-vention (CDC) Web site (http://www.bt.cdc.gov [accessed June 4, 2007]) provides useful information.

Public health workers can contribute to addressing the underlying causes of terrorism and promoting a greater understanding of these issues. These causes include historical, political, economic, social, philosophical, and ideo-logical roots of terrorism. Public health workers should promote programs and other activities that support better understanding and tolerance among people of different backgrounds and nations. They should work to ensure that basic human needs are met and human rights are protected. They can contribute to ending the threat to freedom posed by the curtailment of civil rights and civil liberties by the U.S. government as part of the "war on terror."[8]

As part of its "war on terror," the United States has taken actions that endanger not only civil liberties within the United States but also human rights and peace worldwide. It has indiscriminately attacked civilians whom it labels "terrorists" in Afghanistan, Iraq, and Somalia; has denied *habeas corpus* (a legal action or writ by which detainees can seek relief from unlawful im-prisonment) and the right to counsel and a speedy trial to detainees at Abu Ghraib and at Guantanamo Bay; and "renditioned" detainees to other coun-tries for torture. These actions violate human rights and threaten peace.

References

1. Levy BS, Sidel VW (eds.). Terrorism and Public Health: A Balanced Approach to Strengthening Systems and Protecting People. New York: Oxford University Press, 2003. (Also published in paperback with an updated Epilogue by the American Public Health Association, Washington, DC, 2007.)
2. Hoffman B. Inside Terrorism. New York: Columbia University Press, 1998.

3. Jenkins BM. The Study of Terrorism: Definitional Problems. P-6563. Santa Monica, CA: RAND Corporation, December 1980.
4. Schmidt AP, Jongman AJ. Political Terrorism: A New Guide to Actors, Authors, Concepts, Data Bases, Theories, and Literature. New Brunswick, NJ: Transaction Books, 1988, pp. 5–6.
5. U.S. Code, Title 22, Section 2656f(d).
6. National Counterterrorism Center. Report of Terrorist Incidents—2006. Available at: http://wits.nctc.gov/reports/crot2006nctcannexfinal.pdf (accessed July 20, 2007).
7. Rosner D, Markowitz G. Are We Ready? Public Health Since 9/11. Berkeley, CA: University of California Press, 2006.
8. Sidel M. More Secure, Less Free?: Antiterrorism Policy and Civil Liberties after September 11. Ann Arbor, MI: University of Michigan Press, 2004.

Roles of Public Health Professionals in Preventing War and Its Health Consequences

Like most public health problems, war and its health consequences are preventable. There are several roles that public health professionals can play in preventing war and its consequences. These roles include

- Participating in surveillance and documentation of the health effects of war and of the factors that may cause war
- Developing and implementing education and awareness-raising programs on the health effects of war
- Advocating policies and promoting actions to prevent war and its health consequences
- Working directly in actions to prevent war and its consequences.

Several ethical issues may arise for public health professionals with regard to these roles, especially for medical care workers in war-zone health-related activities that serve to support military efforts (see Chapter 24).

The basic principles of prevention are applicable to the prevention of war and the minimization of its consequences. In this context, we define

- *Primary prevention* as preventing war or causing a halt to a war that is taking place
- *Secondary prevention* as preventing and minimizing the health and environmental consequences of war once it has begun
- *Tertiary prevention* as treating or ameliorating the health consequences of war.

Many of the roles for public health professionals in secondary and tertiary prevention take place in war zones, where there is a narrow line between protecting and serving people on the one hand and supporting the war effort on the other.

Surveillance and Documentation

Public health professionals with access to information on the health and environmental effects of war or militarism, and on factors that may cause war, have the capability and responsibility to gather these data, analyze them, and make them widely available. Such data can be extremely useful if utilized by health professionals and others in conducting education and awareness-raising programs, preventing war or preparation for war, or helping to end a war.

Once a war has begun, public health professionals can play important roles in documenting and publicizing the nature and extent of injuries, physical and mental illnesses, disabilities, and deaths among both civilians and military personnel. These data may be useful for the purposes of limiting the health consequences of the conflict or of bringing about a ceasefire.

Education and Awareness-Raising Programs

Along with gathering and analyzing relevant data, public health professionals can play important roles in activities that inform, educate, and communicate information about the health consequences of war to health professionals, the public, and political leaders. Public health professionals can continue to play these roles after war has begun.

Advocacy

Public health professionals can play important roles in advocating policies and promoting actions that prevent war or minimize the consequences of war. They can usually do this most effectively by working with or on behalf of public health organizations, such as the American Public Health Association. Another avenue for advocacy is through professional organizations for specific disciplines, such as those for physicians, nurses, social workers, other health workers, or their labor unions. Such organizations include the American Medical Association, the American Nursing Association, and the National Association of Social Workers. In addition, health professionals can work within groups with broader memberships, such as the local chapters of Physicians for Social Responsibility, other national affiliates of the International Physicians for the Prevention of Nuclear War, and community or national groups. Other avenues for advocacy by public health professionals are through the governmental agencies in which they work and through intergovernmental agencies, such as those of the United Nations.

There are a variety of objectives for advocacy work by public health professionals. These include

- Promoting nonviolent conflict resolution, both in general and in specific situations
- Advocating increases in public health resources and services
- Advocating decreases in military spending
- Advocating decreases in—and ultimately elimination of—the international arms trade
- Advocating abolition of nuclear weapons (see Chapter 10)
- Advocating for ratification of the Mine Ban Treaty by the United States and other countries that have not yet ratified it (see Chapter 7)
- Advocating, strengthening, and promoting adherence to the Biological Weapons Convention (see Chapter 9)
- Advocating a ban of economic sanctions that may have a major impact on civilians
- Advocating prevention of environmental degradation and overuse of nonrenewable resources in preparation for war or in the conduct of war (see Chapter 5)
- Supporting the United Nations and its activities and promoting financial support of the United Nations.

Even after war has begun, public health professionals can continue to play important roles in advocating policies and promoting activities to minimize the consequences of war, including

- Promoting public health and medical care activities for the protection of civilians
- Preventing the use of chemical, biological, and nuclear weapons (see Chapters 8 through 10)
- Ensuring use by the affected population of appropriate protective devices and medications if such weapons are used (such as barrier methods against chemical and biological weapons, and thyroid tablets to protect against concentration of iodine-131 in the thyroid gland after the use of nuclear and radiologic weapons).

Health professionals can also advocate for effective services for those physically or mentally injured or displaced by war (see Chapters 4, 13, and 22).

Participating Directly in Effective Actions

There are a variety of ways in which public health professionals can act, such as participating in nonviolent conflict resolution. Public health professionals can work in their own or other communities in which violence is likely. They can also participate in activities that foster transparency and trust-building in individual relationships.

There are at least three ways that public health professionals may involve themselves directly in secondary prevention:

- As part of a United Nations peacekeeping force
- As part of another international agency, such as UNICEF
- As part of a nongovernmental (civil-society) organization, such as the International Committee of the Red Cross, the International Rescue Committee, Doctors Without Borders (Médecins Sans Frontières), and Doctors of the World (Médecins du Monde) (see Chapters 22 and 23).

There are a variety of direct-participation roles that public health professionals can play. They can work in many ways to protect the health of civilians (especially women and children), including

- Providing public health services (such as ensuring sanitation and a safe water supply)
- Implementing special measures to ensure provision of public health services (such as ceasefires for immunization days)
- Ensuring access to medical care, including mental health services, for victims and their families
- Maintaining safe zones for hospitals and other health care facilities.

Health professionals can also work to ensure human rights (see Chapter 3):

- Preventing sexual exploitation and other forms of exploitation of women (see Chapter 12)
- Preventing child labor and other forms of exploitation of children, including forcing of children into military roles (see Chapter 11)
- Preventing indentured service and protecting those who refuse to participate in the military (see Chapter 24)
- Protecting the rights of displaced persons (see Chapter 13) and prisoners of war (see Chapter 14).

Protecting the physical environment (see Chapter 5) can be another role for health professionals, including:

- Preventing the use of weapons that damage the environment
- Protecting water supplies
- Ensuring restoration and clean-up of damaged environment.

In terms of tertiary prevention, there are roles that public health professionals can play in caring for victims of war (see Chapters 22 and 23), including assisting and providing health and medical care services for all displaced persons (see Chapter 13) and prisoners of war (see Chapter 14). Health professionals can also help to document the dangers that refugees would face if they were forced to return to their home countries.

Conclusion

War is the one of the most serious threats to public health. Public health professionals can do much to prevent war and its health consequences. Preventing war and its consequences should be part of the curricula of schools of public health, the agendas of public health organizations, and the practice of public health professionals. Activities by public health professionals to prevent war and its health consequences are an essential part of our professional obligations.

The greatest threat to the health of people worldwide lies not in specific forms of acute or chronic diseases—and not even in poverty, hunger, or homelessness. Rather, it lies in the consequences of war. As stated in a resolution adopted by the World Health Assembly, the governing body of the World Health Organization: "The role of physicians and other health workers in the preservation and promotion of peace is the most significant factor for the attainment of health for all."[25]

War is not inevitable. For perhaps 99 percent of human history, people lived in egalitarian groups in which generosity was highly valued and war was rare. War first occurred relatively recently in human history along with changes in social organization, especially the development of nation-states. Even at present, when war seems ever-present, most people live peaceful, nonviolent lives. If we can learn from history, we may be able to move beyond war and create a culture of peace.[26]

References

1. Institute of Medicine, Committee for the Study of Public Health. The Future of Public Health. Washington, DC: National Academy of Sciences, 1988.
2. Rummel RJ. Death by Government: Genocide and Mass Murder Since 1900. New Brunswick, NJ, and London: Transaction Publications, 1994.
3. Zwi A, Ugalde A, Richards P. The effects of war and political violence on health services. In Kurtz L (ed.). Encyclopedia of Violence, Peace and Conflict. San Diego, CA: Academic Press, 1999, pp. 679–690.
4. Garfield RM, Neugut AI. The human consequences of war. In Levy BS, Sidel VW (eds.). War and Public Health. New York: Oxford University Press, 1997.

5. Kloos H. Health impacts of war in Ethiopia. Disasters 1992;16:347–354.

6. Harbom L, Wallensteen P. Patterns of major armed conflicts, 1990–2005. In Stockholm International Peace Research Institute. SIPRI Yearbook 2006: Armaments, Disarmament and International Security. Oxford, UK: Oxford University Press, 2006, p. 108.

7. Holmqvist C. Major armed conflicts. In Stockholm International Peace Research Institute. SIPRI Yearbook 2006: Armaments, Disarmament and International Security. Oxford, UK: Oxford University Press, 2006, pp. 77–107.

8. The Human Security Brief 2006. Vancouver, Canada: University of British Columbia, 2006. Available at: http://www.humansecuritygateway.info/ (accessed June 4, 2007).

9. Stover E, Cobey JC, Fine J. The public health effects of land mines. In Levy BS, Sidel VW (eds.). War and Public Health. New York: Oxford University Press, 1997, pp. 137–148.

10. Stover E, Keller AS, Cobey J, Sopheap S. The medical and social consequences of land mines in Cambodia. JAMA 1994;272:331–336.

11. Ashford MW, Huet-Vaughn Y. The impact of war on women. In Levy BS, Sidel VW (eds.). War and Public Health. New York: Oxford University Press, 1997, pp. 186–196.

12. Mann J, Drucker E, Tarantola D, et al. Bosnia: The war against public health. Medicine and Global Survival 1994;1:140–146.

13. Horton R. On the brink of humanitarian disease. Lancet 1994;343:1053.

14. Reed J, Haaga J, Keely C (eds.). The Demography of Forced Migration: Summary of a Workshop. Washington, DC: National Academy Press, 1998.

15. Hampton J (ed.). Internally Displaced People: A Global Survey. London: Earthscan, Norwegian Refugee Council and Global IDP Survey, 1998.

16. Macrae J, Zwi A. Famine, complex emergencies and international policy in Africa: An overview. In Macrae J, Zwi A (eds.). War and Hunger: Rethinking International Responses to Complex Emergencies. London: Zed Books, 1994, pp. 6–36.

17. Brauer J, Gissy WG (eds.). Economics of Conflict and Peace. Aldershot: Avebury, 1997.

18. Cranna M (ed.). The True Cost of Conflict. London: Earthscan and Saferworld, 1994.

19. Dunne JP, Surry E. Arms production. In Stockholm International Peace Research Institute. SIPRI Yearbook 2006: Armaments, Disarmament and International Security. Oxford, UK: Oxford University Press, 2006, pp 387–430.

20. Sidel VW. The impact of military preparedness and militarism on health and the environment. In Austin JA, Bruch CE (eds.). The Environmental Consequences of War. New York: Cambridge University Press, 2000.

21. Brzezinski M. The Unmanned Army. The New York Times Magazine, April 20, 2003, pp. 38–41, 80–81.

22. Hitt J. Battlefield: Space. The New York Times Magazine, August 5, 2001, pp. 30–35, 55–56, 62–63.

23. Depleted Uranium Education Project. Metal of Dishonor: Depleted Uranium. New York: International Action Center, 1977.

24. Crawley JW. Officials confirm dropping firebombs on Iraqi troops: Results are "remarkably similar" to using napalm. San Diego Union Tribune, August 5, 2003.

25. World Health Assembly. Resolution 34.38. Geneva: World Health Organization, 1981.

26. Fry DP. Beyond War: The Human Potential for Peace. New York: Oxford University Press, 2007.

II

CONSEQUENCES OF WAR

2

The Epidemiology of War

Richard Garfield

Epidemiology, a core science of public health, is increasingly utilized to measure morbidity and mortality related to war and to shed light on the determinants of these health consequences. As 2 to 3 percent of all deaths worldwide are due to intentional injuries, including war-related injuries, the need for epidemiologic analysis to identify determinants and reduce the chance of dying from these causes is great.

War is the fourth most common type of injury death—after unintended injuries, suicides, and homicides.[1] The World Health Organization (WHO) estimated that about 588,000 people in 1998 and 310,000 people in 2000 died from war-related injuries.[1,2] Rates of war-related deaths currently vary from less than 1 per 100,000 people in high-income countries to 6.2 per 100,000 in low- and middle-income countries. Worldwide, the highest rates of war-related deaths by far are found in the WHO African Region (32.0 per 100,000 in 1998), followed by low- and middle-income countries in the WHO Eastern Mediterranean Region (8.2 per 100,000) and European Region (7.6 per 100,000). In 1998, war ranked worldwide as the 13th most common cause of death for infants (children younger than 1 year of age) and as the 5th most common cause for both 5- to 14-year-olds and 15- to 44-year-olds.

The only year for which there currently are detailed worldwide data on deaths due to all four categories of "external causes"—unintended injuries, suicides, homicides, and war-related injury deaths—is 1998. However, research data for the years 2000 and 2002 provide similar findings.[3] Deaths from these causes frequently are not counted by routine reporting systems. Approximately 90 percent of these deaths occur in developing countries. More than 75 percent occur among males. About 50 percent occur among those in the 15- to 44-year-old age group. Half of all of these deaths are due to unintentional injuries, and half are related to motor vehicles. War-related injury deaths account for approximately 5 percent of all injury deaths due to external causes.

Deaths from armed conflict among combatants, already low in 1998 by historical standards, appear to have continued to decrease since then. However, during the same period, the proportion of intentional injury deaths occurring among noncombatants worldwide has appeared to rise.

Beyond WHO, a second source of data has been compiled by several political science and peace organizations that have attempted, since 2000, to count the number of deaths worldwide due to armed conflict.[4] The Uppsala Conflict Data Project (UCDP) in Sweden, the most widely used of these sources, estimated the number of battle deaths from mid-2002 to mid-2003 to be between 33,000 and 62,000, with a most likely estimate of 36,000.[5] While various analysts count the number of armed conflicts differently, they agree that both the number of armed conflicts and the magnitude of conflicts have declined since peaking in about 1996 (Figure 2-1).[6]

Counting battle deaths alone, however, understates the impact of armed conflict. In countries with armed conflict, many other deaths occur—mainly among noncombatants—and there is a wide variation in this excess mortality in the general population.[7] In the least developed countries, especially in Africa where most armed conflicts now occur, the mortality rate in the general population during war may increase up to 10-fold. Estimated excess deaths among noncombatants and battle deaths may exceed 500,000 per year.

A third source of information on war-related injury deaths is comprised of household mortality surveys. In conflicts in Sudan, Congo, Iraq, and elsewhere in the past 20 years, these surveys have been the best source of information—but unfortunately this information is frequently missing from the health system or is exaggerated by political interest groups.[8–11] These surveys must be done carefully, because they are subject to sampling and reporting biases. They can provide important information not available from other sources, such as differences in death rates by region, age, gender, and cause of death. Repeated surveys can provide information on changes in cause-specific mortality rates over time. (See Chapter 15.)

Direct deaths in armed conflict are those deaths that occur as the immediate result of a kinetic injury due to the use of a weapon. Indirect deaths are those that occur as a distant result of weapon use. Examples include deaths due to

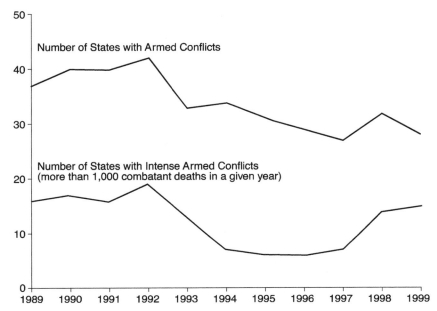

Figure 2-1. Numbers of states with armed conflicts and intense armed conflicts, 1989–1999. (Source: Smith D. Counting Wars: The Research Implications of Definitional Decisions. Paper presented at the Conference on Data Collection on Armed Conflict, Department of Peace and Conflict Research, Uppsala University, June 8–9, 2001.)

malnutrition or infectious disease as a consequence of forced migration. In addition, decreased availability of supplies in health care facilities—resulting from physical barriers, inadequate financial resources, flight of health workers, or increased demand for services due to increased injuries—can lead to indirect deaths. Excess direct and indirect deaths are those beyond baseline levels in a defined period of time.

A Brief History of the Bloody Modern Era

Table 2-1 provides an estimate of the number of conflict-related deaths, by century, from the 16th to the 20th century.[12] These data fail to illuminate the circumstances in which people died. For example, 6 million people are estimated to have died during their capture and transport as slaves over four centuries, and about 10 million indigenous people in the Americas were killed by European colonists.

By all measures, the 20th century was the bloodiest in human history. Reasonable estimates range from 170 million[13] to 231 million[14] deaths directly or

Table 2-1. Estimated Conflict-Related Deaths, by Century

Century	Estimated Conflict-Related Deaths
16th	1,600,000
17th	6,100,000
18th	7,000,000
19th	19,400,000
20th	109,700,000

Source: Garfield RM, Neugut A. Epidemiologic analysis of warfare: A historical review. JAMA 1991;266:688–692.

indirectly resulting from the 25 largest occurrences of collective violence during the 20th century. Conflict-related deaths in wars between combatant forces in the 25 largest military conflicts of the 20th century included 39 million soldiers and 33 million civilians. Many additional deaths occurred during genocides or democides (genocides against one's own ethnic group), in which noncombatants were the primary targets.

Most battle deaths occurred in the first half of the century—during World War I and World War II. Aside from these wars, the Stalinist reign of terror in Russia (from the 1930s to the 1950s) and the Great Leap Forward period in China (from 1958 to 1960) caused the greatest losses of life, both shrouded in uncertainty about the scale of deaths. Altogether, there may have been 100 million conflict-related deaths in the Soviet Union and China among civilians in the 20th century. In addition, famine closely associated with conflict or genocide in the 20th century killed at least 40 million people.

An estimated 5 percent of *all* deaths during the 20th century resulted from the immediate or secondary impact of collective violence—a higher rate than in the 17th, 18th, or 19th centuries, during which an estimated 2 percent of all deaths resulted from collective violence. In the 20th century, there was a 35-fold increase in the number of deaths among soldiers, an increase that greatly exceeded the doubling of the world population (Table 2-2). From 1850 to 1950, the military death rate rose 18-fold. Genocide- and democide-related deaths also increased in the 20th century as centralization of large political and economic systems and emergence of new technologies made mass killings possible.[15]

In the 20th century, 165 collective-violence events each killed more than 6,000 people. Five of these events were responsible for more than 6 million deaths: World War I, World War II, the Russian Civil War, Stalin's rule, and Mao Tse Tung's rule. In each of these events, most deaths occurred among civilians. Together, these five events accounted for about 85 percent of all

Table 2-2. Estimated Average Annual Military Deaths in Wars, Worldwide, by Century

Century	Average Annual Military Deaths in Millions	World Midcentury Population in Millions	Average Annual Military Deaths per Million Population
17th	9,500	500	19.0
18th	15,000	800	18.8
19th	13,000	1,200	10.8
20th	458,000	2,500	183.2

Sources: Garfield RM, Neugut A. Epidemiologic analysis of warfare: A historical review. JAMA 1991; 266:688–692; and Twentieth Century Atlas: Death Tolls for the Major Wars and Atrocities of the Twentieth Century. Available at: http://users.erols.com/mwhite28/warstat2.htm (accessed June 9, 2007).

conflict-related deaths worldwide in the 20th century. In addition, 21 other collective violence events caused between 600,000 and 6 million deaths; 61 caused 60,000 to 600,000 deaths; and 78 caused 6,000 to 60,000 deaths. Most of the events that caused the greatest loss of life occurred early in the 20th century. Only one of the seven largest events occurred after 1950 (famine in China).

Any such accounting of deaths is subject to inaccuracy and subjective interpretation. Reasonably reliable data on deaths resulting from conflict are available only for combatants, and only for those combatants employed by nations. Data for all other population groups affected by conflict come from less complete sources, with counts of victims incomplete at best. Much of our understanding of deaths to noncombatants or combatants not in formal national armed forces comes from reports in the news media, pronouncements from interested parties, or guesses by nongovernmental organizations (NGOs). Because estimates of conflict-related deaths often vary five-fold from one source to another, controversy still surrounds the number of deaths in many 20th-century conflicts. For example, the numbers of deaths in the first two major conflicts of the 20th century—King Leopold's subjugation of the Congo and the Armenian genocide—are still contested.[16]

In 1972, it was estimated that a little less than half of all deaths due to conflict since World War II had resulted directly from the weapons of war.[17] More than two-thirds of these weapons-related deaths were among adult males. Most conflict deaths overall, however, occurred among women and children, mainly as a result of intentional or negligent privations. These deaths occurred most often in camps, as a result of economic sanctions or blockades, and during conflict-related flight and forced dislocation. These patterns continued through the end of the 20th century.

Since World War II, there have been 190 armed conflicts, only one-fourth of which have been between countries (Figure 2-2). Since the end of World War II, wars and deaths have been concentrated in poor parts of the world, especially in Africa and parts of Asia. As a result of these conflicts, an estimated 17 million people have died from direct causes and 34 million people from indirect causes.[18] Most armed conflicts since World War II have lasted less than 6 months. Longer ones often lasted many years, such as the wars in Vietnam that spanned more than two decades. Wars in Afghanistan, Sudan, and Angola also lasted for decades.

The number of ongoing armed conflicts was less than 20 in the 1950s, more than 30 in both the 1960s and 1970s, and more than 50 during the late 1980s. Armed conflicts since 1996 have been fewer in number but, on average, of longer duration. In 1992, there were more than 50 prevalent armed conflicts involving a government; in 2003, that number had fallen to 29. Most armed conflicts now occur *within* rather than *between* countries.

Although conflicts within countries have become most common, conflicts between countries still occur. The war between Iraq and Iran (from 1980 to 1988) resulted in an estimated 700,000 to 1,000,000 combatant deaths and an estimated 50,000 noncombatant deaths.[18] The conflict between Eritrea and Ethiopia (from 1998 to 2000), which was largely fought between two conventional armies using heavy weaponry and trench warfare, resulted in tens of thousands of deaths. There have also been coalitions of multinational forces engaged in conflict by means of massive air attacks—as in the Persian Gulf War against Iraq in 1991 and in the North Atlantic Treaty Organization (NATO) campaign against the Federal Republic of Yugoslavia in 1999.

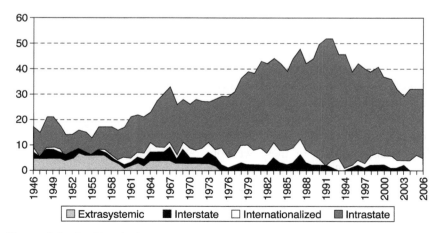

Figure 2-2. Conflicts by boundary type, 1946–2006. (Source: Harbom L, Wallensteen P. Armed Conflict, 1989–2006, Journal of Peace Research 2007; 44, in press.)

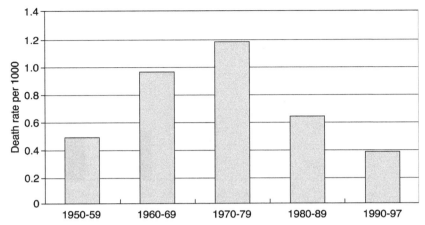

Figure 2–3. Average annual number of war deaths by decade, 1950–1997. (Sources: Human Security Centre. Human Security Report 2005: War and Peace in the 21st Century. New York: Oxford University Press, 2005, p. 31; and Sarkees MR, Wayman FW, Singer JD. Inter-state, intra-state and extra-state wars: A comprehensive look at their distribution over time, 1816–1997. International Studies Quarterly 2003;47:49–70.)

During the past decade, the number of conflict-related deaths has declined more steeply than the decline in the number of conflicts (Figure 2-3). In 1990, an estimated 500,000 conflict-related deaths occurred—slightly fewer than one third of all violent deaths during that year.[19] War-related injury deaths are the least frequent of the three major forms of intentional injury deaths, and they occur predominantly in poorer regions of world; suicide and homicide are more frequent and occur more widely, among both poor and rich countries (Figure 2-4).[20]

This accounting of conflict-related deaths only includes weapons-related deaths, because all other conflict-related deaths are categorized under International Classification of Diseases (ICD) codes for diarrheal diseases, other infectious diseases, malnutrition, and other privation-related causes. Weapons-related deaths are about 30 percent higher for males than for females and reach a peak among 15- to 29-year-olds. The ratio of excess deaths not related to weapons to weapons-related deaths is usually highest in the least developed countries, where public health infrastructure is weakest and where most wars are now fought (Box 2-1). During the war in the Democratic Republic of Congo, for example, there were eight excess deaths not related to weapons for each weapons-related death (see Chapter 17).[21]

From 1995 to 2001, the number of persons killed in conflicts averaged about 100,000 per year. The level of killing varied much by year, with the number of deaths peaking in 1997 and then rapidly declining over the next 4 years.

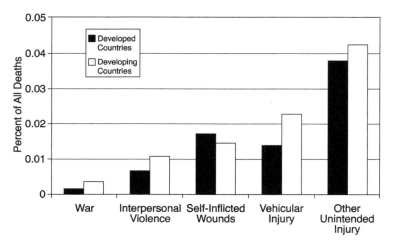

Figure 2-4. Injury deaths, by type, developed and developing countries, 2002. (Source: Revised Global Burden of Disease (GBD) 2002 Estimates: Incidence, prevalence, mortality, YLL, YLD, and DALYs by sex, cause, and region, estimates for 2002 as reported in the World Health Report 2004.)

The number of direct deaths in war peaked in 1994 and has been declining since. In 1994, the Stockholm International Peace Research Institute (SIPRI) started to publish annual estimates of the number of deaths from contemporary wars, confirming that indirect deaths to noncombatants account for most war-

---

Box 2-1 Armed Conflict and Human Development
Richard Garfield

Per-capita income is an inadequate measure of social development. The Human Development Index (HDI) is a better measure because it combines information on income, education, mortality, and life expectancy to characterize both the productivity of a society and the utilization of that productivity in health and education. In general, most deaths during war have been in low- or very-low-HDI countries. Few high-HDI countries have had conflicts on or within their borders.

The Uppsala Conflict Database rates conflicts as minor, intermediate, or major, depending on the number of people killed. Those with more than 1,000 total deaths are rated as major conflicts. For all the years between 1994 and 2003, countries with intermediate conflicts were scored as "1," and those with major conflicts were scored as "2." If a country had more than one conflict, it received more than one score. Summing these scores for the 10-

(continued)

year period generated 12 countries that scored 8 or higher. The HDIs for these countries for 1990 and 2002 were compared.

The countries with the most intense or most durable conflicts in the post-Cold War period showed no uniformity in results. Four were among the 53 countries without HDI scores for one or both periods, making comparison of scores impossible. Two (Russia and the Democratic Republic of Congo) were among the 16 countries with declining HDI scores. Two others without scores (Sierra Leone and Afghanistan) probably also experienced a decline. Among the 106 countries with positive HDI scores, the average HDI rose .066 during the 1990–2002 period. The five countries with conflicts and positive HDI scores were all .060 or greater.

Four of the 12 countries with the greatest levels of conflict during the 1990–2002 period were among the lowest HDI countries in the world, one was medium-low, and two were medium. Five of the 12 countries had medium-high HDI levels in 2002. There were no high-HDI countries among those with high levels of conflict.

More generally, low HDI levels are associated with current or recent conflict. The percentage of countries with conflicts declines as HDI levels rise, and there have been no recent conflicts in high-HDI countries.

The number and global distribution of disasters, such as earthquakes and floods, does not follow the same pattern.[1] Disasters are concentrated in neither high- nor low-HDI countries. Countries with mid-level development experience the most disasters, and an increasing number of disasters. The process of development is actually a cause of the increasing number of disasters, because rapid urbanization, inadequate safety infrastructure, and environmental degradation produce adverse effects additively or possibly synergistically in these countries.

For each person killed in conflict, there may be 10 injured and 100 displaced, especially in countries with the weakest infrastructure, most of which are in Africa. Disasters and wars, as well as the economic challenges arising from both, have uprooted more people than at any time since the end of World War II. Refugees forced to leave their native lands have migrated mainly to high-HDI countries, such as the United States, and mid-HDI countries, such as Iran. Most forced migrants, however, have remained in their home countries, becoming displaced internally to camps, to peri-urban settlements, to other family homesteads, or, as continuous migrants, to many places throughout their home countries. In these ways, conflict can have widespread effects on health, well-being, and social development[2–5] (see Chapter 13).

References

1. International Federation of Red Cross and Red Crescent Societies. World Disasters Report, 1999. Dordrecht: Martinus Nijhoff, 1999.

(*continued*)

Box 2-1 (*continued*)

2. Harris MF, Telfer BL. The health needs of asylum seekers living in the community. Med J Aust 2001;175:589–592.
3. Toole MJ, Waldman RJ. Prevention of excess mortality in refugee and displaced populations in developing countries. JAMA 1990;263:3296–3302.
4. Centers for Disease Control and Prevention. Famine affected, refugee, and displaced populations: Recommendations for public health issues. MMWR Morb Mortal Wkly Rep 1992;41(RR-13).
5. Toole MJ, Waldman RJ. Refugees and displaced persons: War, hunger and public health. JAMA 1993;270:600–605.

related deaths. In 20 conflicts in recent decades, 17 of which were in Africa, 76 percent of all excess deaths could be attributed to indirect causes.[22]

Changing Patterns of Conflict

In the Middle Ages and earlier, war often involved laying of siege, destroying essential goods and services, poisoning water supplies, and/or enslaving the losing army.[23] In wars in Europe after the establishment of nation-states in the 17th century, soldiers of one nation engaged in direct battle almost exclusively with soldiers of a rival nation. Anticolonial wars, often based on guerilla warfare, blurred the distinction between military personnel and civilians. This distinction was further eroded with the breakdown of some countries since the end of the Cold War in 1991. In many internal conflicts—which often pit the state against a section of its civilian population—torture, "disappearances," and other forms of repression have been used in pursuit of political and ideological goals. These tactics have broadened the impact of conflict to the entire civilian population.[24]

Increasingly, military personnel are "irregular," representing a political faction or social group rather than a national army with an accountability structure. In addition, targets of military personnel are more frequently civilians, who may themselves be irregular troops or simply targeted social groups. Targeting of civilians—or of the infrastructure upon which the lives of civilians depend—has become more common. Leverage points to redress this crisis have been lost.[25,26]

During the Cold War, most conflicts—and especially those that caused the most deaths—occurred in wars between countries. Internal conflict was suppressed as part of superpower rivalry. The international forces that stimulated international conflicts and suppressed internal conflicts declined in the 1990s. The potential for international conflict has not disappeared, but the military, political, and informational gaps between possible foes have widened, setting the stage for greater inequalities among those engaged in armed conflict. Thus, the means of waging battle have become asymmetrical. Wars have been fought by one side using ultramodern weapons launched from a distance and the other side using small, easy-to-prepare weapons delivered on the bodies of perpetrators, killing both them and their targets.

After the Cold War ended, small arms became increasingly available and were widely used in armed conflicts.[27] The Geneva Conventions of 1949, the rules of war, require application of the principles of proportionality and distinction. Proportionality involves assessing ways to minimize harm to civilians when a military objective involves targeting that is not exclusively military. Distinction focuses on avoiding civilian targets wherever possible.

Attempts to regulate the brutality of conflicts have not kept pace with the evolving forms of conflict.[28] Most importantly, international humanitarian law and the Geneva Conventions are focused on nation-states waging war and therefore fail to deal adequately with conflicts within states or among multinational coalitions against a single state.

The following threats of conflict each increase the chance of injury or death among noncombatants:

- Depersonalized high-tech weaponry
- Fighting among informal, non-state actors
- Indiscriminate use of weapons.

Along with an increasing number of natural disasters and economic disruptions worldwide, the number and severity of humanitarian crises and the sizes of the populations affected by them have increased. Globalization has also contributed to economic disruption since the end of the Cold War. For the first time in recent decades, some states are experiencing sustained economic declines. Of the 10 countries with the highest mortality rates among children younger than 5 years of age, 7 have experienced recent civil conflict.[29] In only a few of these situations have there been epidemiological studies to assess changes in the rate and distribution of deaths among either combatants or noncombatants.

Historically, most international conflicts have concluded with an end to hostilities after one side was defeated. There have been almost no deaths among military personnel or civilians during most occupations led by the United States or by NATO since World War II. This has not been the case for occupations in Somalia, Afghanistan, and Iraq. In the invasion and occupation of Iraq that began in 2003, not only were there more than 20 times more deaths among noncombatants, but, for the first time in the history of the United States, there were more military deaths after the overthrow of the regime than during the period of major hostilities associated with the invasion (see Chapter 15).

A small group of countries have experienced the most deaths and displacement due to armed conflict or disasters since 1991. In almost all of these countries, there are many more refugees or internally displaced persons than conflict deaths, and many more survivors of disasters than people killed by disasters. Since 1991, conflicts have been responsible for the death of more than 10 percent of the national population in three countries: East Timor, Angola, and Rwanda. The Democratic Republic of Congo, Afghanistan, and Iraq each have had infant mortality rates higher than 10 percent (100 per 1,000 live births).[9, 30–42]

A relatively new development in armed conflicts is the increasing number of violent deaths of civilian United Nations employees and nongovernmental organization (NGO) workers in conflict zones. In the 1985–1998 period, more than 380 deaths occurred among humanitarian workers, with more United Nations civilian personnel killed than United Nations peacekeeping troops.[43]

Torture is a common practice in many conflicts. Because victims are inclined to hide the trauma they have suffered[44] and because there are also political pressures to conceal the use of torture, it is difficult to estimate its prevalence (see Chapter 14).

Conclusion

Armed conflict in the 21st century is very different from that in previous eras of human history. The gradual reduction of conflicts between warring armies of nation-states in recent decades has reduced deaths to combatants to its lowest level worldwide in more than 100 years. At the same time, enormous new challenges have emerged. Civilians are increasingly vulnerable to harm, even where they are not targeted, because of the stunning growth in the capacity of combatants to cause destruction. The protection of civilians in areas with internal conflicts is limited and partial at best. Globalization of some conflicts and changing political goals have made noncombatants anywhere in the world vulnerable like never before and provide little protection against new threats. In recent years, international conventions and national policies designed to protect civilians and combatants from excessive harm have been violated or ignored. Much needs to be done to modernize and improve our ability to identify and reduce the harm caused by armed conflict worldwide.

References

1. Krug E (ed.). World Report on Violence and Health. Geneva: World Health Organization, 2002.
2. International Statistical Classification of Diseases and Related Health Problems, Tenth Revision. Geneva: World Health Organization, 1992–1994.

3. World Health Organization. The Injury Chartbook: A Graphical Overview of the Global Burden of Injuries. Geneva: WHO, 2002.

4. Eck K. A Beginner's Guide to Conflict Data Sets. (Uppsala Conflict Data Project paper no. 1.) Sweden: 2005.

5. Eck, K. "Collective Violence in 2002 and 2003." In Harbom L (ed.). States in Armed Conflict. Uppsala: Department of Peace and Conflict Research, 2004, pp. 143–166. Available at: www.pcr.uu.se/research/UCDP/Hum_Sec_index1.htm(accessed June 28, 2007).

6. Harbom L, Wallensteen P. Armed conflict and its international dimensions, 1946–2004. J Peace Res 2005;42:623–635.

7. Guha-Sapir D, van Panhuis W. The importance of conflict-related mortality in civilian populations. Lancet 2003;351:2126–2128.

8. Burnham G, Lafta R, Doocy S, Roberts L. Mortality after the 2003 invasion of Iraq: A cross-sectional cluster sample survey. Lancet 2006;368:1421–1428.

9. Spiegel DB, Salama P. War and mortality in Kosovo, 1998–1999: An epidemiological testimony. Lancet 2000;355:2204–2209.

10. Depoortere E, Checchi F, Broillet F, et al. Violence and mortality in West Darfur, Sudan (2003–2004): Epidemiolial evidence from four surveys. Lancet 2004;364: 1315–1320.

11. Coghlan B, Brennan RJ, Ngoy R, et al. Mortality in the Democratic Republic of Congo: A nationwide survey. Lancet 2006;367:44–57.

12. Garfield RM, Neugut A. Epidemiologic analysis of warfare: A historical review. JAMA 1991;266:688–692.

13. White M. Historical Atlas of the 20th Century: 30 Worst Atrocities of the 20th Century. 2004. Available at: http://users.erols.com/mwhite28/atrox.htm (accessed June 4, 2007).

14. Leitenberg M. Deaths in Wars and Conflicts Between 1945 and 2000. (Occasional paper no. 29.) Ithaca, NY: Cornell University Peace Studies Program, 2006.

15. Rummel RJ. Death by Government: Genocide and Mass Murder Since 1990. New Brunswick, NJ: Transaction Publications, 1994.

16. Lacey M. The mournful math of Darfur: The dead don't add up. New York Times, May 18, 2005.

17. Eliot G. Twentieth Century Book of the Dead. New York: Scribner, 1972.

18. White M. Historical Atlas of the 20th Century: Death Tolls for the Major Wars and Atrocities of the Twentieth Century. 2005. Available at: http://users.erols.com/mwhite28/warstat2.htm (accessed June 4, 2007).

19. Reza A, Mercy JA, Krug E. Epidemiology of violent deaths in the world. Injury Prev 2001;7:104–111.

20. Murray CJ, King G, Lopez AD, et al. Armed conflict as a public health problem. BMJ 2002;324:346–349.

21. International Rescue Committee. Mortality Study, Eastern D.R. Congo (April–May 2000). Available at: http://www.theirc.org/media/www/mortality_study_eastern_dr_congo_aprilmay_2000.html (accessed June 4, 2007).

22. Small Arms Survey. Yearbook 2005. Chapter 9: Behind the Numbers: Small Arms and Conflict Deaths. Available at: www.smallarmssurvey.org/files/sas/publications/yearb2005.html (accessed June 28, 2007).

23. Keegan J. The Face of Battle. New York: Penguin Books, 1982.

24. Garfield RM. Economic sanctions, humanitarianism, and conflict after the Cold War. Social Justice 2002;29:94–107.

25. Machel G. The Impact of War on Children. London: Hurst and Company, 2001.
26. Rhodes R. Man-made death: A neglected mortality. JAMA 1988;260:686–687.
27. Lumpe L (ed.). Running Guns: The Global Black Market in Small Arms. London: Zed Books, 2000.
28. Robertson G. Crimes Against Humanity: The Struggle for Global Justice. Harmondsworth, UK: Penguin, 1999.
29. Black R, Morris S, Bryce J. Where and why are 10 million children dying every year? Lancet 2003;361:2226–2234.
30. Roberts L, Zantop M. Elevated mortality associated with armed conflict: Democratic Republic of Congo, 2002. MMWR Morb Mortal Wkly Rep 2003;52:469–471.
31. Steering Committee of the Joint Evaluation of the Emergency Assistance to Rwanda. The International Response to Conflict and Genocide: Lessons from the Rwanda Experience. Odense, Denmark: Strandberg Grafisk, 1996.
32. Taylor WR, Chahnazarian A, Weinman J, et al. Mortality and use of health services surveys in rural Zaire. Int J Epidemiol 1993;22(Suppl 1):S15–S19.
33. Garfield R. Health and well-being in Iraq: Sanctions and the impact of the Oil for Food Program. Transnational Law and Contemporary Problems 2001;11:278–297.
34. Welch M. The politics of dead children. Reason 2002;33:52–59.
35. Prunier G. The Rwanda Crisis: History of a Genocide. New York: Columbia University Press, 1995.
36. Ugalde A, Selva-Sutter E, Castillo C, et al. Conflict and health: The health costs of war—Can they be measured? Lessons from El Salvador. BMJ 2000;321:169–172.
37. Garfield RM, Frieden T, Vermund SH. Health-related outcomes of war in Nicaragua. Am J Public Health 1987;77:615–618.
38. Kloos H. Health impacts of war in Ethiopia. Disasters 1992;16:347–354.
39. Cliff J, Noormahomed AR. Health as a target: South Africa's destabilization of Mozambique. Soc Sci Med 1988;27:717–722.
40. Goma Epidemiology Group. Public health impact of Rwandan refugee crisis: What happened in Goma, Zaire, in July 1994? Lancet 1995;345:339–344.
41. Smallman-Raynor M, Cliff A. Civil war and the spread of AIDS in central Africa. Epidemiol Infect Dis 1991;107:69–80.
42. Roberts L, Lafta R, Garfield R, et al. Mortality before and after the 2003 invasion of Iraq: A cluster sample survey. Lancet 2004;364:1857–1864.
43. Sheik M, Gutierrez MI, Bolton P, et al. Deaths among humanitarian workers. BMJ 2000;321:166–168.
44. Weinstein HM, Dansky L, Iacopino V. Torture and war trauma survivors in primary care practice. West J Med 1996;165:112–117.

3

War and Human Rights

George J. Annas and H. Jack Geiger

War is always and everywhere a public health disaster. Because of war's inherent cruelty and savagery, as historian John Keegan has observed, "It is scarcely possible anywhere in the world today to raise a body of reasoned support for the opinion that war is a justifiable activity."[1]

There is a bloody paradox in the world's political and social history. There has never been such universal recognition of human dignity, including the claim that everyone— regardless of race, nationality, religion, gender, sexual orientation, or political belief—is entitled to rights, especially what have been aptly called "life integrity rights."[2] These human rights include the right to life; the right to personal inviolability—not to be hurt; the right to be free of arbitrary seizure, detention, and punishment; the freedom to own one's body and labor; the right to free movement without discrimination; and the right to create and cohabit with family. Life integrity rights embrace, but transcend, the conventional classes of human rights, which include political and civil rights (aspects of freedom or democracy), and social and economic rights (aspects of social justice). They are embodied in a remarkable variety of international human rights and humanitarian laws, conventions, and declarations, including:

- The Charter of the United Nations
- The Universal Declaration of Human Rights
- The International Covenant on Civil and Political Rights
- The Convention on the Prevention and Punishment of the Crime of Genocide
- The Convention against Torture and Other Cruel, Inhuman or Degrading Treatment
- The Convention on the Elimination of All Forms of Discrimination against Women
- The International Convention on the Elimination of All Forms of Racial Discrimination
- The Convention on the Rights of the Child.

These, in turn, are supplemented by specific agreements concerning the conduct of armed conflict (humanitarian law): The Geneva Conventions of 1949 and the Additional Protocols of 1977.

The paradox is that while today's recognition of human rights is unprecedented, with the exception of slavery, human rights have never been violated on so massive a scale, nor with such efficacy and savagery—and the chief instrument of violation is war. The evolution and varieties of warfare over the past century, aided by the technological sophistication, destructive power, and accessibility of new weapons, has all but obliterated the distinction between warfare and mass terrorism (see Box 1–2 in Chapter 1). In the early years of the 21st century, with this paradox unresolved, and accompanied by a poorly defined "global war on terror," the fledgling post–World War II commitment to effective and vigorous protection of human rights is under siege.

"War" is no longer the phenomenon simplistically defined as "a contest between armed forces carried on in a campaign or series of campaigns."[2] The diverse forms of armed conflict now include declared and undeclared wars between nations; full-scale civil wars, including many with genocidal motivations; so-called low-intensity conflicts between competing national political groups (which are often highly intense); and a wide variety of "dirty wars" of repression mounted by governments against their own citizens. The defining characteristic of most of these types of war is a calculated and deliberate assault on civilians in contravention of international humanitarian law. All wars put civilian populations at risk of trauma, illness, or death, and threaten to create humanitarian crises.[3]

Violations of international humanitarian and human rights law can be categorized into five areas, as described in the following sections.

Direct Assaults on Civilians by "Conventional" Means

The wanton killing of civilians in war was defined as a crime by the Hague Convention of 1907. Nonetheless, millions of civilians have been killed in war since then. In the 1930s, the bombing of Ethiopian civilians by Italian planes and of Spanish civilians at Guernica by German planes drew international condemnation as frightening examples of the criminal use of powerful military technology to harm innocent noncombatants, as did Japanese assaults on cities in China. World War II saw the abandonment of scruples by all parties. Examples of assaults on essentially nonmilitary and civilian targets included rocket and bomb attacks on London and Coventry and fire-bombings of Dresden, Hamburg, and Tokyo. Tens of thousands of civilians died, mostly elderly people, women, and children.

The wanton killing of civilians was reaffirmed as a war crime by the Geneva Conventions of 1949—again with little effect. Although the regional and surrogate conflicts of the Cold War replaced massive international confrontations, they were almost uniformly characterized by the indiscriminate bombing and fire-bombing of cities and villages, typified by the armed conflicts in Vietnam and Afghanistan. But the almost automatic assumption that civilians were legitimate and inevitable targets of war was reinforced most during the Cold War by the targeting of cities with intercontinental ballistic missiles and the elaboration of absurd, but massive, "civil defense" plans in both the United States and the Soviet Union.

The end of the Cold War did not change this pattern except, perhaps, to emphasize artillery shelling over bombing as the instrument of choice for attacks on noncombatants and the outright destruction of urban life. The conflict in the former Yugoslavia was marked by the sustained and systematic shelling of many cities.[4,5] These attacks were exceeded in intensity by the Russian assault on Grozny in Chechnya. The highest level of recorded attacks reached was 3,500 shells per day in Sarajevo, and 4,000 *per hour* in Grozny. The first 3 months of conflict in Chechnya killed an estimated 15,000 civilians and made hundreds of thousands of people refugees.[6,7]

Ethnic Cleansing and Extrajudicial Killings

During the 1980s and 1990s, an old and ugly variant of human rights abuse reappeared: conflicts in which the central purpose of military action was the forced removal of civilian populations from their homes and land on the basis of religion, nationality, or ethnic identity. Such actions constitute a crime against humanity under international law (see Chapter 13). Many of the episodes involved mass killing; although they did not approach the methodical slaughter of the Holocaust—industrialized mass murder with the goal of extermination of victimized populations—they were genocidal in spirit. The same was true of the systematic mass murders, forced deportations, detention camps, and enslavement carried out by the Khmer Rouge regime in Cambodia under Pol Pot, a bizarre variant in which victims were characterized not by ethnicity but by urban residence and education.

Other notorious examples of ethnic cleansing are the wars in the former Yugoslavia and in Rwanda. In both conflicts, the instruments of ethnic cleansing were massive assaults on noncombatants; the torture and murder of men, women, and children; the widespread and systematic use of rape to terrorize whole communities; the destruction, by explosives and arson, of homes, farms, industries, and basic infrastructures that provided water, electrical power, food, fuel, sanitation, and other necessities; denial of medical care and other violations of medical neutrality; and siege, blockade, and interference with humanitarian relief. Soldiers and noncombatants alike were starved, tortured, or killed in prison camps, to many of which the International Committee of the Red Cross was denied access.[8] Thousands were victims of arbitrary and extrajudicial execution and were buried in mass graves. Refugees and internally displaced persons were denied protection and deliberately attacked; subjected to beatings, rape, and extortion; forced to walk through minefields; and slaughtered in churches, hospitals, and other sanctuaries (Figure 3-1).

Ethnic cleansing in Yugoslavia and Rwanda are the best-known cases of massive human rights abuses, but attention focused on them has tended to obscure many others, such as those in Sri Lanka, East Timor, Armenia and Azerbaijan, Ossetia and Georgia, China and Tibet, and Iraq and Kurdistan.

In 1988, Iraq destroyed thousands of Kurdish villages. A report on the fate of one such village[9] described murder, forcible disappearance, involuntary relocation, and the refusal to provide minimal conditions of life to detainees. Blatant human rights violations represented by ethnic cleansing will likely continue for decades to come, because dozens of nations have minorities at risk of such onslaughts.[10]

The history of warfare during the past 100 years is replete with smaller-scale, more singular examples of civilian massacres and the punitive destruction of "enemy" villages. The cumulative suffering and loss of life has been enormous. In addition, incidents on the smallest scale, the one-by-one murders by death squads in the so-called dirty wars of repression in El Salvador,[11,12] Nicaragua, Guatemala,[13] Chile,[14] Argentina, Brazil,[15] Haiti,[16] Colombia, Ethiopia, the Philippines, Kashmir,[17] and South Africa over the past six decades, have resulted in hundreds of thousands of dead and "disappeared" civilians (see Chapter 18).

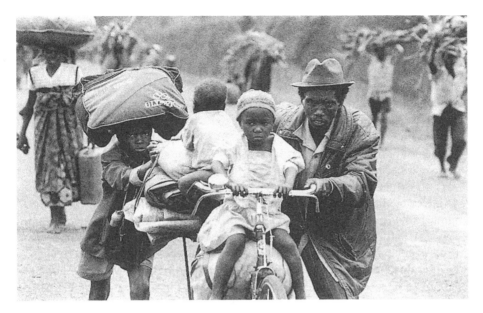

Figure 3-1. A family of Rwandan refugees, their bicycle loaded, make their way along the road to the Benaco Camp in the remote Ngara district, a day's walk from the river where they crossed from Rwanda into Zaire. (Source/photographer: UNICEF/94/0065/ Howard Davies.)

Direct Assaults on Civilians Caused by Indiscriminate Weapons

Indiscriminate weapons are those which, by their effects and defining characteristics, are almost certain (and are usually intended) to harm military combatants and civilians alike and therefore by definition violate the humanitarian law prohibition of wanton killing. They include, but are not limited to, weapons of mass destruction as usually defined: nuclear, chemical, and biological weapons (see Chapters 8, 9, and 10) as well as landmines (see Chapter 7).

The transforming events of 20th-century warfare, the nuclear bombings of Hiroshima and Nagasaki, are described in detail in Chapter 10. That more than 200,000 civilians died from blast, incineration, and radiation is widely recognized; that such mass killing is a violation of human rights is not widely recognized, despite the multiple specific provisions in international law that (1) prohibit attacks that cause unnecessary suffering, (2) require implementation of the principle of proportionality, and (3) affirm the basic immunity of civilian populations and civilians from being objects of attack during armed conflict.

Indirect Assaults on Civilian Populations

Modern military technology, especially the use of high-precision bombs, rockets, and missile warheads, has now made it possible to attack civilian populations in industrialized societies indirectly—but with devastating results—by targeting the facilities on which life depends, while avoiding the stigma of direct attack on the bodies and habitats of noncombatants. The technique has been termed "bomb now, die later."[18]

U.S. military action against Iraq in the 1991 Persian Gulf War and in the Iraq War has included the specific and selective destruction of key aspects of the infrastructure necessary to maintain civilian life and health (see Chapter 15). During the bombing phase of the Persian Gulf War, this deliberate effort almost totally destroyed Iraq's electrical-power generation and transmission capacity and its civilian communications networks. In combination with the prolonged application of economic sanctions and the disruption of highways, bridges, and facilities for refining and distributing fuel by conventional bombing, these actions had severely damaging effects on the health and survival of the civilian population, especially infants and children. Without electrical power, water purification and pumping ceased immediately in all major urban areas, as did sewage pumping and treatment. The appearance and epidemic spread of infectious diarrheal disease in infants and of waterborne diseases, such as typhoid fever and cholera, were rapid. At the same time, medical care and public health measures were totally disrupted. Modern multistory hospitals were left without clean water, sewage disposal, or any electricity beyond what could be supplied by emergency generators designed to operate only a few hours per day. Operating rooms, x-ray equipment, and other vital facilities were crippled. Supplies of anesthetics, antibiotics, and other essential medications were rapidly depleted. Vaccines and medications requiring refrigeration were destroyed, and all immunization programs ceased. Because almost no civilian telephones, computers, or transmission lines were operable, the Ministry of Health was effectively immobilized. Fuel shortages and the disruption of transportation limited civilian access to medical care.[19–21]

Many reports provide clear and quantitative evidence of violations of the requirements of immunity for civilian populations, proportionality, and the prevention of unnecessary suffering. They mock the concept of "life integrity rights." In contrast to the chaos and social disruption that routinely accompany armed conflicts, these deaths have been the consequence of an explicit military policy, with clearly foreseeable consequences to the human rights of civilians. The U.S. military has never conceded that its policies violated human rights under the Geneva Conventions or the guidelines under which U.S. military personnel operate. Yet the ongoing development of military technology suggests that—absent the use of weapons of mass destruction—violations of civilians' human rights will be the preferred method of warfare in the future.

Violations of Medical Neutrality

The Geneva Conventions, customary international law, and medical ethics all mandate

- Medical neutrality
- Protection of medical facilities, personnel, and patients from military attack or interference
- Humane treatment of civilians
- The right of access to care
- Nondiscriminatory treatment of the ill and wounded in time of war.

In the wide range of human rights concerns, medical neutrality is of particular concern to health workers. This is more than a matter of narrow self-interest. Concern for the rights of individual patients and the health of populations is at the core of mandates for health professionals.

Yet in almost every recent armed conflict, violations of medical neutrality have been widespread, systematic, and almost routine. All seven major hospitals in Grozny were destroyed.[6] In the conflict in the former Yugoslavia, hospitals were routinely shelled—in some cases, reduced to rubble—and physicians were special targets of sniper attacks. In Haiti, Kuwait, the West Bank and Gaza Strip, Somalia, and Sudan, hospitals, clinics, and first-aid stations were invaded and patients, medical personnel, and relief workers were assaulted abducted, tortured, and murdered. In El Salvador, where civil conflict was marked by almost every conceivable violation of medical neutrality, health and relief workers were beaten, imprisoned, or murdered for activities as innocent as the vaccination of children. In many conflicts, ambulances are routinely attacked, seized, or blocked. In some civil wars and in so-called "low-intensity conflicts" (somewhat of a misnomer), the destruction of civilian health services has been defended as a legitimate tactic to punish populations suspected of supporting dissident armed forces. In some wars, physicians have been arrested, tortured, or executed for fulfilling their ethical obligation to provide medical care regardless of the patient's political or military affiliation; in others, physicians have actively participated in the torture of dissidents[22] (see Chapter 14).

Contemporary warfare, focused increasingly on assaulting civilian populations and their support structures, is replacing medical neutrality—in practice, if not in law—with strategies in which no civilian systems and no human rights are immune.

War and Intellectual Corruption: Justifying Violations

The Geneva Conventions and other embodiments of human rights protection are undermined by the corrupt view that victory in war is its own justification, so virtually any abuse or atrocity can be rationalized (see Chapter 21). It is a position most frequently articulated as a self-evident necessity by the military, the very institution that is supposed to be constrained by human rights in wartime, and it is strikingly uniform in its expression by soldiers from nations with widely varied political systems.

Is it possible that the existence of laws of war that seek to limit death, pain, and suffering of civilians can actually make war appear more benign than it is, encouraging brutal wars that would not have otherwise been contemplated? Can it ever make sense to go to war to protect civilians from human rights abuses, as has recently been attempted in Kosovo, Bosnia, East Timor, Liberia, and Haiti? These questions are complex and require much more attention than they have received, because war, even when waged for "good" purposes, always terrorizes civilians.

International Laws to Protect Human Rights During War

World War I, with its horrors of trench warfare and chemical weapons, was meant to be the war to end all wars. The failure of the League of Nations to prevent World War II—a global disaster—led to what was hoped were much stronger instruments to prevent war, including the United Nations and specific international human rights laws. The most important human rights documents, including the Universal Declaration of Human Rights, the International Covenant on Civil and Political Rights, and the International Covenant on Economic, Social and Cultural Rights, were all direct products of World War II. The same can be said about the most important humanitarian treaty, the Geneva Conventions of 1949, and the Nuremberg Principles, which were established in war crimes trials of Nazi leaders after World War II. The Nuremberg Principles, which must be distinguished from the Nuremberg Code on human experimentation developed during the Nuremberg Doctors Trial, are the following[23]:

- There are war crimes and crimes against humanity (including murder, torture, and slavery).
- Individuals—not just states—can be held criminally responsible for committing them.
- It is no defense that an individual was "just obeying orders" or following the law of one's country.

The rapid growth of international human rights laws in reaction to the horrors of World War II has been so profound that we need to have some familiarity with what preceded their development before discussing these instruments and their contemporary application and efficacy.

Humanitarian Law

"Humanitarian law" is the unlikely term for the law of war, especially that part of the law of war devoted to rules designed to restrain the actions of the warring parties. The law of war is generally divided into two parts: (1) the law relating to primary prevention by discouraging going to war in the first place (*jus ad bellum*); and (2) the law relating to what may be thought of as secondary prevention, rules for the conduct of war—especially as related to the protection of civilians (*jus in bello*).[24] (See Chapter 21.)

Because war is so terrible, it has, at least since Roman times, required justification, usually set forth in various versions of the "just war" doctrine. This doctrine requires that the war be waged under a public authority, be instigated either for self-defense or to punish a grievous injury, and be pursued only to achieve the just ends—not for vengeance. What constitutes self-defense is open to some interpretation, but the current position of the United States that permits "preemptive" war when a future threat, even one involving weapons of mass destruction, is thought to exist has no "just war" pedigree. Nations need not wait to defend themselves until they are actually attacked, but an attack must be imminent and unstoppable by other means to justify a self-defense war response. Public health principles, which focus on prevention as a means of protecting the health of the public, demand that all reasonable steps be taken to prevent war, including support of international treaties designed to limit the development and use of weapons of mass destruction and support of the United Nations, which was founded primarily to keep the peace.

Secondary prevention or damage control is the goal of *jus in bello*—the attempt to produce rules that limit the destructiveness of an inherently destructive activity. It is strange, and even macabre, to try to develop rules of conduct for mass killings. It is even possible that such rules could make it easier to justify going to war in the first place. Nonetheless, the wholesale slaughter of civilians has been unacceptable since the Thirty Years War (1618–1648) and the work of Dutch jurist Hugo Grotius. Before then, humanitarian rules simply did not exist. Shakespeare's rendition of Henry V's threat to the mayor of a French city, from whom he demanded unconditional surrender or else he would let loose his troops to murder, rape, and pillage, reflects the practice of the Middle Ages[25]:

Take pity of your town and of your people
Whiles yet my soldiers are in my command. . . .
If not, why, in a moment look to see
The blind and bloody soldier with foul hand
Defile the locks of your shrill-shrieking daughters;
Your fathers taken by the silver beards,
And their most reverend heads dashed to the walls;
Your naked infants spitted upon pikes,
Whiles the mad mothers with their howls confus'd
Do break the clouds, as did the wives of Jewry
At Herod's bloody-hunting slaughtermen.
What say you? Will you yield, and this avoid?
Or, guilty in defence, be thus destroy'd?

The Hague Conventions, established before World War I, specifically apply to land warfare and prohibit, among other things, "the attack or bombardment of towns, villages, habitations or buildings which are not defended," as well as "the pillage of a town or place, even when taken by assault." The League of Nations was singularly ineffective in preventing World War II. The Hague rules designed to protect civilians were systemically ignored, not only by Germany and the Soviet Union, but also by Britain in its fire-bombing of German cities (especially Dresden and Hamburg) and by the United States in 1945 in its fire-bombing of more than two dozen Japanese cities and its use of atomic weapons on Hiroshima and Nagasaki.

The basic justification for dropping the atomic bombs was that the laws of warfare applied only to the "civilized nations," and uncivilized peoples could be killed with impunity.[26] As President Harry Truman said 3 days after the bomb was dropped on Hiroshima, "I know that Japan is a terribly cruel and uncivilized nation in warfare. . . ."[27] His position had a long pedigree, including the Crusades, the conquest of the New World, and colonization. A second rationale—that use of atomic weapons on civilian Japanese populations would shorten the war—is simply a restatement of a proposition highlighted earlier in this chapter: War has its own logic, and almost any tactic, regardless of its impact on civilian populations, can be, and often is, justified as militarily necessary.

World War II was followed by the first international war crimes trial in history, conducted at Nuremberg. In his opening statement to the international tribunal, composed of judges from the United States, England, France, and the Soviet Union, Justice Robert Jackson made it clear to all that he understood the critique that the tribunal was designed to render a "victor's justice" based on vengeance "which arises from the anguish of war," rather than justice based on international law. The final judgment not only labeled the waging of aggressive war as a crime against humanity but also catalogued specific acts, including murder, torture, and slavery, as war crimes and crimes against humanity. It was hoped that holding individuals accountable for committing such crimes would help prevent them in the future. It was also hoped, at least by the prosecution team, that the world would establish a "permanent Nuremberg" to be on hand to hold individuals in the future accountable for war crimes and crimes against humanity. In 2000, the International Criminal Court was finally established, based on this model. However, the major military powers, including the United States, have refused to agree to its jurisdiction, primarily because they fear being judged unfairly and arbitrarily by the community of nations for waging aggressive warfare and for using a disproportionate amount of force in so doing.

In short, the legacy of Nuremberg is mixed—perhaps inherently so, since the primary sponsor of Nuremberg, the United States, continues to oppose a "permanent Nuremberg" court; has never publicly acknowledged any doubts about the justice of using atomic weapons on civilian targets; and opposes treaties that would explicitly make first use of nuclear weapons a war crime and a crime against humanity.

The killing of millions of civilians during World War II, as well as the deaths of millions of prisoners of war, led to an expansion of the Geneva Conventions, first with the Geneva Conventions of 1949 (especially Convention IV regarding the protection of civilians), and the two protocols of 1977 (especially Protocol I related to the protection of victims of international armed conflicts). Under Protocol 1, "civilian objects" include all things that are not "military objects"—that is, not "objects which by their nature, location, purpose or use make an effective contribution to military action and whose total or partial destruction, capture or neutralization, in the circumstances ruling at the time, offers definite military advantage." An occupying power is also responsible under Geneva Convention IV and Protocol 1 to ensure that the civilian population is provided with food and medical supplies and, "to the fullest extent of the means available to it," with "clothing, bedding, means of shelter, [and] other supplies essential to the survival of the civilian population."

Human Rights Law

The development of international human rights law based on the horrors of World War II has been more promising. The Charter of the United Nations, signed by the 50 original member nations in 1945, spells out the goals of the United Nations. The first two are "to save succeeding generations from the scourge of war . . . ; and to reaffirm faith in fundamental human rights, in the dignity and worth of the human person, in the equal rights of men and women and of nations large and small." After the Charter was signed, the adoption of an international bill of rights with legal authority proceeded in three steps: a declaration, two treaties, and implementation measures.

The Universal Declaration of Human Rights was adopted by the United Nations General Assembly in 1948 without dissent as "a common standard for all peoples and nations." Its precepts apply in war and peace and provide, among other things, that "Everyone has the right to life, liberty and security of person"; "No one shall be subjected to torture or to cruel, inhuman or degrading treatment or punishment"; "No one shall be subjected to arbitrary arrest, detention or exile"; and "Everyone has the right to freedom of thought, conscience and religion . . . [and to] freedom of opinion and expression." Of special interest to public health is Article 25:

1. Everyone has the right to a standard of living adequate for the health and well-being of himself and his family, including food, clothing, housing and medical care and necessary social services . . .
2. Motherhood and childhood are entitled to special care and assistance.

This was a declaration of principles and thus aspirational; it took a treaty process to make these provisions an obligatory part of international law. Because of another war, the Cold War, two separate treaties were developed, both of which were opened for signature in 1966: the International Covenant on Civil and Political Rights (ICCPR), which the United States supported and which is most directly applicable to war, and the International Covenant on Economic, Social and Cultural Rights, which the United States did not and does not support. The latter contains a more specific right to health, "the right of everyone to the enjoyment of the highest attainable standard of physical and mental health." Given the horrors of poverty, disease, and armed conflicts since World War II, it is easy to dismiss as empty gestures the rights enunciated in these documents.[28] But our disappointments with human rights reflect more our own failures than the failure of the human rights framework. We need not be naïve to continue to believe that the best hope of humankind lies in the protection and promotion of human rights.

How do human rights work in war? Article 4 of the ICCPR provides that, "In time of public emergency which threatens the life of the nation and the existence of which is officially proclaimed," a state may derogate from its obligations under the treaty if contrary measures are "strictly required" for its survival and they are not "inconsistent with their other obligations under international law and do not involve discrimination solely on the ground of race, colour, sex, language, religion or social origin." Even in emergencies, some human rights cannot be compromised by the state, including the right to life; the right not to be tortured or subjected to cruel, inhuman, or degrading treatment or punishment; the right not to be held in slavery; and the right not to be subject to arbitrary arrest or imprisonment. Finally, rights to freedom of thought, conscience, and religion are also protected absolutely. Standards, known as the Siracusa Principles, explain how to apply the emergency derogation provision. They require that when a derogation of the other rights in the ICCPR is made for public emergency, including a public health emergency, the aim must be legitimate and the measure "proportionate to that aim," and "a state shall use no more restrictive means than are required for the achievement of the purpose of the limitation." The principle of proportionality applies directly to warfare; a parallel principle of requiring the use of the "least destructive means necessary" to achieve the military mission has not yet been articulated.

War puts all human rights at risk by its brutal nature. Humanitarian law applies only to armed conflicts and cannot be suspended during hostilities. People around the world continue to suffer, at least in part, because of the lack of effective enforcement mechanisms for human rights and humanitarian law violations. While not a complete solution, the newly established International Criminal Court deserves the support of everyone who believes that human rights and humanitarian law should be taken seriously, and that those who commit war crimes and crimes against humanity should be held accountable for their actions.[29]

References

1. Keegan J. A History of Warfare. New York: Vintage Books, 1993, pp. 56–57.
2. The Shorter Oxford English Dictionary, 3rd ed. London: Oxford University Press, 1964.
3. Geiger HJ, Cook-Degan RM. The role of physicians in conflicts and humanitarian crises. JAMA 1993;270:616–620.
4. Reiff D. On your knees with the dying. In Rabia A, Lifswchultz L (eds.). Why Bosnia? Writings on the Balkan War. Stony Creek, CT: The Pamphleteer's Press, 1993.
5. Magas B. The Destruction of Yugoslavia. London: Verso Press, 1993.
6. Cuny F. Killing Chechnya. New York Review of Books, April 6, 1995, pp. 15–17.
7. Human Rights Watch/Helsinki. Russia: Three months of war in Chechnya. New York: Human Rights Watch/Helsinki Newsletter, February 1995;7(6).
8. Gutman R. A Witness to Genocide. New York: Macmillan, 1993.
9. The Anfal campaign in Iraqi Kurdistan: The destruction of Koreme. New York and Boston: Middle East Watch and Physicians for Human Rights, 1993.
10. Gurr TR, Scaritt JR. Minorities' rights at risk: A global survey. Human Rights Quarterly 1989;11:379–405.
11. El Salvador: Health Care Under Siege. Boston: Physicians for Human Rights, 1990.

12. Geiger HJ, Eisenberg C, Gloyd S, et al. Special report: A new medical mission to El Salvador. N Engl J Med 1989;321:1136–1140.
13. Getting Away with Murder. Boston: Physicians for Human Rights, 1991.
14. Sowing Fear: The Uses of Torture and Psychological Abuse in Chile. Somerville, MA: Physicians for Human Rights, 1988.
15. The Search for Brazil's Disappeared: The Mass Grave at Dom Bosco Cemetery. Washington, DC, and Somerville, MA: Amnesty International, Physicians for Human Rights, and American Association for the Advancement of Science, 1991.
16. Return to the Darkest Days: Human Rights in Haiti Since the Coup. Boston: Physicians for Human Rights, 1992.
17. The Crackdown in Kashmir: Torture of Detainees and Assaults on the Medical Community. Boston and New York: Physicians for Human Rights and Asia Watch, 1993.
18. Geiger HJ, quoted in Kandela P. Iraq: Bomb now, die later. The Lancet 1991;337: 967.
19. Report to the Secretary-General on Humanitarian Needs in Kuwait and Iraq in the Immediate Post-crisis Environment by a Mission to the Area Led by Mr. Martti Ahtisaari, Under-Secretary for Administration and Management. United Nations, March 10, 1991.
20. Report of the WHO/UNICEF Special Mission to Iraq. New York: United Nations Children's Fund, February, 1991.
21. Iraq's Food and Agricultural Situation during the Embargo and the War. Congressional Research Service Report for Congress, February 26, 1991. Washington, DC: The Library of Congress.
22. Medicine Betrayed: The Participation of Doctors in Human Rights Abuses. London: Zed Books and the British Medical Association, 1992.
23. Drinan RF. The Nuremberg Principles in international law. In Annas GJ, Grodin MA (eds.). The Nazi Doctors and the Nuremberg Code. New York: Oxford University Press, 1992, pp. 174–182.
24. O'Brien WV, Arend AC. Just war doctrine and the international law of war. In Bean TE, Sparacino LR (eds.). Military Medical Ethics, Vol. I. Falls Church, VA: Office of The Surgeon General, United States Army; Washington, DC: Borden Institute, Walter Reed Army Medical Center; and Bethesda, MD: Uniformed Services University of the Health Sciences, 2003, pp. 221–249.
25. Shakespeare W. Henry V, III, ii.
26. Lindqvist S. A History of Bombing. New York: New Press, 2000.
27. McCullough D. Truman. New York: Simon & Schuster, 1992, p. 458.
28. Annas GJ. Human rights and health: The Universal Declaration of Human Rights at 50. N Engl J Med 1998;339:1778–1781.
29. Annas GJ. Human rights outlaws: Nuremberg, Geneva, and the global war on terror. Boston U. Law Rev. 2007; 87:427–466.

4

The Impact of War on Mental Health

Evan D. Kanter

Exposure to the horrors of war has profound psychological effects on both military and civilian populations. This chapter focuses on several of these effects, with an emphasis on posttraumatic stress disorder (PTSD), a psychiatric condition that commonly results from war trauma.

Impact on Military Populations

Evolution of a Diagnosis

Recognition of the psychological trauma of war can be found in historical descriptions dating back to Herodotus and in fictional characters from Homer to Shakespeare.[1] During World War I, Wilfred Owen wrote of "men whose minds the Dead have ravished" in his poem "Mental Cases." Despite plain evidence, however, the social order has resisted accepting this reality. Associated with humanity's near-continual involvement in warfare has been a great capacity to suppress awareness of the true consequences of war.

With the development of psychiatry over the past 150 years, the hidden wounds of war have been characterized by many terms. After the U.S. Civil War, it was "soldier's heart." After World War I, it was "shell shock." After

World War II, it was "combat neurosis." Each term represented new clinical insights, yet the devastating impact of psychological trauma was repeatedly forgotten and then rediscovered after each major war. Only in recent decades has the medical and public health community permanently recognized the long-term mental health effects of war.

The concept of PTSD arose in the aftermath of the Vietnam War. The angry insistence and moral force of the Vietnam veterans compelled the public to pay attention. In 1980, PTSD was formally recognized in the *Diagnostic and Statistical Manual of Mental Disorders, Third Edition* (DSM-III) and entered into the clinical lexicon.

The formulation of the diagnosis markedly advanced the pace of epidemiological, clinical, and basic research. This led to greater understanding of the effects of traumatic stress and significant revision of the concept of PTSD. In 1994, the diagnostic criteria were updated in DSM-IV. PTSD was previously considered a normal response to overwhelmingly traumatic events. But now it is clear that most individuals exposed to trauma do not develop PTSD. It is essential to distinguish between PTSD, a psychiatric disorder, and normal stress reactions, in which symptoms may be severe but are transient.

PTSD is not the only psychiatric disorder that may result from exposure to war trauma. Mood disorders, such as major depression, and other anxiety disorders, such as panic disorder, are also frequent sequelae of trauma. PTSD, however, is the prototypic traumatic stress syndrome, and it is the focus of this chapter.

Diagnosis of PTSD

As defined in DSM-IV, PTSD is an anxiety disorder that develops after exposure to a traumatic event characterized by "actual or threatened death or serious injury, or a threat to the physical integrity of oneself or others." The response to the trauma must involve "intense fear, helplessness, or horror." A diagnosis of PTSD then requires the presence of symptoms in each of three categories: re-experiencing, avoidance, and hyperarousal.

Symptoms of re-experiencing include intrusive memories, nightmares, and flashbacks. Both psychological distress and physiological reactivity are triggered by reminders of the trauma. Continual reliving of the trauma interferes with normal functioning and may involve loss of behavioral control. In severe cases, triggers may generalize so that, for example, any loud noise or any face with certain ethnic features may elicit a conditioned fear response.

Avoidant symptoms include avoidance of reminders of the trauma, amnesia for important aspects of the trauma, diminished interest in activities, detachment from others, emotional numbing, and a sense of a foreshortened future. An affected individual may have few or no close relationships and may experience extreme isolation. The person's world shrinks, with progressive loss of activities and social connections in what has been called the "undoing of character."[1]

Hyperarousal symptoms include difficulty sleeping, irritability and outbursts of anger, difficulty concentrating, a constant state of alertness, and an exaggerated startle response. Veterans feel that they are "on guard" all the time. Excessive preoccupation with the safety of one's home and family is characteristic. Family members commonly report the experience of "walking on eggshells" around the veteran. An affected individual may be unable to tolerate crowds due to extreme distress at not being able to notice everything that is occurring.

For a person to be diagnosed with PTSD, symptoms must be present for at least 1 month, and there must be clinically significant distress, such as impairment in social or occupational functioning. A second trauma-related diagnosis, acute stress disorder, was added to DSM-IV to account for symptoms experienced in the first 30 days after a trauma, although the validity of this diagnosis has been questioned. Military psychiatry uses the diagnosis of combat stress reaction. The *International Classification of Diseases, Tenth Revision* (ICD-10) criteria for the diagnosis of PTSD are similar to those of the DSM-IV. In addition, ICD-10 includes the diagnosis of enduring personality change after catastrophic experience, referring to profound long-term effects of traumatic stress.

Associated Features

In addition to 17 symptoms included in the DSM-IV diagnosis of PTSD, there are a variety of commonly associated features, including high levels of depression, suicidal and homicidal ideation, and stress-induced paranoid ideation. Auditory and visual hallucinations may occur that typically are not bizarre but have content consistent with the traumatic events. Difficulty trusting others and issues of guilt, including survivor guilt, are almost universal. Anniversary reactions may be profound, even when the person is not consciously aware of the date. Marked exacerbation of symptoms or re-emergence of dormant symptoms can occur after retraumatization by an event such as a motor vehicle accident or a major surgical procedure.

Functional and Social Morbidity

Poor occupational and social functioning is a hallmark of chronic PTSD. One important dimension of this is the high comorbidity of substance-use disorders, which occur in 50 to 85 percent of those with PTSD.[2] The association is thought to represent self-medication in attempt to control highly distressing symptoms.

Difficulty maintaining employment is typical among veterans with PTSD. A work history reported as "30 jobs in 30 years" is almost diagnostic. The hyperalertness and outbursts of anger result in difficulty getting along with coworkers and supervisors. Concentration deficits affect the ability to complete tasks. A survey of Vietnam veterans showed that PTSD significantly lowered the likelihood of working and significantly decreased hourly wages for those who were working.[3]

Interviews conducted with Vietnam veterans and their spouses or coresident partners 15 years after the war found much higher rates of marital, parental, and family adjustment problems in families of veterans with PTSD than in those without PTSD.[4] Higher levels of family violence were present, and high levels of distress in spouses and partners were found. Behavioral problems in children were evident; one third of male veterans had a child with problems that were clinically significant. Combat exposure overshadowed the effect of any other variable that might predispose to family problems.

Violent behavior is frequent among combat veterans and is much more frequent when PTSD is present. In a sample of Croatian combat veterans, 74 percent demonstrated aggressive behavior, and 37 percent saw a psychiatrist primarily for aggressive behavior.[5] The mean number of violent acts during the previous year for veterans with PTSD was 18.2, compared with 2.7 among veterans without PTSD.

Many families have traditions of military service. With increased understanding of traumatic stress, many veterans have realized that their fathers and grandfathers had PTSD from combat and that this at least partially explained the tension, violence, and emotional distancing that was present in their home environment.[6]

The heavy societal burden of mental health problems among war veterans was demonstrated by a study that used data from the National Comorbidity Survey (1990–1992) to determine the percentage of psychiatric disorders and adverse psychosocial outcomes attributable to combat exposure in U.S. men.[7] It was found that the following were significantly attributable to combat exposure: 28 percent of 12-month PTSD, 7 percent of 12-month major depressive disorder, 8 percent of 12-month substance abuse disorder, 12 percent of 12-month job loss, 9 percent of current unemployment, 8 percent of current divorce or separation, and 21 percent of current spouse or partner abuse. The authors concluded that "combat exposure results in substantial morbidity lasting decades and accounts for significant and multifarious forms of dysfunction at the national level."

Medical Comorbidity

Chronic pain and somatization are commonly seen in combat veterans. Medically unexplained physical symptoms may include musculoskeletal, cardiovascular, neurological, gastrointestinal, and audiological complaints. Fibromyalgia and chronic fatigue syndrome are examples of somatic presentations that have been associated with traumatic stress. The presence and severity of PTSD in Vietnam veterans was correlated with greater self-reported and physician-reported physical health problems.[8] Persian Gulf War veterans with PTSD also endured a greater number of physical symptoms than those with a non-PTSD psychological condition or a medical illness.[9]

The impact of PTSD on physical health goes well beyond somatic anxiety. A growing body of evidence links combat exposure and PTSD with an increased incidence of chronic medical illness, including cardiovascular disease, arthritis, and diabetes.[10] The pathogenetic contribution of PTSD to these diseases may involve alterations in adrenal stress hormones and the immune system. An archival examination of military and medical records from the U.S. Civil War demonstrated that traumatic war experiences were related to signs of disease and risk of early death.[11] Greater exposure to death of military comrades and exposure to war trauma at a younger age were associated with increased signs of physician-diagnosed cardiac, gastrointestinal, and nervous diseases across the lifespan of Civil War veterans.

Suicide

A recent prospective study used data from the 1986–1994 National Health Interview Survey to assess the risk of suicide among veterans in the general U.S. population.[12] The study tracked 320,890 men, of whom 104,026 had served in the U.S. military between 1917 and 1994. Veterans were twice as likely to die of suicide compared with non-veterans in the general population. The study did not address causes of suicide, but psychiatric conditions, including major depression and PTSD, would likely be significant mediators of the effect.

Epidemiology of Combat PTSD

Prevalence

The National Vietnam Veterans Readjustment Survey estimated the lifetime prevalence of PTSD among Vietnam veterans at 31 percent and the current prevalence at 15 percent, 11 to 12 years after the war.[13] A recent reassessment using new data and methods revised the estimate downward to 19 percent lifetime prevalence and 9 percent current prevalence.[14] Even if this lower estimate is correct, it still represents more than 500,000 individuals—a significant psychiatric burden. The reassessment strongly confirmed the dose-response relationship between trauma exposure and PTSD and found no evidence of falsification due to compensation seeking.

Because the concept of PTSD arose after the Vietnam War, popular culture understandably associates PTSD with Vietnam veterans. There is an unfortunate misconception that World War II veterans did not develop PTSD in the same way. During World War II, the U.S. military lost 504,000 personnel from fighting because of psychiatric collapse—enough to staff 50 divisions. At one point, personnel were being discharged from the U.S. Army due to psychiatric problems faster than new recruits were being drafted.[15] The recognition that neuropsychiatric disorders were the leading cause of medical discharge from the military services was the primary impetus leading to the establishment, in 1946, of the National Institute of Mental Health.

After deployment in Iraq, 16 percent of Marines and 17 percent of soldiers surveyed met screening criteria for major depression, generalized anxiety, or PTSD.[16] These data likely underestimate the magnitude of the problem, because (1) PTSD often has a delayed onset, so its prevalence may increase substantially over time; (2) individuals who had been removed from their units, including those removed because of injuries, were not included, and this group might be expected to have higher rates of psychiatric symptoms; and (3) this cohort served early in the Iraq War, and the nature of the fighting subsequently changed in ways that probably increased the risk of PTSD.

Risk Factors

The development of PTSD is a complex biopsychosocial process. Numerous studies have examined characteristics both of the trauma and of the pretrauma and posttrauma environments in order to determine the factors that increase the likelihood of developing PTSD.[17] In addition, trauma-exposed individuals who have not developed PTSD have been studied in order to understand the hardiness and resiliency that they display.

The most important determinant of the probability of developing PTSD is the intensity and duration of trauma exposure. A dose-response relationship between trauma exposure and both incidence of PTSD and severity of PTSD symptoms has been a consistent finding. Other aspects of the trauma that increase the risk of PTSD include unpredictability, uncontrollability, and significant object loss, such as loss of a loved one.

Traumatic events of human design are worse than accidents. For example, interpersonal traumas such as rape or combat carry much higher risk of PTSD than natural disasters. Torture is an extreme example in which there is a specific intention to cause psychological breakdown. In rape trauma, a close relationship to the perpetrator, the use of a weapon, and physical injury increase the risk of PTSD. In combat trauma, the following are especially traumatic: being wounded, witnessing atrocities, witnessing civilian casualties, being responsible for the death of noncombatants, and involvement in "friendly fire" incidents. Soldiers involved in these events have a higher likelihood of developing PTSD. Experiences that dramatically magnify the impact of trauma include being held in captivity and displacement from home (as refugees or internally displaced persons).

The Vietnam Era Twin Registry study of 4,042 male twin pairs demonstrated that genetic factors account for approximately 30 percent of the variance in PTSD symptoms.[18] For reasons that are not understood, female gender has consistently been found to be a predisposing factor; given exposure to the same trauma, women are more than twice as likely to develop PTSD as men.[19] Age at the time of trauma is also a risk factor, with younger individuals being more susceptible. This is an especially important finding, because it is primarily young people who fight wars.

Developmental childhood trauma, such as abuse, neglect, or early parental loss, is also a significant risk factor for PTSD. The relative percentage of individuals with difficult childhoods is increased among military recruits, because military service often offers such individuals opportunities for educational, social, and economic advancement. A commonly expressed reason for joining the military is, "I joined the Army to escape the war [at home]." Other risk factors for PTSD include comorbid psychiatric or medical conditions, subtle neurological dysfunction manifested as neurological soft signs (as in figure copying, the road map test of direction sense, and finger-thumb opposition), lack of education or low intelligence, personality traits such as neuroticism (an enduring tendency to experience negative emotional states), and a history of conduct disorder.

The posttrauma environment also has a critical effect. Family pathologies, such as violence, substance abuse, and mental illness, exacerbate PTSD. Strong social support alleviates severity of symptoms and allows for improved ability to function, given a certain level of symptoms. On the other hand, a negative response of the social group that is stigmatizing, invalidating, rejecting, blaming, or shaming has the opposite effect.

Current Conflicts

The level of combat trauma to which U.S. and allied troops have been exposed in Iraq (see Chapter 15) and Afghanistan is extremely high. For example, one group of 815 Marines returning from Iraq reported a degree of trauma not seen among U.S. troops since the Vietnam War: 97 percent had been shot at, 65 percent had killed an enemy combatant, 28 percent had killed a civilian, 94 percent had seen dead bodies, and 57 percent had handled dead bodies.[16] The wars in Iraq and Afghanistan are being fought without front lines; the threat is everywhere at all times. The inability to distinguish enemy combatants from civilians is extremely distressing and may increase the risk of PTSD. Significant adverse psychological impact may result from the perception that one has been lied to and also from inadequate training or preparedness.

With a volunteer force and prolonged conflict, multiple deployments are common and are a great cause for psychiatric concern. Some soldiers who have diagnosable PTSD or are taking psychiatric medications have been redeployed for further combat. Often, military personnel with significant PTSD symptoms function very well as soldiers. A hyperadrenergic state is conducive to warfare, with the ability to be continually on alert and instantly aggressive. But these attributes are highly dysfunctional at home or in the workplace. After combat, reintegration into society can be extremely challenging. The U.S. Department of Defense has instituted a readjustment counseling program, called "Battlemind," that attempts to address these issues. However, multiple deployments are likely to result in many severe cases of PTSD.

A supportive homecoming may ameliorate some of the pain of readjustment and reintegration for veterans. Early recognition of PTSD cases may lead to better outcomes, since effective treatments are now available. But treatment is of no benefit if it is not sought. In one study, among those who screened positive for a psychiatric disorder, only 23 to 40 percent had sought mental health care.[16] The most common perceived barriers to mental health care were being seen as weak, being treated differently by unit leadership, decreased confidence on the part of unit members, difficulty getting time off work, being blamed for the problem by leadership, and likelihood of harm to one's career.

Traumatic brain injury (TBI) is a "signature wound" of the wars in Iraq and Afghanistan. Due to blast injuries from improvised explosive devices, up to 30 percent of injured soldiers may have suffered some degree of TBI.

Economic Implications of Mental Health Treatment and Disability Compensation

The diagnosis of PTSD has complex political implications, in part because it enables veterans to make claims for compensation of psychiatric disability due to military service—a significant long-term cost of war that is generally not accounted for when weighing decisions to use military force. Currently a U.S. veteran (without spouse or dependents) who is 100 percent disabled and unemployable receives compensation payments from the Department of Veterans Affairs (VA) of $2,471 per month. Over a 50-year period, this could total more than $1.4 million, without adjustment for inflation. Providing PTSD treatment is not only critical for improving health, but it may also ameliorate the economic burden of disability benefits.

The VA is at the forefront of PTSD research and treatment. Its resources include the National Center for Posttraumatic Stress Disorder and more than 100 specialized treatment programs throughout the United States. The magnitude of the influx of new patients that the system will need to absorb has been suggested by postdeployment health assessments of more than 200,000 soldiers and Marines who have returned from the Iraq War. These assessments have revealed that 35 percent of them accessed mental heath services within 1 year of deployment to Iraq, and 12 percent were diagnosed with a mental health problem.[20]

Several reports by the Government Accountability Office (GAO) have raised the question of whether the VA is adequately prepared to manage the health consequences of current warfare, especially with respect to mental health. The GAO found that the VA used "unrealistic assumptions, errors in estimation and insufficient data" to project its overall budget for fiscal years 2005 and 2006, resulting in a $3 billion shortfall.[21] The GAO also examined PTSD treatment and questioned the capacity of the system to absorb the many military personnel expected to have psychiatric problems.[22]

Some who are alarmed by the magnitude of the financial compensation involved have criticized the diagnosis of PTSD. A recently commissioned study by the Institute of Medicine of the National Academy of Sciences emphatically supported the validity of the diagnosis, concluding "that PTSD is a well-characterized medical disorder and that the DSM-IV criteria for diagnosing PTSD are evidence-based, widely accepted, and widely used."[23] In addition, there is little evidence of fraudulent claims.[14]

Military Sexual Assault Trauma

Recognition and treatment of PTSD resulting from military sexual assault trauma (MST) is an emerging area of clinical attention. The extent of sexual violence that occurs in the military has generally been shrouded in secrecy. Victims are frequently treated as if these events never occurred and are told not to talk about them, which can dramatically aggravate the severity of psychiatric symptoms.

Rape occurring during military service is reported by up to 30 percent of women veterans in national surveys. PTSD was present in 60 percent of a sample of women veterans with MST (which includes rape) who were receiving medical or psychiatric treatment in the VA system.[24] Although the prevalence of MST in men is much less than in women, the number of MST-related PTSD cases is similar due to the much larger number of men in the military.

Neurobiology of PTSD

Research into the neurophysiological basis of PTSD has advanced greatly since the diagnosis was established. The evidence conclusively demonstrates that PTSD is a brain disorder—a war wound, no less than a shrapnel wound. Alterations occur in the hypothalamic-pituitary-adrenal axis, the adrenergic system, the serotonergic system, the thyroid, and the immune system. Findings that strongly suggest a hyperadrenergic state in subjects with PTSD include the detection of increased levels of catecholamines in cerebrospinal fluid and the finding of exaggerated responses, such as panic attacks and flashbacks, to administration of the alpha-2-adrenergic antagonist yohimbine.[25] The finding of decreased cortisol levels in PTSD is intriguing, given that increased levels are seen in major depression and in acute stress.[26]

Neuroimaging studies reveal PTSD psychopathology.[27] Alteration of function has been demonstrated in the amygdala, prefrontal cortex, and hippocampus. The amygdala is centrally involved in the coordination of threat response and is necessary for fear conditioning. Functional neuroimaging has demonstrated hyperresponsivity of the amygdala in PTSD. Decreased functioning of the medial prefrontal cortex, which is involved in the extinction of fear conditioning, has been shown. Volume loss and impaired function of the hippocampus, which is involved in explicit memory processes and the encoding of context during fear conditioning, have been demonstrated. In addition, failure of the prefrontal cortex and hippocampus to normally inhibit the amygdala occurs in PTSD.

Treatment of PTSD

Education of patients and families about the effects of psychological trauma is an essential first step in treatment. Coping skills training teaches methods of self-soothing and identifying triggers. Among the variety of approaches are anger management, relaxation techniques, meditation, and mindfulness training.

A variety of psychotherapeutic interventions have demonstrated efficacy.[28] Cognitive-behavioral therapies focus on challenging distorted beliefs and reconstructing negative thought patterns. The premise is that you can change how you feel by changing how you think. Excessive guilt and chronic depression often respond well to this method.

Exposure therapies allow progressive desensitization to traumatic memories in a safe, controlled environment. A common technique is repeated exposure to written or audiotaped accounts of the patient's worst traumatic experience. Patients must be carefully screened, however, because some are unable to tolerate the intensity of this treatment.

Eye movement desensitization and reprocessing (EMDR) combines elements of cognitive and exposure therapy with eye movements or other stimuli that create an alternation of attention back and forth across the person's midline. EMDR has been popular, but controversial, and the significance of the alternating movements has been questioned. Nevertheless, the overall technique has demonstrated efficacy.

Group therapy is often employed for the normalization and validation afforded by dynamic interaction with others who have had similar traumatic experiences. Acceptance-based therapy may be of benefit in tolerating chronic, intractable symptoms. Marital and family therapies play important roles in addressing communication difficulties and behavioral problems in the home.

Pharmacotherapy for PTSD is symptom based.[29] Selective serotonin reuptake inhibitors (SSRIs) are considered first-line treatment. SSRIs may diminish the severity of all three symptom clusters (re-experiencing, avoidance, and hyperarousal). Sertraline and paroxetine are currently the only medications approved by the U.S. Food and Drug Administration for the treatment of PTSD.

The hyperadrenergic state present in PTSD provides a theoretical basis for the use of antiadrenergic agents. The alpha-1-adrenergic antagonist prazosin has demonstrated promising efficacy in suppressing trauma nightmares.[30] Anticonvulsants, such as valproic acid, may be useful in targeting anger dyscontrol and mood swings, perhaps by dampening amygdala hyperactivity. Other classes of antidepressants and new-generation antipsychotics are also frequently used. Sedative medications for anxiety and sleep, including benzodiazepines, do not directly treat the underlying condition but may be useful adjuncts in pharmacotherapy.

Mental Health Impacts of War on Civilian Populations

Modern war is increasingly associated with devastating mental health consequences to civilians. Psychological warfare and terror target civilian populations by means such as antipersonnel landmines, use of child soldiers, "disappearances," torture, and massacres. Systematic mass rape has been used as a weapon of war in Croatia, Bosnia and Herzegovina, and elsewhere with profound psychological effects.

The prevalence of mental disorders among civilian populations increases during wartime and in postconflict settings.[31] A wide variety of psychological symptoms and syndromes has been described. Population-based assessments conducted in Algeria, Cambodia, Ethiopia (Eritrean refugees), and the Middle East (Gaza) demonstrated greatly increased prevalence of mental disorders, including PTSD, other anxiety disorders, mood disorders, and somatoform disorders, among individuals exposed to violence associated with armed conflict.[32] PTSD was present in 40 percent of those assessed in Algeria, 33 percent in Cambodia, 19 percent in Ethiopia, and 28 percent in Gaza. A psychiatric disorder of some type was present in 62 percent of subjects in Algeria, 58 percent in Cambodia, 28 percent in Ethiopia, and 40 percent in Gaza.

Internally displaced and refugee Kosovar-Albanians who returned to Kosovo after the NATO bombing campaign were surveyed in 1999. PTSD symptoms were reported by 17 percent and hatred toward the Serbs by 89 percent. A follow-up survey in 2000 found those who felt hatred toward the Serbs had decreased to 69 percent, but those reporting PTSD symptoms had increased to 25 percent.[33] An epidemiological survey of the population in northern Sri Lanka, where armed conflict has continued for 30 years, found somatization in 41 percent of those interviewed, PTSD in 27 percent, other anxiety disorders in 26 percent, and major depression in 25 percent.[34]

A survey by the Gaza Community Mental Health Center of children aged 10 to 19 years revealed that 33 percent had PTSD symptoms requiring psychological intervention, 49 percent had moderate PTSD symptoms, 16 percent had mild PTSD symptoms, and only 3 percent had no symptoms.[35] Children living in camps had a prevalence of symptoms several times greater than that of children living in towns. Another Palestinian study found that 46 percent of parents reported aggressive behavior among their children, 39 percent reported their children suffered from nightmares, 38 percent reported poor school performance, and 27 percent reported bedwetting.[36] Refugee children were more likely to behave aggressively than non-refugee children. Seventy percent of all parents had not received any psychological support for their children.

Being an internally displaced person or a refugee has consistently been found to increase the prevalence and severity of psychiatric illness and disability. A study of adult Bosnian refugees living in a camp in Croatia found that 39 percent met criteria for major depression, and 26 percent met criteria for PTSD.[37] Among Guatemalan refugees living in Chiapas, Mexico, who were surveyed 20 years after the civil war in Guatemala, 12 percent met criteria for PTSD, 54 percent had anxiety symptoms, and 39 percent had symptoms of depression.[38] The traumatic experiences that were most associated with PTSD were witnessing the disappearance of family members, being close to death, and living in a home with 9 to 15 other people. Among Cambodian refugees who survived the horrors of the Khmer Rouge regime, high rates of psychiatric disorders were found two decades after resettlement in the United States;

the past-year prevalence rate of PTSD was 62 percent and that of major depression was 51 percent.[39]

As in military populations, civilian women are affected by war trauma to a greater degree than men in most studies. Other especially vulnerable populations are children, older people, and disabled people. The use of rape as a weapon of war and the abduction of children by militias are urgent issues that are addressed elsewhere in this book. Journalists covering war and peacekeepers also have been shown to have high rates of PTSD. Psychiatric patients in institutions are an especially vulnerable group, as was evident in the Balkan conflicts of the 1990s. Patients may be abused, as were Serbian patients in Kosovo, or abandoned, as occurred in Bosnia when staff fled the fighting. This failure of large psychiatric institutions has led reconstruction efforts to focus instead on community-based mental health care.

Africa

Africa is the most war-ravaged continent, in terms of both the number of wars between and within nations and the vast number of traumatized civilians there (see Chapter 17). Eight years after the 1994 genocide in Rwanda, 25 percent of the population met criteria for a diagnosis of PTSD.[40] Extremely high rates of mental disorders were also found in specific populations in Uganda, Kenya, and Sudan.[41] The mental health consequences of war and displacement have been a major obstacle to development of the continent.

It has been argued that the diagnostic concept of PTSD, developed in a Western cultural context, is not applicable to populations in the developing world. This argument is undermined by the elucidation of the basic neurobiology of PTSD, which is independent of culture. There is fairly consistent psychopathology among populations from different countries, confirming the validity of PTSD as a diagnosis.[41] What may be very different across cultures, however, is the manner in which mental health services need to be provided for those affected by PTSD and other mental disorders related to war.

A systematic comparison was conducted of civilians exposed to the bombing of the U.S. Embassy in Nairobi, Kenya, in 1998 with civilians exposed to the bombing of the Alfred P. Murrah Federal Building in Oklahoma City in 1995.[42] The two groups exhibited similar psychopathology, including prevalence of PTSD and other psychiatric disorders. In both populations, female gender and preexisting psychiatric disorder were major predictors of bombing-related PTSD. Coping responses in the two groups, however, were quite different. Americans typically utilized psychiatric treatment and were more likely to use medication and alcohol. No Kenyan in the study visited a psychiatrist; instead bombing victims utilized support and debriefing groups as well as religious counseling.

Afghanistan and Iraq

Decades of armed conflict and population displacement in Afghanistan have resulted in a high prevalence of psychiatric symptoms throughout the country. Two well-conducted multi-cluster, population-based studies have been performed. In one study, a survey of 799 adults 15 years of age and older, 62 percent of respondents reported experiencing at least four traumatic events during the previous 10 years.[43] Symptoms of depression were found in 68 percent, symptoms of anxiety in 72 percent, and PTSD in 42 percent. Disabled people and women had poorer mental health status. There was a significant relationship between poor mental health status and traumatic events. Coping strategies included religious and spiritual practices. The other study, with 1,011 respondents 15 years of age and older in Nangarhar Province, found that almost half had experienced traumatic events.[44] Symptoms of depression were observed in 39 percent, symptoms of anxiety in 52 percent, and PTSD in 20 percent. High rates of symptoms were associated with higher numbers of traumatic events experienced. Women had higher rates than men. The main sources of emotional support were religion and family.

There have been many news reports on the current state of mental health in Iraq, but no systematic study has been performed. Iraq's relatively advanced mental health system has been extensively degraded by war and economic sanctions. Ongoing violence and instability impede redevelopment. The 1,500-bed Al-Rashad Hospital, the largest psychiatric hospital in Iraq, was destroyed by looters in April 2003 after U.S. forces broke through walls. The patients fled, including residents of a maximum security ward for violent criminal offenders.

The refugee crisis in Iraq is now among the largest in the world. The United Nations estimates that more than 2 million Iraqis have fled to surrounding countries and another 2 million have been internally displaced (see Chapters 13 and 15). As previously mentioned, displacement from one's home significantly increases the likelihood of PTSD and other psychiatric disorders.

PTSD and the Perpetuation of Conflict

If we know something about the effect of psychological trauma on individuals, we can begin to consider what the societal impact is when many individuals in a population have symptoms of PTSD. These symptoms, which have a neurophysiological basis, include anger outbursts, emotional numbing, isolation and despair, distrust and paranoia, hypervigilance, and preoccupation with an enemy. There is poor regulation of affect, impaired extinction of conditioned fear, and what amounts to decreased "emotional intelligence." The symptoms translate into misunderstanding, bitterness, resentment, aggression, and outright hostility.

It is easy to see then how this grave psychological burden may serve as an engine to perpetuate conflict. Increased understanding of psychological trauma in individuals may help guide the design of treatment approaches and interventions for conflict-affected populations. Advances in trauma theory and neurobiology may be applied to the task of reconstructing war-torn societies.

Psychosocial Intervention

Providing mental health services to civilian populations affected by war poses a tremendous challenge. Resources are likely to be extremely limited. In some cases, there may be no mental health services at all, and there may not have been any services before the war. Moreover, it is not clear how to identify individuals requiring intervention, when to intervene, or what methods of intervention are effective.[45]

Given the many people affected, community-based approaches would seem appropriate. The availability of family and social supports provides considerable protective effect. Efforts at resettlement and vocational training should give attention to strengthening and rebuilding family and village structures. Religious and cultural approaches to coping are very important. Traditional practices and ceremonies should be integrated into rehabilitation and reconstruction efforts. Education about psychological trauma and training of grassroots health workers are likely to be major tasks. The International Society for Traumatic Stress Studies, in collaboration with the RAND Corporation, has issued evidence- and consensus-based guidelines for the mental health training of primary health workers in conflict-affected developing countries.[46]

A cross-sectional, population-based study of the relationship between cognitive and psychiatric effects of war that was conducted in the former Yugoslavia found PTSD and depression to be independent of a sense of injustice arising from perceived lack of redress for trauma.[47] Instead, fear of threat to safety and loss of control over one's life were the most important mediating factors. This has important implications for reconciliation efforts. Truth and reconciliation commissions modeled after the South African example are sophisticated efforts at healing war-torn societies that may be informed by such research.

Conclusion

Psychiatric casualties are the hidden wounds of war. PTSD is an injury to the nervous system that can be severely debilitating. The economic cost of caring for individuals with PTSD is great, and the harmful effects extend to families and communities. The overwhelming impact on society may reverberate for generations.

Our understanding of the psychological trauma of war has increased enormously in the past three decades. Ongoing efforts to improve the recognition and treatment of PTSD and other trauma-related conditions will help mitigate some of the damage. Effective intervention in war-torn societies in the developing world is a challenge that is just beginning to be addressed. Ultimately, the intervention of greatest potential benefit would be the prevention of war.

References

1. Shay J. Achilles in Vietnam: Combat Trauma and the Undoing of Character. New York: Touchstone, 1995.
2. Miller MW, Vogt DS, Mozley SL, et al. PTSD and substance-related problems: The mediating roles of disconstraint and negative emotionality. J Abnorm Psychol 2006;115:369–379.
3. Savoca E, Rosenheck R. The civilian labor market experiences of Vietnam-era veterans: The influence of psychiatric disorders. J Ment Health Policy Econ 2000;3:199–207.
4. Jordan BK, Marmar CR, Fairbank JA, et al. Problems in families of male Vietnam veterans with posttraumatic stress disorder. J Consult Clin Psychol 1992;60:916–920.
5. Begic D, Jokic-Begic N. Aggressive behavior in combat veterans with post-traumatic stress disorder. Mil Med 2001;166:671–676.
6. Byrne CA, Riggs DS. The cycle of trauma: Relationship aggression in male Vietnam veterans with symptoms of posttraumatic stress disorder. Violence Vict 1996;11: 213–225.
7. Prigerson HG, Maciejewski PK, Rosenheck RA. Population attributable fractions of psychiatric disorders and behavioral outcomes associated with combat exposure among US men. Am J Public Health 2002;92:59–63.
8. Beckham JC, Moore SD, Feldman ME, et al. Health status, somatization, and severity of posttraumatic stress disorder in Vietnam combat veterans with posttraumatic stress disorder. Am J Psychiatry 1998;155:1565–1569.
9. Engel CC, Liu X, McCarthy BD, et al. Relationship of physical symptoms to posttraumatic stress disorder among veterans seeking care for Gulf War-related concerns. Psychosom Med 2000;62:739–745.
10. Boscarino JA. Posttraumatic stress disorder and physical illness: Results from clinical and epidemiologic studies. Ann N Y Acad Sci 2004;1032:141–153.
11. Pizarro J, Silver RC, Prause J. Physical and mental health costs of traumatic war experiences among civil war veterans. Arch Gen Psychiatry 2006;63:193–200.

12. Kaplan MS, Huguet N, McFarland BH, Newsom JT. Suicide among male veterans: A prospective, population-based study. J Epidemiol Community Health 2007;61:619–624.

13. Kulka RA, Schlenger WE, Fairbank JA, et al. Trauma and the Vietnam War Generation: Report of Findings from the National Vietnam Veterans Readjustment Study. New York: Brunner/Mazel, 1990.

14. Dohrenwend BP, Turner JB, Turse NA, et al. The psychological risks of Vietnam for U.S. veterans: A revisit with new data and methods. Science 2006;313:979–982.

15. Grossman D. On Killing. Boston: Little, Brown, 1995.

16. Hoge CW, Castro CA, Messer SC, et al. Combat duty in Iraq and Afghanistan: Mental health problems and barriers to care. N Engl J Med 2004;351:13–22.

17. Brewin CR, Andrews B, Valentine JD. Meta-analysis of risk factors for posttraumatic stress disorder in trauma-exposed adults. J Consult Clin Psychol 2000;68:748–766.

18. True WR, Rice J, Eisen SA, et al. A twin study of genetic and environmental contributions to liability for posttraumatic stress symptoms. Arch Gen Psychiatry 1993; 50:257–264.

19. Holbrook TL, Hoyt DB, Stein MB, Sieber WJ. Gender differences in long-term posttraumatic stress disorder outcomes after major trauma: Women are at higher risk of adverse outcomes than men. J Trauma 2002;53:882–888.

20. Hoge CW, Auchterlonie JL, Milliken CS. Mental health problems, use of mental health services, and attrition from military service after returning from deployment to Iraq or Afghanistan. JAMA 2006;295:1023–1032.

21. Government Accountability Office. VA Health Care: Budget Formulation and Reporting on Budget Execution Need Improvement. GAO-06–958. Washington, DC: GAO, September 20, 2006.

22. Government Accountability Office. VA and Defense Health Care: More Information Needed to Determine if VA Can Meet an Increase in Demand for Post-Traumatic Stress Disorder Services, GAO-04–1069. Washington, DC: GAO, September 20, 2004.

23. Board on Population Health and Public Health Practice, Institute of Medicine. Posttraumatic Stress Disorder: Diagnosis and Assessment. Washington, DC: National Academies Press, 2006.

24. Yaeger D, Himmelfarb N, Cammack A, Mintz J. DSM-IV diagnosed posttraumatic stress disorder in women veterans with and without military sexual trauma. J Gen Intern Med 2006;21:S65–S69.

25. O'Donnell T, Hegadoren KM, Coupland NC. Noradrenergic mechanisms in the pathophysiology of post-traumatic stress disorder. Neuropsychobiology 2004;50:273–283.

26. Yehuda R. Advances in understanding neuroendocrine alterations in PTSD and their therapeutic implications. Ann N Y Acad Sci 2006;1071:137–166.

27. Shin LM, Rauch SL, Pitman RK. Amygdala, medial prefrontal cortex, and hippocampal function in PTSD. Ann N Y Acad Sci 2006;1071:67–79.

28. Foa EB. Psychosocial therapy for posttraumatic stress disorder. J Clin Psychiatry 2006;67(Suppl 2):40–45.

29. Davidson JR. Pharmacologic treatment of acute and chronic stress following trauma: 2006. J Clin Psychiatry 2006;67(Suppl 2):34–39.

30. Raskind MA, Peskind ER, Kanter ED, et al. Reduction of nightmares and other PTSD symptoms in combat veterans by prazosin: A placebo-controlled study. Am J Psychiatry 2003;160:371–373.

31. Murthy RS, Lakshminar, R. Mental health consequences of war: A brief review of research findings. World Psychiatry 2006:5;25–30.

32. De Jong J, Komproe I, Ommeren M. Common mental disorders in postconflict settings. Lancet 2003;361:2128–2135.

33. Lopes Cardozo B, Kaiser R, Gotway CA, Agani F. Mental health, social functioning, and feelings of hatred and revenge of Kosovar Albanians one year after the war in Kosovo. J Trauma Stress 2003;16:351–360.

34. Somasundaram D, Jamunanatha CS. Psychosocial consequences of war: Northern Sri Lankan experience. In de Jong J (ed.). Trauma, War and Violence: Public Mental Health in Socio-cultural Context. New York: Plenum, 2002.

35. Sarraj EE, Qouta S. The Palestinian experience. In Lopez-Ibor JJ, Christodoulou G, Maj M, et al. (eds.). Disasters and Mental Health. Chichester: Wiley, 2005.

36. Mousa F, Madi H. Impact of the humanitarian crisis in the occupied Palestinian territory on people and services. Gaza: United Nations Relief and Works Agency for Palestinian Refugees in the Near East (UNRWA), 2003.

37. Mollica RF, Sarajlic N, Chernoff M, et al. Longitudinal study of psychiatric symptoms, disability, mortality, and emigration among Bosnian refugees. JAMA 2001; 286:546–554.

38. Sabin M, Lopes Cardozo B, Nackerud L, et al. Factors associated with poor mental health among Guatemalan refugees living in Mexico 20 years after civil conflict. JAMA 2003;290:635–642.

39. Marshall GN, Schell TL, Elliott MN, et al. Mental health of Cambodian refugees 2 decades after resettlement in the United States. JAMA 2005;294:571–579.

40. Pham PN, Weinstein HM, Longman T. Trauma and PTSD symptoms in Rwanda: Implications for attitudes toward justice and reconciliation. JAMA 2004;292:602–612.

41. Njenga FG, Nguithi AN, Kang'ethe RN. War and mental disorders in Africa. World Psychiatry 2006;5:38–39.

42. North CS, Pfefferbaum B, Narayanan P, et al. Comparison of post-disaster psychiatric disorders after terrorist bombings in Nairobi and Oklahoma City. Br J Psychiatry 2005;186:487–493.

43. Cardozo BL, Bilukha OO, Crawford CA, et al. Mental health, social functioning, and disability in postwar Afghanistan. JAMA 2004;292:575–584.

44. Scholte WF, Olff M, Ventevogel P, et al. Mental health symptoms following war and repression in eastern Afghanistan. JAMA 2004;292:585–593.

45. Stein BD, Tanielian TL. Building and translating evidence into smart policy: Continuing research needs for informing post-war mental health policy. World Psychiatry 2006:5;34–35.

46. Eisenman D, Weine S, Green B, et al. The ISTSS/RAND guidelines on mental health training of primary healthcare providers for trauma-exposed populations in conflict-affected countries. J Trauma Stress 2006;19:5–17.

47. Basoglu M, Livanou M, Crnobaric C, et al. Psychiatric and cognitive effects of war in former Yugoslavia: Association of lack of redress for trauma and posttraumatic stress reactions. JAMA 2005;294:580–590.

5

The Impact of War
on the Environment

Arthur H. Westing

The environmental consequences of war can be categorized as (1) unintentional, (2) intentional, and (3) intentional for purposes of amplification through the release of "dangerous forces." Environmental damage is also caused by military activities during times of peace. This chapter focuses on the adverse environmental impacts of war and military activities during both wartime and peacetime. (Not covered here are any benefits of war and other military activities on the environment; these derive primarily from the sparing of habitats, and the wildlife they contain, during war because they are temporarily inaccessible to other forms of human exploitation.)

Unintentional Wartime Impacts

Unintentional environmental damage in wartime—which is also termed ancillary, incidental, or collateral damage—is generally anticipated.[1] Such damage often results from the profligate use of high-explosive munitions against enemy personnel and matériel or from the use of tanks and other heavy off-road vehicles. Both of these forms of ancillary environmental damage can be especially disruptive of local habitats and the animals that live in and depend upon those habitats. Air and water pollution can result from battle-related activities in an area. In addition, displacement of persons from a war zone and their concentration into refugee camps can damage the environment and habitats of animals and plants (see Chapter 13).

Aside from the battlefields, the environmental impact of military activities during wartime is generally greater than during peacetime, with more-disruptive activities often excused as "necessities of war." Construction of base camps, fortifications, and lines of communication often leads to environmental disruption. Further ancillary wartime environmental damage can derive from the heavy exploitation of timber, food, and feed by armed forces, both within and beyond war zones.

The use of depleted uranium (DU) to increase the mass and hardness of military shells has led to environmental contamination in Iraq (in 1991 and since 2003), in Kosovo (in 1999), and in Bosnia and Herzegovina (in 1994–1995). Concerns over the toxic and radioactive properties of DU, which is largely uranium-235, led to a major postwar environmental assessment in Kosovo by the United Nations Environment Program (UNEP).[2] No DU contamination was detected in battlefield ground surface, soil, rocks, water, air, plants, milk, buildings, or other objects. However, as precautionary measures to avoid possible health risks, UNEP recommended fencing off targeted areas until they were cleaned up, advising local residents to not handle residual DU munitions, and periodically testing local groundwater and drinking water.

Intentional Wartime Impact

Conventional weapons, which consist of explosives, incendiaries, and guns of various sizes, have accounted for the overwhelming majority of adverse environmental consequences owing to war. During World War II, for example, there was extensive carpet bombing of cities in Europe and Japan (Figure 5-1). This not only accounted for many deaths and injuries, but also caused widespread devastation of urban environments. Another example is the bombing of rural areas during the Vietnam War, which led to severe disruption of forests and agricultural fields. The resultant bomb craters remained for several decades afterward, often filled with stagnant water, providing breeding sites for mosquitoes that transmit malaria and other mosquito-borne diseases (Figure 5-2).

Conventional warfare can be environmentally and socially devastating. However, the level of devastation depends more on the objectives, will, and tenacity of the parties to the conflict than on the modernity of the armed forces involved or the sophistication of their weapons. Improvements in weaponry over the ages have not led to any discernible increase in the damage brought about by warfare; they have only increased the efficiency with which warfare is perpetrated. For example, one of the most environmentally and socially

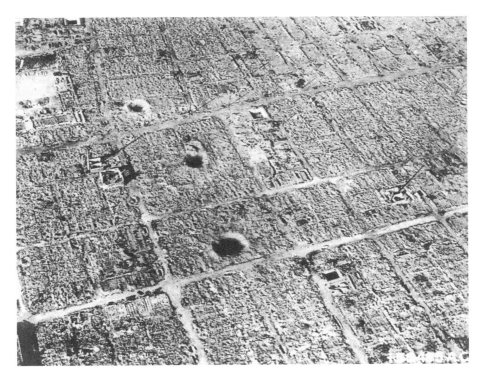

Figure 5-1. Damage to Osaka in 1945 as a result of a series of attacks by American B-29 bombers. Their bombloads included a high percentage of incendiaries, which destroyed the city's large wooden houses by fire. (Source: Library of Congress, Negative LC-USZ 62-104726.)

devastating wars in recent centuries—the Chinese Rebellion of 1850–1864—was fought with quite primitive arms by today's standards. In this war, the Tai Ping (Great Peace) Movement failed to overthrow the ruling Manchu Dynasty.[1] The Tai Ping forces employed intense violence and performed much pillaging; the Manchu forces used similar or greater levels of terror and violence. Government forces used large-scale "scorched-earth" tactics to starve into submission forces in the rebellious regions. The countryside, especially of the lower Yangtze River region (Anhui [Anhwei] Province and parts of surrounding provinces), was devastated; 100 years later, it had still not fully recovered.

Forest Clearing

Forests are often destroyed during wartime, mainly to deny cover and concealment to an enemy, and, to a much lesser extent, to deny timber resources to

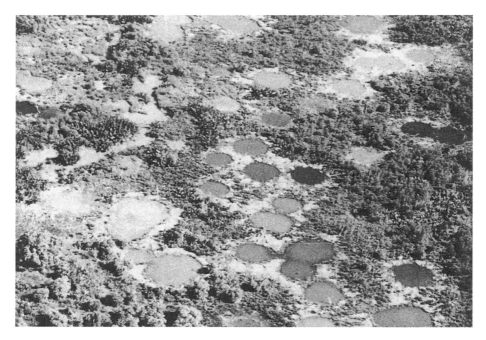

Figure 5-2. Bomb-destroyed mangrove forest, Bien Hoa Province, South Vietnam, 1971. (Photograph by Arthur H. Westing.)

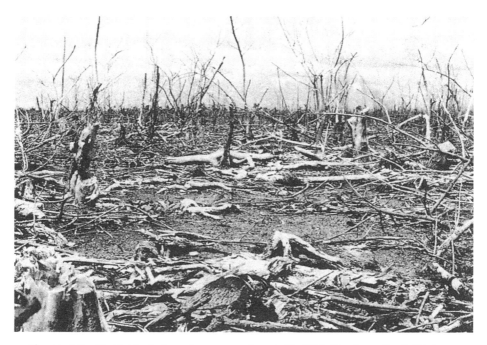

Figure 5-3. Herbicide-destroyed mangrove forest, Gia Dinh Province, South Vietnam, 1970. (Photograph by Arthur H. Westing.)

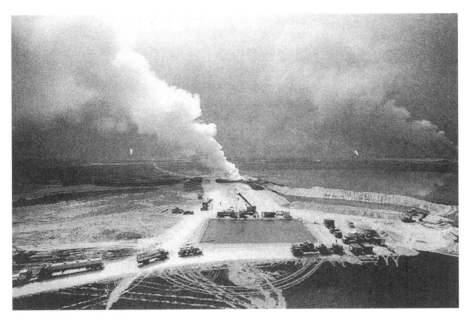

Figure 5-4. Burning oil wells at the Al Burgan oil field in Kuwait. (Photograph by Jim Hodson.)

an enemy. Huge forests can be devastated by spraying them with herbicides, using heavy tractors equipped with forest-clearing blades, performing saturation bombing, and setting self-propagating wildfires.

Herbicides (chemical anti-plant agents) were used widely for forest clearing by the United States during the Vietnam War from 1961 to 1975 (Figure 5-3). The U.S. military sprayed 72 million liters of herbicides onto almost 2 million hectares, including Agent Orange (2,4-dichlorophenoxyacetic acid [2,4-D] and 2,4,5-trichlorophenoxyacetic acid [2,4,5-T] contaminated with dioxin, a potent carcinogen and teratogen), which may have caused many cases of cancer and birth defects. It also used heavy tractors to clear more than 300,000 hectares of forest and dropped about 7 million tons of bombs in saturation bombing actions.[3–5] Devastation of forests in order to deny an enemy cover and concealment can greatly damage upland forest ecosystems and can lead to utter destruction of coastal ecosystems. When the vegetation of a forest ecosystem is destroyed, its wildlife are often decimated because of loss of their natural habitat. At the same time, soil and associated nutrients are eroded and washed away. Depending on the severity of attack, the type of vegetation, and the local site conditions, natural recovery of an assaulted forest ecosystem can take years or even decades.

Stream Manipulation

Many important rivers flow through more than one country. A nation at war against a nation that is downstream can divert or contaminate the water of a river before it reaches the downstream population. Such an act could represent a major calamity, especially in an arid region.

Releases of Oil

During the Persian Gulf War of 1991, Iraqi forces retreating from Kuwait ignited approximately 630 oil wells, producing dense clouds of dark, soot-laden smoke (Figure 5-4).[6] The huge amounts of smoke, consisting of soot and various combustion gases, that was released into the atmosphere persisted for several months and led to adverse health effects in people, livestock, and wildlife. They also released liquid oil onto land and into the Persian Gulf from about 20 collecting centers, at least three oil tankers, and various storage tanks and pipelines. Many sabotaged oil wells continued to discharge oil for many months. The resultant oil releases may have amounted to 60 million barrels. On land, approximately 200 small oil lakes were created, leading to the death of much wildlife and to diverse other environmental problems, including contamination of groundwater. About 6 million barrels of oil were released into the Persian Gulf, severely contaminating Kuwaiti offshore waters and about 400 km (250 miles) of coastline (primarily of Saudi Arabia), thereby disrupting marine habitats and killing much migratory avian, mammalian, and reptilian wildlife. A study of 1,599 U.S. soldiers after their return from Kuwait found that they experienced eye and upper respiratory tract irritation, shortness of breath, coughing, rashes, and fatigue more frequently than other soldiers did during a baseline period; these symptoms were associated with reported proximity to the oil fires, and their occurrence declined among soldiers after they left Kuwait.[7]

Another study of 1,560 veterans who served in the Persian Gulf War demonstrated that self-reported exposure was associated with asthma, bronchitis, and major depression, but there was no association between these health problems and modeled exposures; the authors concluded that their findings did not support the hypothesis that the veterans' respiratory symptoms were caused by exposure to oil-fire smoke.[8]

Denial of Access

Landmines are used to deny military forces access to specific areas, thereby hindering, slowing, or channeling the movements of enemy forces and sapping their morale (see Chapter 7). Antitank and antipersonnel landmines as well as cluster-bomb submunitions (CBUs) have often been heavily and widely used by regular and insurgent forces. Landmines and cluster bombs are especially gruesome means of warfare. In addition, operations to clear such explosive remnants of war can be seriously disruptive. Such operations are time-consuming, technically difficult, expensive, exceedingly dangerous, and rarely fully successful. In former battle zones, therefore, farming, herding, and forestry may be hazardous pursuits. Furthermore, metal fragments from various weapons may become embedded in wood, making it unsafe to saw into it. And all of these adverse effects on the environment are dwarfed by the impacts of the production and use of nuclear weapons (see Chapter 10).

Use of Nonrenewable Fuels and Other Materials by the Military

During both war and preparation for war, the military forces of many nations consume huge amounts of fossil fuels and other nonrenewable materials. Energy consumption by military equipment can be substantial. For example, an armored division of 348 battle tanks operating for 1 day consumes more than 2.2 million liters of fuel, and a carrier battle group operating for 1 day consumes more than 1.5 million liters of fuel. In the late 1980s, the U.S. military annually consumed 18.6 million tons of fuel (more than 44 percent of the world's total), and emitted 381,000 tons of carbon monoxide, 157,000 tons of oxides of nitrogen, 78,000 tons of hydrocarbons, and 17,900 tons of sulfur dioxide.[9]

Intentional Release of Dangerous Forces

Under certain conditions, military forces can manipulate a component of the natural or built environment in order to release dangerous pent-up forces.[10] Often called "environmental warfare," this possibility could become especially tempting if the hostile manipulation involved application of a relatively modest effort (triggering energy) that would release substantially more energy to destroy a specific target. Environmental warfare can involve attacks on impoundments of fresh water, nuclear power stations, and even forests. In a similar fashion, attacks on some industrial facilities can release toxic chemicals over wide areas.

Impoundments of Fresh Water

Hundreds of major dams that impound huge quantities of water have been constructed in many countries. Many of these dams could be breached with relative ease, by direct attack or sabotage, releasing the impounded water and causing much death and destruction. Such hostile action was used in several conflicts, including World War II and the Korean War. Recovery from the environmental and social impacts of such actions can take decades. The most devastating example was the intentional release of waters of the Yellow River during the Second Sino-Japanese War.[11] In 1938, attempting to stop an advance of the Japanese army, the Chinese dynamited the Huayuankow Dike near Chengchow. Several thousand Japanese soldiers drowned, and the advance of the Japanese Army into China along this front was halted. In the process, however, the flood waters also ravaged major portions of Henan, Anhui, and Jiangsu provinces, and several hundred thousand Chinese people drowned. In addition, several million hectares of farmland, 4,000 villages, and 11 cities were destroyed. The river was not brought back under control until 1947.

Nuclear Facilities

Almost 200 clusters of nuclear power stations, as well as many nuclear re-processing plants and nuclear waste repositories, are present in more than 30 countries. These facilities are vulnerable to assault by overt attack or sabotage, with the possible release of iodine-131, cesium-137, strontium-90, and other radioactive elements. After an assault, the most heavily contaminated zone would be a threat to life, the next most contaminated zone would be a threat to health, and a larger, less contaminated zone would be agriculturally unusable. The radioactive area after such an assault might defy effective decontamination and could be a threat to health for many decades—as was the case after nuclear weapon testing on and near Pacific islands in the 1940s and 1950s and after the nuclear power plant incident at Chernobyl in Ukraine in 1986.

Spreading Wildfires

Under certain habitat and weather conditions, military forces could start forest fires that would be self-propagating and enormously destructive of forests and their animal and plant life. In killing the vegetation of a forest ecosystem, such incendiary warfare could cause substantial damage to wildlife and forest nutrients. Recovery could take decades. Under certain conditions, such incendiary warfare in grassland (prairie) and tundra ecosystems could also cause widespread damage (and persistent damage in tundra ecosystems).

Peacetime Impacts

Most nations ("states," in diplomatic terminology) continuously maintain armed forces for several reasons, including (1) to deter attacks from outside their borders or, failing that, to defend against such attacks; (2) to threaten attacks on other nations in support of foreign policy objectives or, failing that, to carry out such attacks; and/or (3) to deter or quell internal uprisings, recognizing that most wars in recent decades have been civil wars fought between governments and insurgents.

The environmental consequences of the maintenance of armed forces can result from the following[9,12]:

- Establishing military fortifications and other military facilities
- Equipping and supplying armed forces with weapons and other military equipment and supplies, and, in turn, disposing of such equipment and supplies once they become obsolete or otherwise unwanted
- Training armed forces and testing their weapons
- Routinely deploying armed forces nationally, within other nations, and within areas beyond any national jurisdiction.

The environmental impacts of peacetime military activities are approximately proportional to the fraction of gross domestic product that they represent in a nation, which is now about 3 percent for both developed and developing nations.

From 1945 to 1990, the United States produced approximately 70,000 nuclear weapons; several other nations also produced large numbers of these weapons. This production of nuclear weapons led to major environmental contamination. For example, the area around Chelyabinsk, Russia, was heavily contaminated with radioactive materials from a nearby nuclear weapons production facility. The level of ambient radiation in and near the Techa River in that area was up to 28 times the normal background radiation level.[13] Similarly, leakage of radioactive materials from storage of wastes from nuclear weapons production at Hanford, Washington, led to extensive radioactive contamination. Open-air testing of nuclear weapons by the United States, the Soviet Union, and other countries also resulted in environmental contamination, with increased rates of leukemia and other cancers among populations located downwind from these tests (Box 5-1).

The dismantling and disposal of nuclear weapons has also led to environmental contamination. Overall, the United States has dismantled about 60,000 nuclear warheads since the 1940s. More than 12,000 plutonium pits (steel or beryllium spheres containing plutonium-239 that trigger nuclear fission when compressed by explosives) are stored in containers at a nuclear weapons plant in Texas. Plans are underway to produce as many as 80 new pits annually, and the George W. Bush administration has advocated building a modern pit facility capable of producing 250 to 900 pits annually by 2018. (See Chapter 10.)

Box 5-1 Malignancies Associated with Radioactive Fallout
Barry S. Levy and Victor W. Sidel

The world's population has been exposed to low levels of fission products from the testing of nuclear weapons in the atmosphere. Epidemiological associations have been demonstrated between leukemia and nuclear fallout in the general population, especially among people living in areas downwind from open-air testing locations.

The strongest association has been with acute and myeloid types of leukemia among children. In addition, the entire U.S. population had increased leukemia rates during and for several years after open-air nuclear testing took place; the rates fell sharply afterward.[1] Veterans who received high gamma radiation doses while participating as military personnel in the U.S. atmospheric nuclear weapons testing program from 1945 to 1962 have had higher mortality from lymphopoietic cancers (relative risk [RR]: 3.72; 95% confidence interval [CI]: 1.27–10.83).[2] U.S. Navy veterans who participated in atmospheric nuclear testing in 1958 in the Pacific have had increased mortality from cancer (RR: 1.42; 95% CI: 1.03–1.97), and specifically from liver cancer (RR: 6.42; 95% CI: 1.17–35.3), but no increase in leukemia or lymphoma mortality.[3] Servicemen and male civilians from the United Kingdom who participated in the their country's atmospheric nuclear weapons tests and experimental programs in the 1950s and early 1960s have had an increased risk of leukemia, excluding chronic lymphatic leukemia (RR: 1.83; 90% CI: 1.15–2.93).[4]

A weak association has been found between bone marrow dose of radiation due to radioactive fallout from the Nevada nuclear test site and all types of leukemia in Utah. The greatest risk of developing acute leukemia was found in people in the high-dose group who were younger than 20 years of age at the time of exposure and who died before 1964.[5] People exposed to more than 2.0 sieverts (Sv) of ionizing radiation from nuclear weapons tests in Kazakhstan between 1949 and 1963 had almost double the risk of leukemia (odds ratio: 1.91; 95% CI: 0.38–9.67). There was also an excess relative risk for leukemia of 10 percent per 1 Sv of additional exposure.[6] People in Norway and Sweden who were exposed to radioactive fallout from nuclear testing in northwest Russia had an increased risk of thyroid cancer during childhood and adolescence.[7] The populations of both the United States and the Marshall Islands exposed to radiation from U.S. nuclear weapons testing have had, as a result, an increased occurrence of thyroid cancer that increased with radiation dose to the thyroid.[8][9]

Populations were also exposed to radiation after the April 1986 accident at Chernobyl, Ukraine. Populations in Europe who were most highly exposed to Chernobyl fallout have had a slightly higher leukemia incidence and an increasing leukemia risk with estimated cumulative excess radiation dose.[10]

(continued)

Children younger than 10 years of age who lived within 150 kilometers (90 miles) of Chernobyl have had an increase in thyroid cancers, most likely caused by direct external or internal exposure to short-lived radioactive isotopes, such as iodine-131 and iodine-133.[11]

Public health professionals have a responsibility to help ensure that testing of nuclear weapons, especially in the atmosphere, does not resume.

References

1. Archer JW, Berent S. Controversies in neurotoxicology. Neurol Clin 2000;18: 741–764.
2. Dalager NA, Kang HK, Mahan CM. Cancer mortality among the highest exposed US atmospheric nuclear test participants. J Occup Environ Med 2000;42:798–805.
3. Watanabe KK, Kang HK, Dalager NA. Cancer mortality risk among military participants of a 1958 atmospheric nuclear weapons test. Am J Public Health 1995; 85:523–527.
4. Muirhead CB, Bingham D, Haylock RG, et al. Follow up of mortality and incidence of cancer 1952–1998 in men from the UK who participated in the UK's atmospheric nuclear weapons tests and experimental programmes. Occup Environ Med 2003;60:165–172.
5. Stevens W, Thomas DC, Lyon JL, et al. Leukemia in Utah and radioactive fallout from the Nevada test site: A case-control study. JAMA 1990;264:585–591.
6. Abylkassimova Z, Gusev B, Grosche B, et al. Nested case-control study of leukemia among a cohort of persons exposed to ionizing radiation from nuclear weapons tests in Kazakhstan (1949–1963). Ann Epidemiol 2000;10:479.
7. Lund E, Galanti MR. Incidence of thyroid cancer in Scandinavia following fallout from atomic bomb testing: An analysis of birth cohorts. Cancer Causes Control 1999;10:181–187.
8. Institute of Medicine and National Research Council. Exposure of the American People to Iodine-131 from Nevada Nuclear Tests: Review of the National Cancer Institute Report and Public Health Implications. Washington, DC: National Academy Press, 1999, p. 6.
9. Takahashi T, Schoemaker MJ, Trott KR, et al. The relationship of thyroid cancer with radiation exposure from nuclear weapon testing in the Marshall Islands. J Epidemiol 2003;13:99–107.
10. Hoffmann W. Has fallout from the Chernobyl accident caused childhood leukaemia in Europe? A commentary on the epidemiologic evidence. Eur J Public Health 2002;12:72–76.
11. Shibata Y, Yamashita S, Masyakin VB, et al. 15 years after Chernobyl: New evidence of thyroid cancer. Lancet 2001;358:1965–1966.

Source: This box was adapted from Levy BS, Sidel VW. War. In Frumkin H (ed.). Environmental Health: From Global to Local. San Francisco: Jossey-Bass, 2005, pp. 274–275.

Chemical weapons can contaminate the environment, not only during war but also during the preparation for war. The potential for exposure exists for workers involved in the development, production, transport, or storage of these weapons and for community residents living near facilities where these weapons are developed, produced, transported, or stored. In addition, disposal of these weapons, involving disassembly and incineration, can represent hazards. (See Chapter 8.)

Biological agents, which consist of bacteria, viruses, and other microorganisms and their toxins, not only can produce illness in people but can also lead to long-term contamination of the environment that may affect people, other animals, and plants. For example, Gruinard Island, off the coast of Scotland, remained contaminated for many decades as a result of a test use of anthrax spores by the United Kingdom and the United States in 1942. During the 1950s and 1960s, secret, large-scale, open-air tests at the U.S. Army Dugway Proving Ground may have introduced the microorganisms that cause Q fever and Venezuelan equine encephalitis into the deserts of western Utah. In 1979, the accidental release of anthrax spores near Sverdlovsk, in the Soviet Union, resulted in at least 79 cases of inhalation anthrax and at least 68 deaths.[14] (See Chapter 9.)

Hazardous wastes from military operations are potential contaminants of air, water, and soil. At Otis Air Force Base in Massachusetts, groundwater was contaminated with trichloroethylene, classified by the International Agency for Research on Cancer (IARC) as a probable carcinogen, and other toxins. In adjacent towns, lung cancer and leukemia rates have been 80 percent above the state average. At the Rocky Mountain Arsenal in Colorado, 125 chemicals were dumped during 30 years of nerve gas and pesticide production, creating "the most contaminated square mile on earth," according to the Army Corps of Engineers. At McChord Air Force Base in Washington State, benzene, classified as a definite human carcinogen by IARC, was found on the base in concentrations as high as 503 parts per billion (ppb), almost 1,000 times the state's limit of 0.6 ppb.[15]

Legal Constraints

Several multilateral treaties are relevant to the protection of the environment in times of war—including both incidental and intentional consequences. Most of these treaties, which have high levels of acceptance among nations, are applicable only to international warfare, whereas most recent wars have been civil wars.

Two principles underlie the law of war:

- The right of belligerents to choose methods of warfare is not unlimited, as embodied in the 1899 Hague Convention II, the 1907 Hague Convention IV, and the 1977 Geneva Protocol I.
- Those military actions that are not precisely regulated are to be controlled by the principles of humanity and the dictates of the public conscience, as embodied in the 1949 Geneva Convention IV and the 1977 Geneva Protocol I.

Eliminating or Avoiding War

Adherence to the 1928 Renunciation of War Pact would eliminate environmental damage associated with international war. In addition, there are several instruments intended to prevent any war from occurring in certain geographic regions, including (1) the 1920 Spitsbergen Treaty, meant to protect the Svalbard archipelago (between Norway and the North Pole), including Bear Island, from military activities; (2) the 1921 Aaland Islands Convention, meant to similarly protect the Aaland archipelago (in the Baltic Sea between Sweden and Finland); and (3) the 1959 Antarctic Treaty, meant to protect Antarctica and, more ambiguously, its surrounding waters. These three regions cover a combined land area of 14 million square kilometers (km^2), or 9 percent of global land area.

A status of neutrality is a further attempt to avoid war. Austria, Malta, Switzerland, and Vatican City enjoy internationally recognized neutrality, while Costa Rica, Finland, Ireland, and Sweden have made unilateral declarations of neutrality.[16] These eight nations cover a combined area of 1 million km^2, or 1 percent of global land area. In addition, 185 or more natural heritage sites of outstanding universal value, located within 130 countries, are now internationally recognized by the 1972 World Heritage Convention. Such sites are not to be subjected to deliberate harm from war or other activities.

Conventional War

The most important constraint on military disruption of the environment derives from the 1977 Geneva Protocol I. This treaty establishes that the natural environment shall be protected from means of international warfare that may be expected to cause widespread, long-lasting, and severe damage—a novel addition to the law of war. The 1998 International Criminal Court Statute classifies such action as a war crime.

Both the 1977 Geneva Protocol I and Protocol II limit attacks on agricultural areas, a constraint on incidental environmental damage. The 1981 Incendiary Weapons Protocol III includes a modest limitation on attacking forests or other plant cover with incendiary weapons.

The 1899 Hague Convention II and the 1907 Hague Convention IV both require that, during an occupation, the occupying nation may make only usufructory (temporary) use of the forests and agricultural lands of the occupied nation. In addition, the United Nations Security Council determined that Iraq was liable for any direct environmental damage and depletion of natural resources caused by its invasion and occupation of Kuwait in 1990 and 1991.

The use of antipersonnel landmines is restricted by both the 1981 Mine Protocol II and the 1996 Mine Protocol II. And the possession of antipersonnel landmines is prohibited by the 1997 Mine Ban Treaty. (See Chapter 7.)

Naval War

Legal limits to damaging the ocean environment through military activities, during times of peace or war, are minimal. All of the several environmental protection instruments for the ocean specifically exempt military activities from their strictures, under a principle usually referred to as "sovereign immunity."[17] The 1907 Hague Convention VIII provides some minimal constraints regarding sea mines that are of potential advantage to the marine environment. The United Nations Security Council, in what may have been its first recognition of wartime environmental damage, called upon both belligerents during the Iran–Iraq War of 1980–1988 to refrain from any action that could endanger marine life in the Persian Gulf.

Several instruments attempt to establish nuclear weapon–free maritime zones, which together add up to 191 million km^2 of ocean (53 percent of global ocean area). They are:

- The 1967 Latin American Nuclear Weapon Treaty (68 million km^2, or 19 percent)
- The 1985 South Pacific Nuclear Free Treaty (118 million km^2, or 33 percent)
- The 1995 Southeast Asia Nuclear Weapon Free Treaty (5 million km^2, or 1 percent).

Nuclear War

No multilateral treaty proscribes nuclear war (see Chapter 10). Yet, as noted previously, several instruments attempt to establish zones of complete peace, which together add up to 15 million km^2 (10 percent of the global land area). In addition, there have been attempts to establish zones specifically free of nuclear weapons. The total area of these is substantial—224 million km^2 (mainly ocean), representing 44 percent of the entire globe, including 55 nations. The 1967 Latin American Nuclear Weapon Treaty establishes a total area of 88 million km^2 (including 20 million km^2 of land in 32 nations). The 1985 South Pacific Nuclear Free Treaty establishes a total area of 126 million km^2 (including 8 million km^2 of land in 13 nations). And the 1995 Southeast Asia Nuclear Weapon Free Treaty establishes a total area of 9 million km^2 (including 4 million km^2 of land in 10 nations).

Finally, the 1971 Seabed Treaty prohibits the placement of nuclear weapons on or under the ocean floor of the high seas (beyond territorial waters), for a total area of about 352 million km^2 (97 percent of global ocean area). However, the most diverse and productive marine ecosystems are found to a great extent in the excluded territorial waters—that is, within that strip of coastal ocean that is 22 kilometers (12 nautical miles) wide.

Biological Warfare

The 1925 Geneva Protocol prohibits the use of biological weapons, and the 1972 Biological Weapons Convention prohibits even the possession of biological weapons. (See Chapter 9.)

Chemical Warfare

The 1925 Geneva Protocol prohibits the use of chemical weapons, the 1993 Chemical Weapons Convention prohibits even the possession of chemical weapons, and the 1972 Biological and Toxin Weapon Convention prohibits the possession of certain (toxin) chemical weapons. The 1998 International Criminal Court Statute classifies such action as a war crime. (See Chapter 8.)

Environmental Warfare

Manipulating the natural or built environment for hostile purposes is constrained to some extent. Both the 1977 Geneva Protocol I and Protocol II prohibit attacks on dams and nuclear power stations that would release so-called dangerous forces. And the 1977 Environmental Modification Convention also constrains such hostile actions, although quite inadequately.[18]

Conclusion

Given the wide range of adverse impacts that war and the preparation for war have on the environment, the only effective way to prevent these adverse consequences on the environment may be to prevent war itself. Health professionals can play vital roles by documenting these adverse consequences and their actual and potential effects on human health.

References

1. Westing AH. Warfare in a Fragile World: Military Impact on the Human Environment. London: Taylor & Francis, 1980, pp. 16, 249.
2. United Nations Environment Program. Depleted Uranium in Kosovo: Post-conflict Environmental Assessment. Nairobi: United Nations Environment Program, 2001, p. 185.
3. Westing AH. Ecological Consequences of the Second Indochina War. Stockholm: Almqvist & Wiksell, 1976, p. 119.
4. Westing AH. Herbicides in warfare: The case of Indochina. In Bourdeau P, Haines JA, Klein W, Krishna Murti CR (eds.). Ecotoxicology and Climate. Chichester, UK: John Wiley, 1989, pp. 337–357.
5. Westing AH. Chemical warfare against vegetation in Vietnam. Environmental Awareness 2002;25:51–58.
6. Westing AH. Environmental dimension of the Gulf War of 1991. In Brauch HG, Marquina A, El-Sayed Selium M, et al. (eds.). Security and Environment in the Mediterranean. Berlin: Springer Verlag, 2003, pp. 523–524.
7. Petruccelli BP, Goldenbaum M, Scott B, et al. Health effects of the 1991 Kuwait oil fires: A survey of US army troops. J Occup Environ Med 1999;41:433–439.
8. Lange JL, Schwartz DA, Doebbeling BN, et al. Exposures to the Kuwait oil fires and their association with asthma and bronchitis among Gulf War veterans. Environ Health Perspect 2002;110:1141–1146.
9. Renner M. Environmental and health effects of weapons production, testing, and maintenance. In BS Levy, VW Sidel (eds.). War and Public Health (updated edition). Washington, DC: American Public Health Association, 2000, pp. 117–136.
10. Westing AH. Environmental Hazards of War: Releasing Dangerous Forces in an Industrialized World. London: Sage Publications, 1990, p. 96.
11. Westing AH. Weapons of Mass Destruction and the Environment. London: Taylor & Francis, 1977, p. 54.
12. Ehrlich AH, Birks JW (eds.). Hidden Dangers: Environmental Costs of Preparing for War. San Francisco: Sierra Books, 1990, p. 246.
13. Keller B. Soviet city, home of the A-bomb, is haunted by its past and future. New York Times, July 10, 1989, pp. A1–A2.
14. Meselson M, Guillemin J, Hugh-Jones M, et al. The Sverdlovsk anthrax outbreak of 1979. Science 1994;266:1202–1208.
15. Renner M. Assessing the military's war on the environment. In Brown LR, Durning A, Flavin C, et al. (eds.). State of the World 1991. New York: Norton, 1991.
16. Westing AH. Towards eliminating war as an instrument of foreign policy. Bulletin of Peace Proposals 1990;21:29–35.
17. Westing AH. Environmental dimensions of maritime security. In Goldblat J (ed.). Maritime Security: The Building of Confidence. (Document No. UNIDIR/92/89.) Geneva: United Nations Institute for Disarmament Research, 1992, pp. 91–102.
18. Westing AH. Environmental Modification Convention: 1977 to the present. In Burns RD (ed.). Encyclopedia of Arms Control and Disarmament. New York: Macmillan Library Reference, 1993, pp. 947–954.

III

TYPES OF WEAPONS

6

Conventional Weapons

Wendy Cukier

Weapons categorized as "conventional" include small arms and light weapons (SALWs), explosives, and incendiaries, as well as the systems used to distribute them. Conventional weapons and the armed forces that use them account for about 80 percent of global military expenditures and about 80 percent of the world arms trade. Whereas guns were implicated in 60 to 90 percent of direct war-related deaths for 2003, other conventional weapons accounted for the remaining 10 to 40 percent.[1]

Both major, or "heavy," conventional weapons and SALWs are used in the vast majority of international and civil wars. For example, in the war in Afghanistan, the U.S. military needed both major conventional weapons and SALWs to dominate the conflict. In the Iraq War, a wide range of conventional weapons has been used, from the insurgents' improvised explosive devices (IEDs) to the advanced unmanned aircraft of Coalition forces. The same has been true in armed conflicts in Colombia, Chechnya, Israel, Sri Lanka, Colombia, and the Philippines. Whereas SALWs caused most deaths in these conflicts, major conventional weapons were also widely used.[2]

Small Arms

Among conventional armaments, the weapons of choice are small arms (fire-arms). Small arms are weapons that can be carried and used by an individual, including revolvers, pistols, rifles, shotguns, submachine guns and assault rifles. Although there have been attempts to differentiate "military" from "civilian" small arms, these definitions are fraught with problems, because many manufacturers supply both markets, adapting military designs to civilian markets or, in some cases, promoting weapons based on their military or police use. In 101 conflicts fought between 1989 and 1996, SALWs were generally the weapons of preference and sometimes the only weapons used.[3] SALWs are small, cheap, and easy to carry and maintain.

There are many sources for legal and illegal guns. Influxes of guns and ammunition fuel existing conflicts and increase the risk that instability will turn into conflict. Supplies of weapons to war zones increase the duration, intensity, and lethality of conflict.

Heavy Conventional Weapon Systems

Heavy conventional weapon systems contrast greatly with SALWs. Seven categories of heavy conventional weapon systems are defined in the United Nations Register of Conventional Arms[4]:

1. *Battle tank:* A tracked or wheeled, self-propelled armored fighting vehicle with high cross-country mobility and a high level of self-protection, weighing at least 16.5 metric tons unladen weight, with a high-muzzle-velocity, direct-fire main gun of at least 75 mm caliber.
2. *Armored combat vehicle:* A tracked or wheeled, self-propelled vehicle, with armored protection and cross-country capability, either (1) designed and equipped to transport a squad of four or more infantrymen or (2) armed with an integral or organic weapon of at least 20 mm caliber or an antitank missile launcher.
3. *Large-caliber artillery system:* A gun, howitzer, artillery piece combining the characteristics of a gun and a howitzer, mortar, or multiple-launch rocket system capable of engaging surface targets by delivering primarily indirect fire, with a caliber of 100 mm or larger.
4. *Combat aircraft:* A fixed-wing or variable-geometry winged aircraft armed and equipped to engage targets by employing guided missiles, unguided rockets, bombs, guns, cannons, or other weapons of destruction.

5. *Attack helicopter:* A rotary-wing aircraft equipped to employ antiarmor, air-to-ground, or air-to-air guided weapons and equipped with an integrated fire control and aiming system for these weapons.
6. *Warship:* A vessel or submarine with a standard displacement of 850 metric tons or more, armed or equipped for military use.
7. *Missile or missile system:* A guided rocket or ballistic or cruise missile capable of delivering a payload to a range of at least 25 km (about 15 miles), or a vehicle, apparatus, or device designed or modified for launching such munitions.

These conventional weapons systems are essentially the means of distributing bombs, missiles, bullets, and a range of explosive and incendiary devices.

Injury patterns also differ according to whether the bombs are manufactured or improvised. "Manufactured explosives," which include those usually used by military forces, are mass-produced and quality-tested as weapons. They are almost always high-order explosive (HE) devices and include bombs (usually air-dropped, unpowered, explosive devices), grenades, shells, depth charges, warheads (in missiles), and antipersonnel landmines. Low-order explosive (LE) devices include pipe bombs, gunpowder, and pure petroleum-based bombs (Molotov cocktails). They are often improvised and used by non-state actors, including those who are called "terrorists."

Modern weapons use both kinetic and potential energy to achieve maximum lethality. Kinetic-energy systems rely on the conversion of kinetic energy to work. Potential-energy systems use explosive energy directly in the form of heat and blast or by acceleration of metal as a shaped charge, explosively formed penetrator (EFP), or case fragments to increase their kinetic energy and damage volume. The quantity of energy released determines the extent of the damage produced.

In 2005, the traditional "big five" arms-exporting countries—the United States, Russia, France, Germany, and the United Kingdom—still dominated global sales of major conventional weapons, with an estimated 82 percent of the market. Not only do these countries provide weapons to countries engaged in a variety of armed conflicts, but they also often supply both sides in a conflict.

Explosives

During war, antipersonnel landmines (see Chapter 7) and fragmenting munitions (mortars, bombs, and shells) are more likely than bullets to injure civilians.[5] The nature of the injuries is dependent on the design of weapons

---

Box 6-1 Protecting Civilians
Geneva Convention IV

The most specific requirements for protecting civilians appear in Article 51 of Protocol I of Geneva Convention IV: Protection of the Civilian Population:

1. The civilian population and individual civilians shall enjoy general protection against dangers arising from military operations. To give effect to this protection the following rules, which are additional to other applicable rules of international law, shall be observed in all circumstances.
2. The civilian population as such, as well as individual civilians, shall not be the object of attack. Acts or threats of violence the primary purpose of which is to spread terror among the civilian population are prohibited.
3. Civilians shall enjoy the protection afforded by this section, unless and for such time as they take a direct part in hostilities.
4. Indiscriminate attacks are prohibited. Indiscriminate attacks are:
   a. Those which are not directed at a specific military objective;
   b. Those which employ a method or means of combat which cannot be directed at a specific military objective; or
   c. Those which employ a method or means of combat the effects of which cannot be limited as required by this protocol; and consequently, in each such case, are of a nature to strike military objectives and civilians or civilian objects without distinction.
5. Among others, the following types of attacks are to be considered as indiscriminate:
   a. An attack by bombardment by any methods or means which treats as a single military objective a number of clearly separated and distinct military objectives located in a city, town, village or other area containing a similar concentration of civilians or civilian objects; and
   b. An attack which may be expected to cause incidental loss of civilian life, injury to civilians, damage to civilian objects, or a combination thereof, which would be excessive in relation to the concrete and direct military advantage anticipated.
6. Attacks against the civilian population or civilians by way of reprisals are prohibited.

---

and their use. The increased rate of civilian deaths in the past several decades has been linked to the involvement of groups with little training in and little regard for the fourth Geneva Convention, which protects civilians (Box 6-1). It is also linked to the specific design of weapons, which are often "indiscriminate" in their targets, and the form of warfare, which has shifted from battlefields to urban centers. Weapons that fragment easily injure more than one person. When shells, bombs, and mortars are used, there is less visual contact between users and victims, and more destructive force.

The use of explosives is also common in "terrorist" acts. Explosives were used in 43 of 355 terrorist attacks in 2001, 83 of 198 in 2002, and 102 of 208 in 2003.[6] When bombs are successfully planted on airplanes, there are few survivors.[7] Plastic and volatile explosives such as SEMTEX are the predominant weapons used by terrorists in aviation-related incidents.[8] The September 11, 2001, attacks on the World Trade Center and the Pentagon represented the first time that airplanes were used as missiles, explosives, and incendiary devices. Each airplane was loaded with an estimated 60,000 pounds of jet fuel and was traveling at 300 or more miles per hour on impact. Almost 3,000 people died in those attacks, the most fatalities in a recorded terrorist event.[9]

Armed conflict produces a variety of secondary effects that lead to more deaths. Attacks with conventional weapons destroy health-supporting infrastructure, such as food and water supply systems, health services, sewage treatment plants, and transportation and communications systems, with lasting effects on health and social and economic development. Millions of people are displaced, and death rates among these forced migrants can be very high. Conflict also diverts resources from the provision of essential services. Moreover, easy access to weapons contributes to violations of human rights and humanitarian law. It undermines governance and increases threats from armed groups and organized crime.

Powerful explosions have the potential to inflict many different types of injuries on victims; however, the pattern of injury inflicted on the body is relatively consistent regardless of the context. The most common injury for survivors of explosions is penetrating blunt trauma. Blast lung is the most common fatal injury among initial survivors. Explosions in confined spaces (such as mines, buildings, or large vehicles) and/or structural collapse are associated with the greatest morbidity and mortality. Blast injuries can occur to any body system. Up to 10 percent of all blast survivors have significant eye injuries. Although initial discomfort can be minimal, patients may seek care days, weeks, or even months after the event. Symptoms include eye pain or irritation, foreign body sensation, altered vision, and periorbital swelling. Contusions may occur. Clinical findings in the gastrointestinal tract may be absent until the onset of complications. Victims can also experience tinnitus and/or temporary or permanent deafness from blasts.

Specific types of injuries are associated with specific explosives. Knowledge of the potential mechanisms of injury, early signs and symptoms, and natural courses of these problems greatly aids the management of blast injuries. In most bomb attacks, there are many more injured than killed. In addition, those with close exposure to the traumatic event, especially individuals threatened with possible injury or death, are likely to have adverse psychological responses[10] (see Chapter 4).

The main objective of political attacks on civilians is often to create psychological terror, which, in turn, can cause chaos and panic.[11] Letter bombs kill about 3 percent of those affected, but they create widespread fear.[12] Secondary devices render an area insecure, thereby hampering rescue efforts and injury control. The indirect effects of "terrorist" acts are also wide ranging, including significant disruptions to tourism and economic development. (See Box 1-2 in Chapter 1.)

Incendiaries

The use of incendiaries in war has a long history, with examples depicted on Assyrian bas-reliefs as early as 1200 B.C.E. A mixture of sulfur, pitch, resin, naphtha, lime, and saltpeter was developed in Greece in the 7th century A.D. and was said to have been used by the Eastern Roman Emperors, most commonly against Muslims. The weapon was known to the Crusaders as "Greek Fire"; it was difficult to extinguish and was similar to modern napalm. Flamethrowers were first used in World War I. During World War II, widespread carpet bombing with incendiaries occurred. Napalm was used by the U.S. military during the Vietnam War (see Chapter 19) and was used in former Yugoslavia and in Iraq by U.S. and British forces. The use of incendiaries is not prohibited by international law, but the use of incendiaries against civilian targets is generally considered illegal. The Protocol on Prohibitions or Restrictions on the Use of Incendiary Weapons (Protocol III, or the Incendiary Weapons Protocol) is annexed to the 1980 Convention on Prohibitions or Restrictions on the Use of Certain Conventional Weapons Which May Be Deemed to Be Excessively Injurious or to Have Indiscriminate Effects. Although the United States ratified the Convention, it did not agree to be bound by Protocol III.

Interventions

During the 1990s, trade of conventional weapons was the subject of heightened political attention from governments and nongovernmental organizations (NGOs). In the disarmament forums at the United Nations, discussions on disarmament of conventional weapons have focused on (1) limitations on conventional weapons; (2) transparency in international arms transfers and the establishment of a United Nations Register on Conventional Arms; (3) regional approaches to building military confidence and security among nations;

and (4) the strengthening of international humanitarian and disarmament law with respect to inhumane weapons, including antipersonnel landmines.

When prohibiting the use of certain conventional weapons, such as napalm and other incendiaries, was first raised in the United Nations General Assembly in the late 1960s, there were numerous proposals for banning other weapons that also were deemed to cause unnecessary suffering or indiscriminate effects, such as antipersonnel mines and booby traps. Considerable work was done in the late 1960s and the 1970s, including some under the auspices of the International Committee of the Red Cross and diplomatic conferences on protocols to the Geneva Convention of 1949 (relating to humanitarian law in armed conflicts). In 1977, the General Assembly decided to convene a United Nations conference with the aim of reaching an agreement on prohibitions or restrictions on the use of certain conventional weapons. In 1980, a United Nations conference at Geneva adopted the Convention on Prohibitions or Restrictions on the Use of Certain Conventional Weapons Which May Be Deemed to Be Excessively Injurious or to Have Indiscriminate Effects (Convention on Conventional Weapons, or CCW); the convention was opened for signature in 1981 and came into force in 1983. Annexed Protocol I prohibits the use of any weapons that injure with fragments that are not detectable by x-rays. Protocol II prohibits or restricts the use of mines (excluding antiship mines), booby traps, and other delayed-action devices. Protocol III prohibits or restricts the use of incendiary weapons (weapons designed with the primary purpose of setting fire to objects or causing injury by means of fire).

In 1992, the United Nations Register of Conventional Arms was established. In 1993, the Secretary-General reported on the Register to the General Assembly, bringing into the public domain the information submitted by 87 nations—including most of the major supplier countries—on arms imports and exports in the seven categories of heavy conventional weapon systems previously described.

Efforts are being made to broaden the scope of the CCW. NGOs are calling on governments to have the CCW specifically address cluster munitions, which widely spread bomblets or submunitions, thereby threatening both civilians and military personnel during attacks. Cluster munitions also leave behind unexploded ordnance, which can pose a threat to civilians for decades after a conflict.

In addition, efforts are being made to better regulate materials that can be used for IEDs by criminals and "terrorists." For example, in 1998, a United Nations Economic and Social Council (UNESCO) resolution recommended that nations that had not already done so consider reviewing laws and regulations concerning explosives and their component parts to make those instruments more effective in combating crime.[13]

Definitions of war and peace are less clear now than ever before. The boundaries between political violence and criminal violence are often blurred. For example, several countries in southern Africa and in Central America had a seamless transition from politically motivated violence to criminal violence in the early 1990s,[14] without mortality rates declining significantly after the political violence officially ended. (See Chapter 18.) Postwar violence is related to many factors, principal among which is the inadequacy of mechanisms for reintegrating combatants into society. But another critical reason for postwar violence is the continued circulation of SALWs. When weapons are not collected after armed conflict, interpersonal violence substitutes for violence between warring factions.

Calculating the deaths from SALWs in conflict zones is difficult because of inadequate data and definitional issues. Deaths in armed conflicts are usually not officially categorized according to the instrument of death. In most conflicts, however, SALWs are a significant cause of both combatant and noncombatant (civilian) deaths. The Small Arms Survey, an annual study by the Graduate Institute for International Studies (GIIS) in Geneva, estimates that, in 2003, there were about 80,000 victims of small arms in conflicts worldwide.

Government arms purchases often exceed legitimate security needs and divert resources from health and education. The U.S. Congressional Research Service estimated that, collectively, countries in Asia, the Middle East, Latin America, and Africa spent $22.5 billion on arms during 2004, 8 percent more than they did in 2003. This sum would have enabled those countries to put every child in school and to reduce child mortality by two-thirds by 2015, fulfilling two of the U.N. Millennium Development Goals.[15]

In addition to the deaths from direct conflict, guns are responsible, indirectly, for many of the deaths from hunger and preventable diseases that occur during conflict. And although there has been much focus on deaths from small arms during war, there are many more deaths worldwide from firearms in the hands of civilians in countries *not* engaged in conflict.

Gun violence drains resources from services for other health problems. Consider the following example. A 16-year-old Congolese boy suffered a shattered jaw from a bullet shot by rebel soldiers. It took a year for him to raise the money from friends and family members to have it treated. He traveled to Nairobi, Kenya, for an operation in which surgeons inserted a steel plate into his jaw. The surgery took 9 hours and cost $6,000—an amount equivalent to the cost of 1 year of primary education for 100 children, full immunizations for 250 children, and 1½ years of education for a medical student. In Uganda, as another example, the government health budget allocates US$77 per capita per year for health care; in contrast, the average cost of treating a single gunshot wound is US$284.

In conflict zones, more injured victims die during transport than at treatment facilities. The medical transportation infrastructure and local personnel trained in first aid cannot carry the burden created by increased arms proliferation. Other secondary effects include problems related to the blood supply. Blood availability and transfusion are key issues in developing countries. In addition, emergency responses to large-scale violence often do not accommodate conscientious testing for human immunodeficiency virus (HIV) infection, which may result in additional long-term problems.

Violence fueled by firearms also threatens the reinstatement of democratic governance, which many people consider essential to sustainable peace. The continued availability of weapons often produces other lasting consequences, such as the breakdown of civil order and dramatic increases in lawlessness, banditry, and illicit drug trafficking. Firearms can change the balance of power and may raise the level of violence. Even if, in the short term, their use is for self-defense, the long-term effect may be to limit, if not negate, other ways of addressing conflict resolution by peaceful means. In Central America, for example, the United Nations has been very successful in peacekeeping, but the proliferation of SALWs presents a challenge to long-term stability and reconciliation.[16] High rates of gun ownership are generally related to high rates of gun-related violence in both conflict zones and areas nominally at peace (Table 6-1).

Table 6-1. Firearm Deaths, by Country

Country	Year	Firearm Deaths (Minimum)	Firearm Death Rate per 100,000 Population (Minimum)	Percentage of Firearm Deaths that are Homicides
Colombia	2002	22,827	56	93
Venezuela	2000	5,689	34	95
South Africa	2002	11,709	27	97
El Salvador	2001	1,641	26	98
Brazil	2002	38,088	22	97
Puerto Rico	2001	734	19	91
Jamaica	1997	450	19	98
Guatemala	2000	2,109	19	NA
Honduras	1999	1,677	16	NA
Uruguay	2000	104	14	22
Ecuador	2000	1,321	13	80
Argentina	2001	4,327	11	38
United States	2001	29,753	10	38

Source: Cukier W, Sidel VW. The Global Gun Epidemic: From Saturday Night Specials to AK-47s. New York: Praeger, 2006.

The Global Gun Supply

The international market for firearms is large and complex, in terms of both the markets served and the players in the distribution chain (from production through to use). Almost 100 countries are engaged in some aspect of firearm manufacture, although much of the production is concentrated in a few countries—including the five permanent members of the United Nations Security Council (the United States, Russia, China, the United Kingdom, and France) and several other European, Asian, and Latin American countries (Table 6-2).

In many cases, the production of firearms is controlled by the government. Some firearms manufacturers are state controlled and are tied very closely to defense industries; others focus on "consumer markets"—an extremely diverse group in scale of operations and range of products offered.

Although the United Nations often uses embargoes to try to stop the flow of weapons to conflict zones, the global arms trade is often not transparent, and there are many opportunities for small arms sales in contravention of limited international standards. For example, an illicit arms broker—an intermediary who arranges or facilitates the transfer of weapons but does not necessarily take possession of the weapons—often cannot be prosecuted under national arms export or import laws because the weapons never enter the country where the broker is operating. Brokers are therefore able to operate with impunity. Each of the 13 United Nations arms embargoes imposed in the past decade has been systematically violated; however, very few of the many embargo violators named in United Nations sanctions reports have been successfully prosecuted. Fewer than 40 countries have controls on arms brokers, and even fewer have the necessary extraterritorial controls.[17]

Table 6-2. Leading Countries in Gun Exports

Country	Estimated Value of Gun Exports ($US Millions)
United States	533
Italy	250
Brazil	164
Germany	159
Belgium	145
Russia	41–130
China	100

Source: International Action Network on Small Arms (IANSA). Bringing the global gun crisis under control. London: IANSA, 2006. Available at: http://www.iansa.org/campaigns_events/gun-control-2006.htm (accessed September 13, 2007).

Legal firearms are diverted to illegal markets, fueling armed conflicts and crime worldwide. Almost every small firearm considered "illegal" began as a legal one. Misuse and diversion occur through three broad categories of mechanisms: (1) misuse of legally held firearms by their lawful owners (countries, organizations, or individuals); (2) diversion of legal firearms into the "gray market," including weapons sold by legal owners to unauthorized individuals, weapons sold illegally, and weapons stolen or diverted through other means; and (3) illegal manufacture and distribution of firearms (accounting for only a small fraction of the illicit gun trade).

Diversions from national stockpiles are major sources of SALWs used in internal conflicts in several parts of the world. Corruption, theft, and seizure account for many illegal weapons transfers. Distribution networks for illegal weapons are complex and varied. Some are well organized and sophisticated, delivering containers of hundreds or thousands of weapons at a time; others are operated by small-scale criminal entrepreneurs. The "trail of ants"—small shipments of guns carried across borders—can produce a steady stream of weapons. For example, groups such as the Irish Republican Army received firearms from U.S. gun shows and dealers by a variety of mechanisms. More firearms are possessed by civilians than by governments and police. Diversion of these firearms, especially in the United States, fuels illicit firearms markets and deaths worldwide.

Several nations near South Africa have strict domestic controls on firearms and correspondingly lower crime rates than in South Africa itself, where gun controls are far more lenient. As a result, countries adjoining South Africa, such as Lesotho and Botswana, must contend with much gun smuggling across their borders from South Africa.[18] In North America, guns are exported from the United States to the gray markets of Canada and Mexico. In Mexico, U.S. guns account for 80 percent of illegal firearms[19]; in Canada, about 50 percent of all illegal handguns used in crimes come from the United States. However, proximity to a country with less stringent gun controls is not a prerequisite to importing guns.

The "culture of violence" is both a cause and an effect of the availability of SALWs. Widespread arms possession, created and normalized during the militarization of societies, can contribute to individuals' resorting to guns for resolving problems. For example, in areas in Cambodia with high levels of weapons possession, people threaten others with guns in arguments over traffic violations.[20] Increased availability of weapons also fuels the culture of violence. Relief workers in many parts of the world have noted increased numbers of thieves carrying guns, as well as escalation of violence in social disputes. This "culture of violence" has also been observed in South Africa.[21]

There is a complex dynamic between the supply and demand for firearms. More weapons tend to promote armed violence, which, in turn, promotes fear, which drives the demand for more weapons and thus more violence. Addressing feelings of insecurity is critical to efforts to stem the demand for firearms. Countries and regions with the highest rates of firearm ownership and firearm-related violence are less able to address these problems than countries with low rates. Stricter controls on firearms both reflect and shape values and gun culture—which may explain why countries with relatively low rates of gun ownership and crime are more able to move quickly to strengthen laws when tragedy strikes.

The Rise of a Global Movement

Governments and nongovernmental (civil society) organizations (NGOs) have begun working together to control the proliferation and stop the misuse of firearms worldwide. Many countries and NGOs, including the International Action Network on Small Arms (IANSA), assert that much more needs to be done to prevent the diversion and misuse of firearms.

Gun violence is a preventable problem. Although measures that strike at the roots of violence are critically important, reducing the availability of small arms reduces the lethality of political, criminal, and self-directed violence. Unlike other weapons, firearms serve purposes deemed legitimate in many cultures, so they are difficult to regulate. In addition, most illegal guns begin as legal firearms, in the hands of the military, the police, or civilians. Given the portability of guns and the relaxation of many national borders, guns easily flow from unregulated to regulated countries. Strict gun regulation in one country can be undermined by weak controls in a neighboring jurisdiction. Therefore, international standards are necessary.

Several resolutions passed by United Nations bodies stress the importance of regulation of possession of firearms by civilians as a strategy to reduce conflict, crime, and human rights violations. The 1997 Resolution of the United Nations Crime Prevention and Criminal Justice Commission provided important guidelines for national laws, reminding us that guns move from unregulated to regulated areas and that controls over guns are needed to prevent postconflict violence, crime, youth violence, and violence against women. The basic components of an effective regimen for regulating firearms include screening and licensing firearm owners, controlling and tracking sales through registration of firearms, defining safe storage to reduce the chances of gun theft, controlling ammunition, and banning weapons not suitable for civilians, such as military assault weapons.

Since the 2001 United Nations Conference on the Illicit Trafficking in Small Arms and Light Weapons in All Its Aspects, the problem of regulating civilian possession of guns is getting more attention. Although explicit ref-

erences to the regulation of civilian possession and use of firearms were de-
leted from the 2001 Conference Program of Action due to pressure from the
United States, several conference recommendations have implications for
the regulation of civilian possession of guns, such as the agreement to criminalize illegal possession of small arms, which suggests standards for legal
possession. In the end, the U.S. government and governments of a few other
countries, blocked the consensus needed for follow-up. However, a vote taken
at the meeting of the United Nations First Committee in 2006 provided a
mandate for follow-up work on a global arms trade treaty. The United Nations
Special Rapporteur on Human Rights stressed that countries have obligations
to adequately regulate civilian possession of firearms under international human rights law. Many regional agreements have emerged, which include har-
monization of legislation regarding civilian possession.

Although some countries have totally prohibited civilian ownership of all
guns, most countries accept that some firearms serve legitimate purposes. The
challenge, then, is to allow small arms to be used for legal purposes while reducing the likelihood that they will be misused, in conflicts among civilians
or for criminal purposes.

Demand for small arms is linked to many economic, cultural, and security
factors. Strategies to reduce demand vary among societies. They include the
following:

- Reducing economic inequality
- Bringing about security sector reform so that citizens are prepared to
  trust the police and the justice system
- Raising awareness of the risks of gun ownership
- Investing in children
- Providing healthy options for youth
- Addressing the culture of violence.

At the same time, the international community has been developing global
norms and standards to regulate the sale and transfer of weapons both within
and between countries. Much effort has been focused on defining the conditions under which weapons should be sold. There is broad recognition that
international transfers of weapons should not take place if they are likely to be
used in human rights violations, to fuel conflict, or to hinder development.
Measures specifically targeted at brokers who exploit gaps in laws are essential. Leakage of weapons from national stockpiles is a major problem;
these stockpiles must be securely managed to prevent theft or diversion of
guns onto the criminal market. Surplus weapons must be destroyed, and so
must those seized by police or collected in disarmament programs. Systems to
mark and trace small arms possessed by governments or civilians are needed

in order to trace guns to source and enforce these measures. In addition, given the tendency of political violence to transform into criminal violence, guns must be removed after armed conflicts through disarmament, demobilization, and reintegration strategies and the establishment of regulatory frameworks.

At the national level, there need to be minimum standards of firearm regulation to reduce the possibility that people will obtain guns and misuse them. Many regional agreements prohibit possession of certain weapons by civilians when the risk is thought to outweigh the utility; examples include fully automatic and selective-fire military assault rifles. These agreements also set minimum standards for licensing firearm owners, registering firearms, and requiring safe storage.

Acknowledgment: This chapter is based in part on Cukier W, Sidel V. The Global Gun Epidemic: From Saturday Night Specials to AK 47s. New York: Praeger, 2006.

References

1. Graduate Institute of International Studies (GIIS). Small Arms Survey 2005: Weapons at War. New York: Oxford University Press, 2005.
2. Goldring N. Two sides of the same coin: Establishing controls for SALW and major conventional weapons. Available at: http://cpass.georgetown.edu/Articles/Goldring ConventionalWeapons.pdf (accessed June 8, 2007).
3. Coupland R. The effect of weapons on health. Lancet 1996;347:450–451.
4. United Nations. General and Complete Disarmament: A Second Review Conference of the Parties to the Convention on the Prohibition of Military or Any Other Hostile Use of Environmental Modification Techniques, A/RES/46/36, 6 December 1991. Available at: http://www.un.org/documents/ga/res/46/a46r036.htm (accessed June 8, 2007).
5. Coupland RM, Samnegaard HO. Effect of type and transfer of conventional weapons on civilian injuries: Retrospective analysis of prospective data from Red Cross hospital. BMJ 1999;319:410–412.
6. Cukier W, Chapdelaine A. Small arms, explosives and incendiaries. In Levy BS, Sidel VW (eds.) Terrorism and Public Health: A Balanced Approach to Strengthening Systems and Protecting People. New York: Oxford University Press, 2003, pp. 155–174.
7. McMullin D. Lockerbie insurance, air security, hardened luggage containers can neutralize explosives. Sci Am 2002;266:15–16.
8. Safeer HB. Aviation security research and development plan. Atlantic City, New Jersey: U.S. Department of Transportation, Federal Aviation Administration, March 1992.
9. McCarthy M. Attacks provide the first major test of USA's National Anti-Terrorist Medical Response Plans. Lancet 2001;358:941.
10. Stephenson J. Medical, mental health communities mobilize to cope with terror's psychological aftermath. JAMA 2001;286:15.

11. Stein M, Hirshberg A. Medical consequences of terrorism. Surg Clin North Am 1999;79:1537–1552.
12. Missliwetz J, Schneider B, Oppenheim H, Wieser I. Injuries due to letter bombs. J Forensic Sci 1997;42:981–985.
13. United Nations Economic and Social Council. Regulation of Explosives for the Purpose of Crime Prevention and Public Health and Safety. Resolution 1998/17. July 28, 1998.
14. Renner M. Small arms. In Taipale I (ed.). War or Health?: A Reader. London: Zed Books, 2002, pp. 88–103.
15. Amnesty International, Oxfam International, and International Action Network on Small Arms (IANSA). Arms Without Borders: Why a Globalised Trade Needs Global Controls. 2006. Available at: http:www.Oxfam.org/en/files/bn0610_arms_without_borders/download (accessed June 8, 2007).
16. Chloros A, Johnston J, Joseph K, Stohl R. Breaking the cycle of violence: Light weapons destruction in Central America. (BASIC Occasional Papers on International Security, No. 24.) London: BASIC, 1997.
17. International Action Network on Small Arms (IANSA). Bringing the Global Gun Crisis Under Control. London: IANSA, 2006.
18. Cukier W, Sidel V. The Global Gun Epidemic: From Saturday Night Specials to AK-47s. New York: Praeger, 2006.
19. Sinthay N, Ashby J. Possibilities to reduce the number of weapons and the practice of using weapons to solve problems in Cambodia. Phnom Penh: STAR Kampuchea, 1998.
20. Cock J. Fixing our sights: A sociological perspective on gun violence in contemporary South Africa. Society in Transition 1997;1–4:70–81.
21. Goldring N. A glass half full: The UN Small Arms Conference. Prepared for the Council on Foreign Relations, Roundtable on the Geo-Economics of Military Preparedness, September 26, 2001.

7

Landmines

Susannah Sirkin, James C. Cobey, and Eric Stover

Despite remarkable progress toward their eradication, landmines still constitute a harrowing human-made epidemic and are aptly described as "weapons of mass destruction in slow motion."[1] Although the exact number is not known, it is estimated there are more than 80 million landmines strewn across fields, forests, and footpaths in at least 78 countries. Annually, an estimated 15,000 to 20,000 new casualties (deaths and nonfatal injuries) are reported— more than 40 per day, almost 2 per hour.[2,3] The countries with the four highest numbers of incident casualties in 2004 and 2005 (in descending order of frequency) were Colombia, Cambodia, Afghanistan, and Iraq. Also believed to have high casualty rates (in alphabetical order) were Angola, Burma, Burundi, Chechnya, the Democratic Republic of Congo, India, Iran, Laos, Nepal, Pakistan, the Palestinian Territories, Somalia, Sri Lanka, Sudan, Turkey, and Vietnam.[4]

Mines cannot distinguish between steps of soldiers and those of children. They recognize no ceasefire; long after the fighting has stopped, they continue to devastate populations, threatening livelihoods and causing trauma and disability well into a postwar generation. In 2004 and 2005, more than half of the countries recording new mine injuries had not experienced armed conflict during that period. It is estimated that half of landmine victims who die of their injuries die before they reach appropriate medical care. More than 90 percent of landmine victims today are civilians, largely rural poor people. One-fourth are children (Figure 7-1), making landmines one of the six preventable major causes of death to children worldwide. A mine costs as little as $3 to manufacture but as much as $1,000 to uncover and remove from the ground.[2,4,5]

Mines not only maim and kill; they also render large tracts of land uninhabitable, with a loss of livelihood for millions. Those most likely to encounter antipersonnel mines are poor people in rural areas.[6] Peasants foraging for wood and food or tilling their fields are particularly at risk. Children herding livestock are vulnerable because they often traverse wide tracts of land in search of fresh pastures. Refugees and internally displaced persons returning to their homes after years or decades of war fear deadly mines poised to detonate on roads and byways, or even in their front yards.[1,7] Mines strewn over huge areas of Cambodia, where as many as 4,466 square kilometers (1,724 square miles) of land are believed to be contaminated by landmines and other unexploded ordnance, constitute one of the worst manmade environmental disasters of the century.[8,9] Deminers in Afghanistan have determined that many mountainous areas of that country will be contaminated for 50 years or more.[10] The presence of mines in more than 1,250 "danger zones" in the

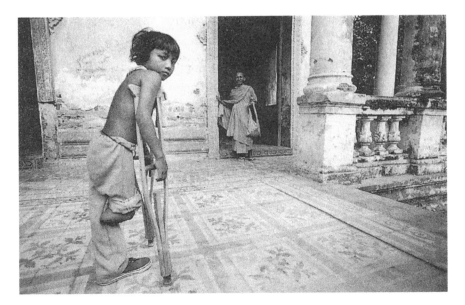

Figure 7-1. A disabled boy maimed by a landmine stands in a courtyard of a UNICEF-assisted rehabilitation center located in the Wat Tan Temple in Phnom Penh. (Source/Photographer: UNICEF/5907/Roger Lemoyne.)

Democratic Republic of Congo instills fear across a population already traumatized by the 5-year civil war in that large country[11] (see Chapter 17).

Health professionals were at the forefront of efforts to expose the deadly legacy of landmines, calling attention to tens of thousands of fatalities and injuries in the 1980s and early 1990s in Cambodia, Afghanistan, Mozambique, and Somalia.[12,13] The assertion by Physicians for Human Rights (PHR) and Human Rights Watch (HRW) in 1991[14] that this inhumane and indiscriminate weapon should be outlawed was soon echoed by relief workers, deminers, veterans, and leaders of the International Committee of the Red Cross (ICRC), galvanizing an unprecedented mine-ban movement that eventually linked governments, victims themselves, and thousands of nongovernmental (civil society) organizations (NGOs) on all continents.

The mine-ban movement led, in 1997, to the Convention on the Prohibition of the Use, Stockpiling, Production and Transfer of Anti-Personnel Mines and on Their Destruction (the Mine Ban Treaty). This treaty should be considered a landmark public health measure for the prevention and treatment of war-related injuries and deaths. By 2005, states parties to this unprecedented international agreement (that is, nations that have ratified it) had destroyed close to 40 million stockpiled antipersonnel mines, cleared tens of thousands of square kilometers of mine-infested land, and provided hundreds of millions of dollars to support rehabilitation in more than 50 countries.[5] The International Campaign to Ban Landmines (ICBL), together with its coordinator Jody Williams, received the Nobel Prize for Peace in 1997 for this visionary global grassroots effort.[15,16]

The Use of Mines

Antipersonnel mines were first used in World War II, when German and Allied troops emplaced them to prevent enemy soldiers from removing larger antitank mines. British and Italian forces scattered mines extensively in North Africa. German Field Marshall Erwin Rommel made up for a shortage of men and weapons by resorting to massive use of mines in his offensive across the Sahara in 1942. In the early 1960s, the United States perfected a sophisticated class of antipersonnel mines, known as remotely delivered mines (or "scatterables"), to stop the flow of men and matériel from North to South Vietnam through Laos and Cambodia.[12] American pilots dropped so many of these mines that they referred to them as "garbage." Weighing only 20 grams, they could flutter to the ground without detonating but still contained enough explosive to tear off a person's foot.

During the period of increased internal armed conflict in many countries beginning in the 1970s, the antipersonnel mine, like the automatic rifle, became a weapon of choice for many government and guerrilla armies around the world. Cambodian soldiers and guerrillas were so enamored of mines that they referred to them as their "eternal sentinels"—never sleeping, always ready to attack. Cambodia now has the highest percentage of inhabitants disabled by landmines of any country in the world.[1] In Cambodia, there are 45,000 survivors of landmine explosions, many of whom are amputees; approximately 800 Cambodians each year are killed or injured by landmines.[17]

Mines are cheap, easy to carry, extremely durable, and thought by military planners to be highly effective in stopping large ground assaults by conventional forces. From 1970 to 2000, they were readily available from a vast global network of government and private arms suppliers. The main producers were China, the former Soviet Union, Italy, and the United States, although dozens of countries produced and sold them. The 1989 edition of *Jane's Military Vehicles and Logistics* listed 76 pages of different kinds of mines in use, and that list was not comprehensive.[18] More recently, an outsider to the Mine Ban Treaty, the United States, has pursued its development of "smart mines," which are supposed to "self-destruct" within a period of 4 to 15 days.[19,20]

In addition to egregious injury, what makes mines especially abhorrent is the indiscriminate destruction they cause. Unlike bombs or artillery shells, which are designed to explode when they approach or hit their target, mines lie dormant until a person, a vehicle, or an animal triggers the mechanism. Modern mines often have nonmetallic casings that render much mine detection gear useless. Many models have camouflaged casings that make visual identification extremely difficult. Some antipersonnel mines are about the size of a thermos-bottle top, so a soldier can easily strew scores of them during a single patrol. Brightly colored "butterfly" mines, widely used in Afghanistan and elsewhere, have been mistaken for toys, detonating in children's hands.

The Mine Ban Treaty

Until the entry into force in 1999 of the Mine Ban Treaty, international law specifically permitted the use of mines to achieve military objectives. In 1980, the United Nations adopted a protocol to the Convention on Certain Conventional Weapons (CCW) restricting the use of "mines" (defined as any munitions placed under or near the ground or other surface area and designed to be detonated or exploded by the presence, proximity, or contact of a person).[22,23] It called on military commanders to warn civilians of the presence of minefields, maintain maps of mine placement, and remove mines after they were no longer required. The CCW was amended in 1996. For countries that have not signed the Mine Ban Treaty, the CCW is still in force, although it has been routinely violated over the years by its signatories, including the Soviet Union, which scattered mines across Afghanistan in houses, mosques, roads, and grazing land, and China, which supplied most of the mines used by the Khmer Rouge in Cambodia.[24,25]

The ineffectiveness of the CCW, the slow pace of United Nations negotiations to restrict or ban landmines, and the conviction that this weapon should be outlawed on moral, human rights, and humanitarian grounds led to the formation in 1992 of the ICBL. Initiated by the Vietnam Veterans of America Foundation, PHR, HRW, the Mines Advisory Group, Handicap International, and Medico International, the ICBL issued a call for a ban in several publications and began to recruit other groups and experts to the cause. That same year, the United States imposed a 1-year moratorium on the sale, export, and transfer of antipersonnel land mines, supporting legislation introduced by Senator Patrick Leahy (D-VT) and Congressman Lane Evans (D-IL).[26] In 1993, the export moratorium was extended for another 3 years. In 1994, President Bill Clinton called for a ban on landmines before the United Nations General Assembly.

The ICBL soon picked up the support of virtually every major humanitarian and relief organization, religious denomination, disarmament group, and medical association and rallied thousands of survivors who trekked across their mine-ridden countries on crutches and in makeshift wheelchairs. Cambodians gathered 340,000 signatures in a "peace walk" across the country, presenting them to the ICBL Conference in Phnom Penh in 1995. Factory workers at Fiat, the Italian automobile company, mobilized publicly and shut down the manufacture and export of landmine components at their plants. Media coverage of landmines and their impact in Asia and Africa was especially relentless. By 1996, the leadership of the governments of Belgium (the first country to unilaterally ban landmines), Norway, Canada, Austria, South Africa, and other countries created the momentum for a treaty on a fast track—outside the normal United Nations arms negotiation process. Canada's Foreign Minister Lloyd Axworthy then stunned the participants at the first Ottawa landmines conference in 1996 by announcing that within 1 year his country would convene a meeting to sign a ban treaty, side-stepping the dilatory U.N. Conference on Disarmament process.[27]

The 1997 treaty, frequently referred to as the Ottawa Convention, is a comprehensive international instrument that effectively bans the use, production, and trade of antipersonnel landmines. It includes measures for stockpile destruction, mine clearance, and victim assistance. In 1997, 122 nations signed the treaty in Ottawa. When the requisite 40th ratification was attained 2 years later, the treaty became binding under international law—more rapidly than any previous disarmament convention.[28] Significantly, the three leading military powers, China, the United States, and Russia, have not signed the treaty. Observers believe, however, that the treaty has created an environment in which trade and use of antipersonnel landmines are effectively taboo, even though these holdout nations officially reserve the right to produce and use these weapons—or, as in the case of the United States, seek to reclassify more sophisticated models as something other than landmines.[29]

In April 2006, U.N. Secretary General Kofi Annan stated that "the global trade in landmines has virtually halted." As of June 2006, 152 countries were states parties to the Mine Ban Treaty, constituting well over three-fourths of all countries. The fact that the United States has not ratified the treaty has been used by other countries as an excuse for not ratifying it.[30] Remaining challenges in implementation of the treaty include monitoring compliance by governments and curbing uncontrolled use of the weapon by nongovernmental forces that are not bound by the treaty.[5, 31]

Medical Consequences of Mine Casualties

Mines kill on impact or inflict ravaging wounds, usually resulting in traumatic or surgical amputation. These small weapons produce damage either by blast or by driving dirt, bacteria, clothing, and metal and plastic fragments into tissue and bone, often causing serious secondary infections.[32,33] The severity of the injury is determined by the type of mine and the proximity and location of the victim relative to the explosion. Damage is rarely confined to one leg; lesser but still severe damage is frequently caused to the other leg, the genitals, arms, chest, and face. The impact of the exploding mine can destroy blood vessels well up the leg, forcing surgeons to amputate much higher than the site of the primary wound. In many cases, amputation is required because those helping the victim fail to loosen tourniquets on the wounded limbs at regular intervals. Blinding in one or both eyes is common, as is conductive deafness, especially for children.[6,7,34,35] If a mine is handled and detonates, it can blow off fingers, hands, and arms and shatter parts of the face, chest, and abdomen.[36] The ICRC reported that war surgeons consider mine injuries to be among the worst they ever have to treat, inflicting wounds more severe than those caused by most other conventional weapons.

Medical studies of combatants injured by mines indicate that immediate first aid to stop the bleeding and administration of antibiotics to prevent serious infection, such as gangrene, followed by meticulous debridement and prompt surgical care are crucial to saving lives and reducing disabilities.[37] Early evacuation from the minefield is critical. Medical facilities operated by the United States military in Vietnam (1965–1973) and those operated by the Israeli military in Lebanon (1982)[38] achieved treatment results previously unsurpassed in war surgery. This success was due to the short transportation distances, availability of helicopters, and well-equipped medical facilities. In most wars, however, battlefield first aid, evacuation, and treatment facilities are far from ideal, with resultant high morbidity and mortality. In developing countries, where landmine injuries continue to threaten lives and livelihoods, inadequate health care systems make prompt and proper care well beyond the reach of most victims.

Many mine-blast victims die in the fields or on the way to the hospital due to loss of blood. In a 1991 study of civilian casualties in Cambodia, PHR and Asia Watch (now Human Rights Watch/Asia) found that mine-blast victims from rural areas spent an average of 12 hours from time of injury until they reached a hospital with surgical facilities.[15] An ICRC study of 757 patients being treated for mine injuries in two hospitals in an unspecified country found that most patients were admitted 6 to 24 hours after injury.[39] This delay in care can result in sepsis and severe shock.

Even when civilians injured by mines reach medical facilities, they often fail to receive proper care because blood and medical supplies, such as surgical instruments, x-ray film, anesthesia, and antibiotics, are in short supply or unavailable. Victims of mine blasts are also more likely to require amputation[13,36] and to remain in hospital longer than those wounded by other munitions. They usually require multiple operations and blood transfusions. However, hospitals in or near war zones are usually understaffed and have few, if any, orthopedic surgeons, let alone general surgeons with extensive experience in treating blast-related injuries.

Public Health Challenges and the Role of Health Professionals

Landmine victims frequently overwhelm underresourced hospital facilities. In Mozambique, landmine victims, representing only 4 percent of admissions, required 25 percent of hospital resources.[40] In Angola, 20 people per day were hospitalized with mine injuries at a time when fragile health systems were attempting to recover from decades of war and neglect. The burden of care and rehabilitation for mine victims has frequently diverted resources from vaccination, sanitation, and nutrition programs in postconflict environments (see Chapter 25). Countries struggling to develop basic health infrastructure cannot easily serve the needs of mine victims. In Afghanistan in 2004, only 10 percent of mine-impacted communities had health facilities of any kind. In the Democratic Republic of the Congo, health workers reported not having received a state salary for more than a decade (see Chapter 17). In Iraq, health facilities have been damaged and looted, forcing the closure of two of the three rehabilitation hospitals there[5] (see Chapter 15).

Once a mine amputee leaves the hospital, a lifelong series of challenges awaits. If survivors are lucky, they will receive the necessary artificial limbs or appliances needed to achieve mobility and productivity. International humanitarian agencies, including the ICRC and Handicap International, produce prostheses for those injured by mines around the world. Most are now being produced in local workshops using cheap, durable, but flexible materials, such as polypropylene. Landmine amputees, however, usually require repeated fittings and new prostheses over a lifetime, and these may be unavailable or inaccessible to survivors once they return home. Many survivors return to their villages without such devices and must then confront stigma and discrimination from family members and other villagers, who often view them as an economic burden. Male survivors, whose value in farming or herding cultures is usually directly related to their physical strength and mobility, are frequently unemployable. Disabled women are often deemed unfit for marriage.

The psychosocial consequences of landmine injuries are just beginning to be understood in mine-affected countries and cultures. Anecdotal reports of psychological trauma indicate that emotional pain may endure well beyond the physical suffering. Six years after stepping on a mine in northern Uganda, a woman told a reporter, "The physical pain fades with time, but no temporal measure can heal the emotional wounds left after an explosion. When victims lose their sense of sight or hearing, or when stumps replace limbs and a once stout man is permanently reduced to his knees, not even the smartest surgeon in the world can arrest the emotional bleeding."[41] Qualitative research has also shown that landmine amputees on four continents report being systematically denied access to adequate health care, housing, education, social contact, and economic opportunities due to their disabilities and feel unvalued by their families and friends.[42]

Landmine survivors indicate that the psychological trauma and loss of self-esteem resulting from their injuries can be overcome if, in addition to coming to terms themselves with the loss of limbs or other injuries, they receive medical care, social support, respect for their rights and dignity, and the means to become productive members of their society.[42] Increasingly, rehabilitation projects in mine-ridden countries include job training and creation of employment opportunities. The ICRC now operates more than 60 physical rehabilitation projects in 25 countries. New rehabilitation programs and training projects for people with disabilities have opened in recent years in Thailand, Uganda, Sri Lanka, Jordan, Pakistan, Nepal, and elsewhere. However, more than 10 years after the signing of the Mine Ban Treaty, the promise of assistance to victims worldwide is far from fulfilled.[43]

As many as 400,000 landmine survivors require care and rehabilitation, and the number continues to grow. Yet reporting of incidents that occur in remote areas and in underresourced settings is not systematic, and up-to-date information on incidents and needs continues to be elusive. At the first review conference of the Mine Ban Treaty in 2004, governments acknowledged the need for accurate data on new casualties that could lead to identification of areas for mine clearance and greater access to services. With the launch of the Geneva International Centre for Humanitarian Demining (GICHD), collection of data has become more standardized. Research tools, such as those developed by the World Health Organization and PHR, have enhanced abilities to study the impact of landmines and to allocate appropriate resources accordingly.[44,45] Standardization of data collection and compilation of data nationally and globally need to be improved.

The provisions of the Mine Ban Treaty for victim assistance are unique among disarmament agreements:

> Each State Party in a position to do so shall provide assistance for the care and rehabilitation and social and economic reintegration of mine victims and for mine awareness programmes. Such assistance may be provided, inter alia, through the United Nations system, international, regional or national organizations or institutions, the International Committee of the Red Cross, national Red Cross and Red Crescent societies and their International Federation, non-governmental organizations, or on a bilateral basis.

The ICBL, which now mobilizes worldwide to monitor and advocate for the fulfillment of the treaty's promise, has convened working groups to develop guidelines and best practices, urged governments to establish comprehensive programs, and advocated for adequate funding and commitment from governments and donors. Detailed guidelines for the care and rehabilitation of survivors, produced by the ICBL Working Group on Victim Assistance, exhort donors and program implementers to do the following[46]:

- Provide health care and community workers with training in emergency first aid
- Ensure that medical facilities meet minimal standards for care of injuries
- Produce prosthetic and assistive devices that are safe, durable, and reparable locally
- Develop and sustain community-based peer support groups
- Emphasize training of local workers and incorporate them into the design of programs
- Support legislation protecting the rights of people with disabilities
- Train data collectors to address traumatized survivors with sensitivity.

Although these standards require much of nations and the international community, national support of assistance to landmine victims is a rapidly emerging norm of customary international law.

The Future

In the 1990s, there was unprecedented attention to the landmine crisis and to the commitment of governments and civil society to eliminate landmines worldwide. Ultimately, only a total halt on use and the systematic removal of all mines that have been placed in areas where people need to live, work, and travel will lead to their elimination. Stepping up the pace of mine removal is costly and requires a commitment to developing local capacity and investing in new demining technologies. In the meantime, health professionals and development workers will continue to engage in mine awareness and education for populations living in or returning to contaminated environments (Box 7-1).

There is a danger that the intensity of concern about landmines will diminish as the 1997 Nobel Peace Prize to the ICBL, the novelty of the Mine Ban Treaty, and the engagement of celebrity figures, such as Diana, Princess of Wales, fade from memory. Serious investment in demining and victim assistance will be required well into the 21st century.

The major military powers and other countries that have not signed the Treaty may still be tempted to use landmines, if they find it expedient to do so. Before September 11, 2001, supporters of the Treaty in the United States, including more than 50 state and national associations of health professionals, endorsed the U.S. Campaign to Ban Landmines and called upon the United States to sign the Treaty.[47]

In August 2006, U.S. Senators Patrick Leahy (D-VT) and Arlen Specter (R-PA) introduced the "Victim-activated Landmine Abolition Act of 2006" (S.3768). Although the bill does not ban the use of landmines, it prohibits the United States from producing landmines and other related weapons. If enacted, this legislation would bring about "a legislative freeze of the production of landmines and other weapons that are set off by a victim." It would also prevent the United States from producing new antipersonnel mine systems.[48] In June 2007, the United States Campaign to Ban Landmines expanded its mandate to call for a ban on cluster munitions, which mimic landmines in the indiscriminate and unacceptable harm to civilians that they cause.

At the time of the Nobel Prize announcement, health professionals were credited with being "the first witnesses of the carnage of mines and given the responsibility of repairing what is often irreparable."[49,50] But they were also credited for their documentation of the devastating effects of landmines in countries with minimal health infrastructure and their uniquely effective role

Box 7-1 Mine Risk Education
Avid Reza, Reuben Nogueira-McCarthy, and Mark Anderson

Mine action programs are intended to reduce the threat and the risks of landmines and explosive remnants of war (ERW). These risks include both the physical risk to individuals and communities and the risk to socioeconomic development caused by landmines and ERW. Mine action programs are based on an integrated approach that includes five complementary activities[1]:

- Mine risk education (MRE)
- Humanitarian demining, including mine and ERW survey, mapping, marking, and clearance
- Victim assistance, including rehabilitation and reintegration
- Stockpile destruction
- Advocacy against the use of antipersonnel mines.

MRE programs are an essential part of an integrated mine action strategy, primarily because of their versatility, flexibility, and involvement in many different spheres of community development. As a stand-alone activity, MRE programs may also play an important role in protecting communities and building their capacity to address their mine problems, especially in the absence of a comprehensive mine clearance, survey, or marking operation. In both respects, MRE refers to "activities which seek to reduce the risk of injury from mines/ERW by raising awareness and promoting behavioral change; including public information dissemination, education and training, and community mine action liaison."[2]

MRE activities include the following[3]:

1. *Public awareness* through information dissemination using mass media, posters, and public information campaigns. Although this approach alone is not considered effective, it is one of the only ways to communicate mine-safety messages during an emergency situation characterized by armed conflict and large-scale population movements. Logistical constraints and safety concerns prevent other mine-action activities, such as demining, from being performed during emergencies, leaving information dissemination as the only tool available for preventing these injuries.

2. *Education and training*—sharing knowledge through teaching and learning in both formal and nonformal settings. Examples are teacher-to-child education in schools, parent-to-child and child-to-parent education in the home, peer-to-peer education in work and recreational environments, and landmine safety training for humanitarian aid workers.

3. *Community mine action liaison,* a community-based method that consists of exchanging information among officials, mine-action organizations,

(continued)

and communities on the presence and risk of mines and ERW. This approach is intended to improve the capacity of the affected community to develop local risk-reduction strategies and to integrate MRE more effectively into a comprehensive mine action program.

The mine action strategy of the Cambodia Mine Action Centre (CMAC) is a good example of a community-based, integrated approach to preventing injuries from mines and ERW, especially unexploded ordnance (UXO).[4] Its core activities include mine and UXO clearance; mine and UXO surveys and marking; mine and UXO risk education and reduction; and training as well as research and development in mine action. The goal of the CMAC mine and UXO risk education and reduction activity is to provide awareness to decrease the risk of injuries and deaths due to mines and UXOs. In 2001, CMAC, with the support of United Nations Children's Fund (UNICEF) and Handicap International Belgium, designed a strategy for a more sustainable and community-oriented approach to mine awareness—rather than just providing mine awareness information and education. CMAC's risk-education and risk-reduction strategy is based on ongoing assessments of the needs of the affected communities with participation of the existing community structures and local officials in prioritizing mine action activities. In addition, the planning of MRE is linked to demining, victim assistance, and community development program planning.

Although it appears that MRE has an important role to play in preventing mine and ERW injuries, there has been very little research evaluating the effectiveness of MRE as a stand-alone or integrated activity. Most evaluations have instead consisted of operational research.[5] Very few outcome evaluations have been conducted, and most of the studies have focused on assessing the impact of MRE on mine awareness. In order to determine what types of MRE are most effective, outcome evaluations are needed to assess the effectiveness of MRE interventions on changing behavior and reducing mine injuries. Public health practitioners could contribute significantly to mine action by using their knowledge and expertise in program evaluation to assist mine action programs to determine which activities are most effective for preventing injuries due to mines and ERW.

References

1. United Nations Mine Action Service. International Mine Action Standards (01.10): Guide for the Application of International Mine Action Standards, 2003. Available at: http://www.mineactionstandards.org/imas.htm (accessed June 9, 2007).
2. United Nations Mine Action Service. International Mine Action Standards (12.20): Implementation of Mine Risk Education Programmes and Projects, 2003. Available at: http://www.mineactionstandards.org/imas.htm (accessed June 9, 2007).
3. United Nations Children's Fund, Geneva International Centre for Humanitarian Demining. International Mine Action Standards for Mine Risk Reduction Education—Best Practice Guidelines: An Introduction to Mine Risk Education, 2005.

(continued)

Box 7-1 (*continued*)

Available at: http://www.mineactionstandards.org/guides.htm (accessed June 9, 2007).
4. Cambodian Mine Action Centre. Mine Action Strategies: Integrated Work Plan 2006. Available at: http://www.cmac.org.kh/Menu_MineAction_IWP2006.asp (accessed June 9, 2007).
5. Geneva International Centre for Humanitarian Demining. Mine Action: Lessons and Challenges, 2005. Available at: http://www.gichd.org/publications/mine-action-lessons-and-challenges/ (accessed June 9, 2007).

in alerting U.S. and international policy makers and the general public to this issue.

A mine-free world depends on health professionals' continuing to document the consequences of landmines and to advocate for the total and permanent elimination of landmines worldwide.

Acknowledgment: The authors thank Susanna Facci Calì for assistance in preparation of this chapter.

References

1. Office of International Security and Peacekeeping Operations, United States Department of State. Hidden Killers: The Global Problem with Uncleared Landmines. Washington, DC: U.S. Department of State, 1993.
2. Landmine Survivors Network (LSN). Landmine Facts. Available at: http://www.landminesurvivors.org (accessed June 9, 2007).
3. International Committee of the Red Cross (ICRC): Landmine victim assistance, 2004. Available at: http://www.icrc.org/Web/Eng/siteeng0.nsf/htmlall/focus_mines_assist_041118 (accessed June 9, 2007).
4. Pearn J. Children and war. J Paediatr Child Health 2003;39:166–172.
5. Landmine Monitor Core Group. Landmine Monitor Report 2005: Towards a Mine-Free World. New York: Human Rights Watch, 2005.
6. Bilukha OO, Brennan M, Woodruff BA. Death and injury from landmines and unexploded ordnance in Afghanistan. JAMA 2003;290:650–653.
7. Physicians for Human Rights and The Arms Project (a division of Human Rights Watch). Landmines: A Deadly Legacy. New York and Boston: Human Rights Watch and Physicians for Human Rights, 1993.
8. Lewis F. Make a misstep and you're dead. New York Times, May 4, 1992, p. A17.
9. Cambodian Mine Action Center. Landmine Impact Survey, 2002. Available at: http://www.sac-na.org/pdf_text/cambodia/toc.html (accessed July 18, 2007).
10. National Mine Action Programs. Special report: The future of mine action. J Mine Action 2002;6:1–112.
11. Landmines kill 1,800 in DR Congo in three years. Agence France Presse, Kinshasa, April 4, 2006.

12. Asia Watch and Physicians for Human Rights. Landmines in Cambodia: The Coward's War. New York: Asia Watch and Physicians for Human Rights, 1991.
13. Physicians for Human Rights. Hidden Enemies: Land Mines in Northern Somalia. Boston: Physicians for Human Rights, 1992.
14. Towards an international ban on landmines. New Scientist 1991;132:26–30.
15. Cameron MA, Lawson RJ, Tomlin BW (eds.). To Walk Without Fear: The Global Movement to Ban Landmines. Toronto: Oxford University Press, 1998.
16. Nobel Award citation. Available at: nobelprize.org/nobel_prizes/peace/articles/williams/index.html (accessed June 9, 2007).
17. Vines A. The crisis of anti-personnel mines. In Cameron MA, Lawson RJ, Tomlin BW (eds.). To Walk Without Fear: The Global Movement to Ban Landmines. Toronto: Oxford University Press, 1998.
18. Foss CF, Gander TJ (eds.). Jane's Military Logistics. Coulston, UK: Jane's Information Group, 1989.
19. Human Rights Watch. Position Paper on "Smart"(Self-Destructing) Landmines, February 27, 2004. Available at: http://hrw.org/english/docs/2004/02/27/7681.htm (accessed June 9, 2007).
20. Adams BN. Broken Wings: The Legacy of Land Mines. Greenville, SC: Greenville County Museum of Art, 1997.
21. Would you trust an "intelligent" antipersonnel landmine? Lancet 2005;366:690.
22. The 1997 Convention on the Prohibition of the Use, Stockpiling, Production and Transfer of Anti-Personnel Mines and on Their Destruction. Available at: http://www.icbl.org/treaty/text/english (accessed June 9, 2007).
23. The Convention on Certain Conventional Weapons (CCW). Available at: http://www.un.org (accessed June 9, 2007).
24. Coupland RM, Korver A. Injuries from antipersonnel mines: The experience of International Committee of the Red Cross (ICRC). BMJ 1991;303:1509–1512.
25. Stover E, Charles D. The killing minefields of Cambodia. New Scientist 1991;132:27.
26. United States House of Representatives. National Defense Authorization Act for Fiscal Year 1993. 102nd Congress, 2nd session, October 1, 1992; pp. 255–257.
27. Lawson RJ, Gwozdecky M, Sinclair J, Lysyshyn R. The Ottawa process and the international movement to ban anti-personnel landmines. In Cameron MA, Lawson RJ, Tomlin BW (eds.). To Walk Without Fear: The Global Movement to Ban Landmines. Toronto: Oxford University Press, 1998, pp. 160–161.
28. Shawn R, Williams J. After the guns fall silent: The enduring legacy of landmines. Washington, DC: Vietnam Veterans of America Foundation, 1995.
29. Flynn M. Landmines: Clearing the way. Bulletin of the Atomic Scientists September/October 2005;61:5.
30. Agence France Presse. Speech in NY marking the first International Day for Mine Awareness and Assistance in Mine Action. April 5, 2006.
31. Discussion meeting in Tbilisi, Georgia, between Dr. Cobey and military leaders of Georgia and Azerbaijan, 1998.
32. Traverso LW, Fleming A, Johnson DE, Wongrukmitr B. Combat casualties in northern Thailand: Emphasis on land mine injuries and levels of amputation. Mil Med 1981;146:682–685.
33. Khan MT, Husain FN, Ahmed A. Hindfoot injuries due to landmine blast accidents. Injury 2002;33:167–171.
34. Hardaway RM. Vietnam wound analysis. J Trauma 1978;18:635–643.

35. Schwab L. Preventable blindness and antipersonnel landmines. Community Eye Health J 1997;10:35–37.
36. International Committee of the Red Cross. Caring for landmine victims. Available at: http://www.icrc.org/ (accessed June 9, 2007).
37. Hsieh CH, Huang KF, LiLiang PC, et al. Below-knee amputation using a medial saphenous artery-based skin flap. J Trauma 2006; 61:353–357.
38. Danon YL, Nili E, Dolev E. Primary treatment of battle casualties in the Lebanon war. Israel J Med Sci 1982;20:300–302.
39. Asia Watch. Afghanistan: The forgotten war. New York: Human Rights Watch, February 1991.
40. Sheehan E, Croll M. Landmine Casualties in Mozambique. London: The Halo Trust, 1993.
41. Gone with the blast: The landmine problem. New Vision, Uganda, May 24, 2006.
42. Ferguson A, Richie BS, Gomez M. Psychological factors after traumatic amputation in landmine survivors: The bridge between physical healing and full recovery. Disabil Rehab 2002;26:931–938.
43. Moszynski P. Landmine casualties are falling, but the wounded need more help. BMJ 2004;329:1256.
44. The Nairobi Summit on a Mine Free World, 2004. Available at: http://www.reviewconference.org (accessed June 9, 2007).
45. Physicians for Human Rights. Measuring the Magnitude of Landmine Injuries: A Guide to Assist Governments and Non-governmental Organizations in Collecting Data about Landmine Victims, Hospitals, and Orthopedic Centers. Boston: Physicians for Human Rights, September 1999.
46. International Campaign to Ban Landmines (ICBL). Available at: http://www.icbl.org/ (accessed June 9, 2007)
47. United States Campaign to Ban Landmines. Medical Call to President Bush. Available at: http://www.banminesusa.com (accessed July 18, 2007).
48. Friends Committee on National Legislation. Issues: Landmines. Bipartisan Legislation Introduced in the House and Senate Bans U.S. Procurement of Landmines. Available at: http://www.fcnl.org/issues/item.php?item_id=1995&issue_id=9 (accessed June 9, 2007). (Latest information can be found at: http://www.banminesusa.com/news/874_clusterRestrictions.html [accessed July 18, 2007].}
49. Hansen T. The International Campaign to Ban Landmines. Peace Rev 2004;16:365–370.
50. Clements C. Cited in Physicians for Human Rights. Health Professionals Lauded for Their Role in Campaign to Ban Landmines [press release]. Cambridge, MA: Physicians for Human Rights, October 1997.

8

Chemical Weapons

Ernest C. Lee and Stefanos N. Kales

Chemical warfare has existed for thousands of years. The Chinese used arsenical smoke as a weapon as early as 1000 B.C.E.[1] In the 20th century, chemical agents were used against military and civilian targets on numerous occasions. The world still remains vulnerable to the deliberate use of chemical weapons. To better appreciate the public health threats posed by chemical agents, a basic understanding of their properties is helpful.

The Basics of Chemical Agents

Chemical agents are compounds designed to kill or disable people through toxic or poisonous mechanisms. They are relatively simple to make and use. Their effects are often dramatic and immediate. Both combatant and noncombatant populations can be the targets of these weapons. Environmentally persistent chemical agents can also be used to deny terrain or to contaminate food and water. Like nuclear and biological weapons, chemical weapons have psychological, political, operational, and strategic impacts.

Chemical attacks can be delivered by almost any type of conventional weapon system or spray device, or by nontraditional means, such as the plastic bags used by the Aum Shinrikyo cult to launch sarin attacks in Japan in the mid-1990s.[2] Intentional release of industrial chemicals is also another possible means of chemical attack; information about the presence of specific chemicals may be available from workers in a chemical plant. In contrast, delivery by chemical *weapons* is more likely to involve unidentified substances.

Chemical agents have shorter latency periods between exposure and the onset of symptoms than do biological agents. Chemical exposures are quickly recognizable due to the rapid onset of similar symptoms in a group of persons or the close proximity of a group of persons to a chemical release.[3] However, real-time identification of specific chemicals through clinical, laboratory, or environmental testing is difficult. Given the rapid action of chemical agents, the window for effective therapy is often narrow if serious chemical intoxication has occurred. Therefore, empirical treatment of chemical casualties is of paramount importance and requires some understanding of toxic mechanisms, presenting symptoms, and principles of triage and emergency management.

General Properties and Exposure Variables

Chemical agents can be absorbed by several routes, depending on the physical state of the toxin (vapor, aerosol, liquid, or solid) and existing ambient conditions (temperature and humidity). In vapor or aerosol form, chemical agents usually enter the body via the respiratory tract through oral and nasal mucosa, large and small airways, and pulmonary alveoli. After inhalation, they may produce respiratory injury or be absorbed systemically, with subsequent toxic effects elsewhere. Vapors and liquid droplets can be absorbed through the skin and mucous membranes. Solid-state compounds can also produce harmful effects through skin exposure, or, if dispersed as fine powders, they can affect the respiratory tract and mucous membranes. Agents may penetrate the skin to form temporary reservoirs and spread systemically, causing adverse effects.

Chemical agents may be divided into two major physical categories based on their rate of environmental decomposition after release:

1. Persistent agents that present a danger for days to weeks by remaining a contact hazard or by vaporizing slowly to produce an inhalation hazard
2. Nonpersistent agents that rapidly disperse and present a hazard for minutes to hours.

The potential number of persons adversely affected during a chemical attack is determined by the setting (indoor or outdoor), the proximity of individuals to the release and their density, and ambient conditions such as wind, rainfall, humidity, and temperature. Wind can be exploited to spread airborne chemicals and thus increase the number of individuals exposed; wind can also disperse toxins more rapidly. Rain reduces the effectiveness of chemical agents by washing away, diluting, and promoting hydrolysis. High temperatures decrease the persistence of chemical agents but produce higher vapor concentrations; low temperatures increase persistence. Because of these variables, the prediction of direct and secondary effects of chemical weapons is complex.

Major Classes of Chemical Agents

Because of the many chemical agents and the difficulties in rapid identification, empirical assessment and management of those affected by recognition of syndromes is recommended. Within this framework of major "toxidromes," chemical agents can be divided into four major groups: asphyxiants, cholinesterase inhibitors, respiratory tract irritants, and vesicants/skin caustics (Table 8-1).[3] As a general principle for all significant chemical exposures, after extrication, exposed victims should be decontaminated. First responders should have appropriate personal protective equipment to avoid exposure from the environment as well as secondary exposures from their patients. Immediate management is directed at the ABCs of Airway, Breathing, and Circulation.

Asphyxiants

Asphyxiants may be classified as either simple or chemical. Simple asphyxiants, such as nitrogen, carbon dioxide, and inert gases, physically displace oxygen in air when released in sufficient concentrations in relatively closed or confined spaces. Inhalation results in oxygen deficiency and hypoxemia. Chemical asphyxiants, such as cyanides, carbon monoxide, and hydrogen sulfide, interfere with oxygen transport or cellular respiration or both, causing subsequent tissue hypoxia. Asphyxiants are absorbed via inhalation; cyanides can also be readily absorbed by the mucous membranes and skin. Mild symptoms include fatigue, headache, nausea, and dizziness. Severe symptoms range from dyspnea to cardiac ischemia, altered mental status, seizure, syncope, and coma. Asphyxiants cause prominent cardiovascular and neurological signs. Respiratory failure may occur from central nervous system depression. Standard military protective masks equipped with charcoal impregnated with metal salts provide adequate protection against field concentrations of cyanide vapors[4] (Figure 8-1) Specific management of asphyxiants starts with extrication to fresh air and the administration of 100 percent oxygen. Cyanide poisoning is additionally treated with antidotes: sodium nitrite and thiosulfate (used in the United States) or hydroxocobalamin (used in Europe).

Table 8-1. Features of Selected Major Chemical Exposures

Features	Asphyxiants	Cholinesterase Inhibitors	Respiratory Tract Irritants	Vesicants
Most likely agent in accidental release	Carbon monoxide	Organophosphorus pesticides	Chlorine and its derivatives, ammonia	—
Most likely agent in act of terrorism	Cyanide	Sarin and VX	Chlorine, phosgene	Sulfur mustard
Hallmark	Tissue hypoxia in cardiovascular system and central nervous system; usually, absence of respiratory tract irritation; no increase in secretions	Cholinergic syndrome with pupil constriction (miosis) and increased exocrine secretions; increasing effects on central nervous system with increasing exposure	Respiratory tract irritation and symptoms, usually more prominent than irritation of eyes and skin	Eye injuries and skin burns with vesicle formation, followed by respiratory tract irritation and, in the case of exposure to high concentrations, systemic effects
Typical Presentations				
Mild symptoms	Headache, fatigue, anxiety, irritability, dizziness, nausea	Miosis, dim vision, eye pain, rhinorrhea, irritability, headache, chest tightness, sweating	Nose and throat irritation, sore throat, cough, chest tightness, eye irritation	Conjunctivitis, limited erythema, epistaxis, sore throat, cough

120

Moderate-to-severe symptoms	Dyspnea, altered mental status, cardiac ischemia, syncope, coma, seizure	Salivation, Lacrimation, Urination, Defecation, Gastrointestinal cramping, and Emesis (SLUDGE); wheezing, muscle weakness, fasciculations, cognitive impairment, incontinence, coma, seizure Exposure to VX or high vapor concentrations of other nerve agents	Laryngitis, wheezing, stridor, laryngeal edema, acute lung injury	Corneal damage, vesicles and bullae, nausea, wheezing, stridor, laryngeal edema, acute lung injury
Hyperacute onset—sudden collapse	High concentrations of cyanide or hydrogen sulfide and oxygen deficiency within a confined space		—	—
Acute onset—typically within minutes to hours after exposure	Most exposures to asphyxiant gases (carbon monoxide, cyanide) and oxygen deficiency	Vapor exposure, ingestion of liquid form, or moderate-to-large dermal exposure	Riot-control agents, irritants highly and intermediately water soluble (ammonia, hydrochloric acid, chlorine)	Lewisite, phosgene oxime, high concentrations of sulfur mustard
Delayed onset—typically 4 to 6 hours after exposure	Low-to-moderate concentrations of substances that metabolize to primary asphyxiants—methylene chloride (carbon monoxide), acrylonitrile, and propionitrile (cyanide)	Limited exposure of skin to droplets but not vapor	Poorly soluble gases (phosgene, nitrogen dioxide)	Sulfur mustard

Source: Kales SN, Christiani DC. Acute chemical emergencies. N Engl J Med 2004;350:801.

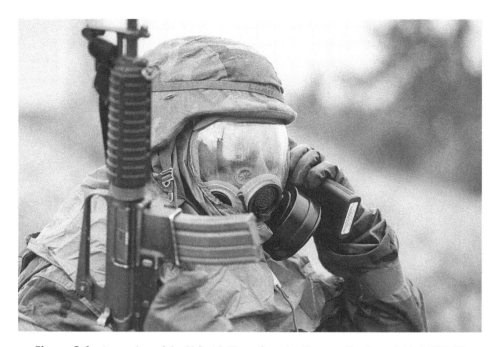

Figure 8-1. A member of the U.S. Air Force Security Forces talks through his MCU-2P chemical/biological protective mask as he communicates with other team members via radio during a combat employment readiness exercise. (Source: Department of Defense photograph by Tech. Sgt. Lance Cheung, U.S. Air Force.)

Cholinesterase Inhibitors

Carbamate pesticides, organophosphorus pesticides, and weaponized organophosphorus compounds (such as sarin, soman, tabun, and VX) all inhibit acetylcholinesterase, resulting in cholinergic overstimulation and subsequent muscarinic and nicotinic effects.[3,5–7] Cholinesterase inhibitors may be absorbed by inhalation, by ingestion, and through the skin. If nerve agent vapor exists alone, a specialized mask may provide adequate protection; however, if liquid agent is present, a mask, chemical protective suit, gloves, and overboots are required.

Muscarinic symptoms include rhinorrhea, salivation, bronchorrhea, and ophthalmic symptoms such as tearing, miosis, dim vision, and headaches. Large does may cause abdominal cramping, nausea, emesis, diarrhea, and fecal or urinary incontinence. Nicotinic symptoms include muscle weakness, fasciculations, and paralysis. Initially, tachycardia and hypertension may occur. Central nervous systems effects can range from irritability and mild cognitive impairment to convulsions and coma. Multiple mechanisms can contribute to respiratory failure, which can be fatal. Although depression of erythrocyte and serum cholinesterase activity confirms intoxication, treatment should not await these results, because they are not rapidly available. Antidotes include atropine, pralidoxime (or other oxime drugs), and benzodiazepines. Atropine works primarily at muscarinic sites, with dosing adjusted to minimize dyspnea, airway resistance, and respiratory secretions. Pralidoxime reactivates acetylcholinesterase. Benzodiazepines, such as diazepam, are the only effective anticonvulsant drugs for the treatment of persons poisoned with cholinesterase inhibitors.[3,5–7]

Organophosphorus chemical weapons (nerve agents) differ from organophosphorus insecticides, to which they are structurally related. Nerve agents are watery and volatile and act rapidly, but their effects are of shorter duration and require a smaller total dose of atropine. In contrast, insecticides are oily and less volatile. They have a slower onset of toxicity but longer duration of effects and require a large cumulative dose of atropine.[3,6,8,9]

Over time, the organophosphorus component of a nerve agent irreversibly forms a covalent bond with acetylcholinesterase, in a process known as "aging," and the enzyme becomes resistant to reactivation by pralidoxime.[1,7] Therefore, after appropriate decontamination, pralidoxime must be given promptly to prevent aging. Aging time can range form minutes (soman) to hours (sarin). In contrast, aging is not clinically relevant for organophosphorus insecticides, because these agents age at a very slow rate; however, oximes are still given to reactivate cholinesterases.[10]

Respiratory Tract Irritants (Choking Agents)

Respiratory tract irritants primarily attack the airways and lungs, causing respiratory tract inflammation, bronchospasm, and lung injury (noncardiogenic pulmonary edema). This group includes phosgene, diphosgene, chlorine, and chloropicrin as well as "tear gas" (lacrimogenic agents).[3,11–13] (Tear gas, usually considered nonlethal, was used by U.S. military forces in Vietnam to force into the open people who had been hiding.) Appropriate chemical masks can protect against these agents. Highly water-soluble irritants, such as ammonia, are absorbed in the upper respiratory tract, triggering symptoms that give early warning of toxicity. Less water-soluble irritants, such as phosgene, are able to penetrate more deeply with minimal or no symptoms, causing lung injury with a delayed onset.[3] In water, phosgene is hydrolyzed, forming hydrochloric acid and carbon dioxide. Phosgene causes acute lung injury, which interferes with gas exchange and ultimately leads to hypoxia. It can also cause irritation of the eyes and upper respiratory tract.[3,4,14] During the acute phase, exposed personnel may exhibit only minimal signs and symptoms; however, acute lung injury can later develop suddenly. Diuretics should be avoided, because they can exacerbate intravascular hypovolemia.[4] After decontamination of the skin and eyes, initial treatment consists of rest and oxygen. Rest is crucial, because physical exertion exacerbates lung inflammation. Bronchodilators should be used to treat bronchospasm, if present.[4] The use of corticosteroids, other than for the treatment of severe bronchospasm, is controversial.

Vesicants/Skin Caustics (Blister Agents)

There are three major families of vesicants: mustard, arsenical vesicants such as lewisite, and the halogenated oximes. Vesicants burn and blister any part of the body they contact.[4] Ophthalmic and cutaneous effects of exposure are the most prominent. Ophthalmic effects include conjunctivitis, corneal damage, and vision loss.[3,15,16] Skin lesions include vesicles and bullae, which are fragile and can rupture, promoting wound infection. Blister fluid, however, is not contaminated with the vesicant agent. Moist skin areas, such as the groin and axillae, are more susceptible to lesions. Inhalation of vapors can lead to respiratory epithelial necrosis, with complications including hemorrhagic edema and secondary pneumonia. These complications usually occur within 48 hours after exposure and are the most common cause of death.[3,17]

Mustard is an alkylating agent that affects DNA chains and is an inflammatory activator. Mustard agents can cause vomiting and diarrhea when ingested, and hematopoietic suppression, including bone marrow failure, may occur within days to weeks after exposure.[3]

Vesicants can penetrate the skin by contact with either vapor or liquid. Latency depends on the class of the agent: several hours for mustard, shorter duration for lewisite, and negligible for oximes.[4] A specialized mask, chemical protective suit, gloves, and overboots are required for protection. Because mustard is absorbed by many materials, protective equipment must be changed regularly. Treatment consists of rapid decontamination (preferably within 2 minutes) before irreversible chemical reactions with the skin occur. Airway protection is required for moderate to severe exposures. Additionally, specialized ophthalmic, burn, and critical care may be required. Ophthalmic treatment consists of topical anticholinergic agents, antibiotics, and petrolatum to prevent eyelid adhesion. Burn care includes debridement, topical antibiotics, and analgesics.[3,15,18,19]

Basic Management

Public Health Preparedness

Unlike military personnel, who can focus preparation on the relatively few chemicals agents capable of meeting military requirements, civilian health personnel may face attacks by non-state entities whose agent selection principles could differ from military ones. Furthermore, the timing of attacks on civilian populations may be more unpredictable. Most major U.S. cities have a Metropolitan Medical Response System (MMRS), which is usually better equipped to respond to chemical agent attacks than typical emergency medical service response teams.[20]

A variety of chemical agent detectors have been designed to alert first responders to imminent danger. Detectors must function in real-world environments where price, portability, and time are critical factors. Often, the most challenging aspect for chemical agent identification is differentiating weapon agents of interest from other chemicals in the environment. Various technologies employed include spectroscopy, flame photometry, photoionization, and use of calorimetric indicators, electrochemical detectors, acoustical wave sensors, and immunoassays.[20] Detectors must be subjected to extensive scrutiny, because excessive false-positive results can lead to response fatigue; in contrast, a single false-negative finding can result in the loss of human life.

Special Populations

Chemical attacks on civilian populations pose a unique challenge to public health workers. Many emergency response plans have been largely based on military chemical casualty care doctrines, which are designed to protect a healthy adult combatant in a battlefield scenario. However, the general population also contains groups that are more vulnerable to chemical effects, including children, older people, and individuals with underlying illness of varying types and degrees of severity. Although management of chemical effects on pediatric patients does not differ markedly from that for adult patients, physiological differences between children and adults must be considered. Children's smaller mass reduces the dose of chemical agent required to cause detrimental effects, while their higher respiratory rates and minute volumes increase the dose of chemical agent delivered at a constant concentration of toxic vapor. Children also have less mature metabolic systems for detoxification. In addition, children exposed to a chemical agent may present to a health care provider in a different manner that an adult. For example, children in cholinergic crisis induced by nerve agents may not necessarily manifest miosis. Finally, because children, on average, have more years of life left than their adult counterparts, there is more time for latent effects of chemical agent exposure to become manifest; therefore, children are theoretically more vulnerable to the longer-term effects of alkylating agents, such as mustard, which is mutagenic as well as carcinogenic.[21,22]

Older populations should be considered when planning for response to a chemical attack. On average, older persons have a higher prevalence of underlying chronic diseases. Additionally, liver volume, hepatic blood flow, and hepatic clearance capacity decline with age.

Delayed and Long-term Effects

The probability of delayed effects in persons exposed to certain chemical agents depends on the dose, exposure duration, and individual susceptibility. Delayed effects include mutations, cancer, and birth defects; however, only limited research is available concerning these adverse effects. Public health planning should also include measures designed to mitigate long-term psychological sequelae among attack survivors.

Contingency Planning

Given the potential magnitude of harm that can be inflicted on a population, advanced preparation needs to be made for a large-scale chemical attack. Military and federal government resources can be valuable to local emergency planners. The Defense Threat Reduction Agency (DTRA) has developed software tools to model nuclear, chemical, biological, and radiological releases. Such simulation technology provides a fast, effective, and inexpensive means to prepare plans for dealing with potential attacks.

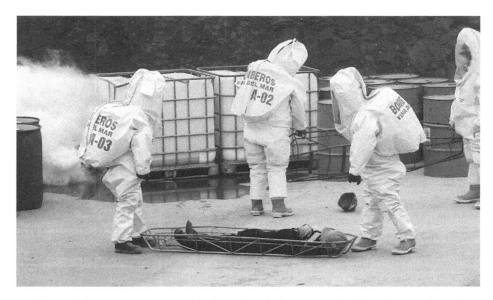

Figure 8-2. Exercise in protection from chemical weapons in Chile. (Source: Organization for the Prohibition of Chemical Weapons.)

Various emergency response agencies should communicate and work together in formulating contingency plans for chemical attacks and a chain of command that is mutually agreed upon. To this end, joint training exercises are essential. Resources, such as decontamination equipment, personal protective equipment, and antidotes, must be prepositioned to strategic locations. Maps of major industrial sites that could be targets of attacks should be maintained by hazardous material response teams and MMRSs, along with information regarding treatment for respective hazardous material or energy exposures. Emergency contingency plans should be logistically and economically feasible as well as sustainable. Hospitals as well as first-response units should have decontamination equipment, personal protective equipment, and adequate training in the use of this equipment (Figure 8-2). Panic that may ensue after an attack will likely lead to many people seeking medical attention that is not needed, overwhelming triage personnel if they are not adequately trained. Large-scale, multimodality patient simulation can be used to train clinicians and nonclinicians for potential attack scenarios.[23]

The Use of Chemicals Agents in War and Terrorist Attacks

Although guns and conventional explosives have been the terrorist weapons of choice, some terrorist groups show interest in acquiring the capability to use chemical, biological, radiological, or nuclear materials. Terrorism attacks have become more lethal and are often designed to kill as many people as possible. Some terrorist groups are driven by ethnic hatred, political beliefs, or religious ideology. Certain groups may lack a concrete goal other than to punish their enemies by killing as many of them as possible.

The Aum Shinrikyo religious cult launched two attacks in Japan using sarin. In the first attack, a truck was used to release an aerosol cloud of sarin into a residential neighborhood of Matsumoto in June 1994.[1,2] As a result, 7 people died and another 200 required hospitalization for at least one night. In a second attack, terrorists carried diluted sarin solution in plastic bags into subway trains and punctured the bags, releasing sarin vapor into three convergent lines of the Tokyo subway system. This attack was the largest disaster ever caused by nerve gas in peacetime. It was a failure in many respects; Aum Shinrikyo had used many highly skilled technicians and spent tens of millions of dollars developing a chemical attack that killed fewer people than conventional explosives could have. However, examination of the aftermath illustrates how even a botched attack easily overwhelmed an ill-prepared disaster management system. Although only 12 people died, approximately 1,000 were injured. In addition, because of the panic that the attack caused, 4,971 patients who had no signs of adverse effects were evaluated by health care facilities on the day of the attack.[25,26]

Several problems with hospital plans and disaster management were revealed. The main hospital involved had not established a definite plan of how to channel large numbers of affected people through its three entrances. As a result, affected people, family members, media crew, and onlookers streamed into the hospital from all three entrances, creating a chaotic situation. Many medical records were lost. Because the cause of the illness was not known until about 3 hours after the release, many hospital staff members were secondarily exposed. Hospitals lacked decontamination facilities and proper ventilation. Staff members did not have immediate access to chemically resistant personal protective equipment. One hospital alone expended 700 ampules of pralidoxime chloride and 2,800 ampules of atropine sulfate; because its original stockpile of antidote was depleted, the hospital had to airlift in additional supplies.[24]

Although use of chemical agents against noncombatants has only recently drawn attention, they have been used by military forces for centuries. The ancient Spartans used noxious smoke and flame against cities during the Peloponnesian War. Leonardo da Vinci proposed a powder of arsenic sulfide. During the Russo-Japanese War, Japanese soldiers used arsenical rag torches.[27]

Most chemical agents used in World War I were discovered during the 18th and 19th centuries. Both the French and the British tested various chemicals weapons on the battlefield. The French used ethyl bromoacetate grenades against the Germans during the German invasion of Belgium and France.[27] The Germans pursued offensive chemical weapons. In October 1914, German forces fired 3,000 projectiles filled with dianisidine chlorosulfate, a lung irritant, at the British in Neuve-Chapelle; however, the explosion of the shells nullified their chemical activity. The Germans later developed munitions containing xylyl bromide and fired more than 18,000 of them at Russian positions near Bolimov, located in the plains west of Warsaw; in this case, cold temperatures prevented vaporization of the gas, and the attack was largely unsuccessful.[28–30]

The first successful German chemical attack occurred in April 1915 in Ypres, Belgium. German forces waited for favorable wind conditions and then released large amounts of chlorine gas from cylinders.[31] The Allies responded with chlorine attacks. Thus began a deadly competition to develop better protective masks, more potent chemicals, and more effective delivery systems (Figure 8-3). The Germans escalated to the use of phosgene and diphosgene, while the French resorted to hydrogen cyanide and cyanogen chloride. In order to bypass protection rendered by masks, the Germans introduced mustard, a persistent vesicant capable of harming body areas not protected by gas masks.

In 1943, a U.S. freighter that was carrying 100 tons of mustard gas in 100-pound bombs was bombed by German planes while it was waiting to be

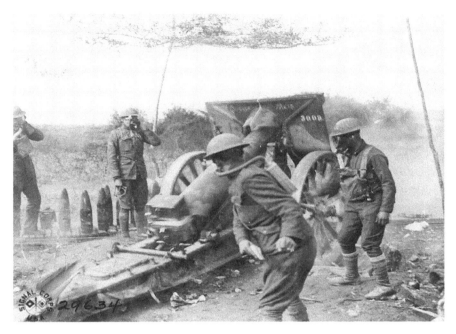

Figure 8-3. Members of the 108th Field Artillery firing in mission-oriented protective posture, Argonne, France, October 1918. This battery was under fire of enemy gas shells at the time this photograph was taken. (Source: National Archives.)

unloaded at the seaport of Bari, Italy. As a result, 628 people were affected, of whom 69 died within two weeks of the bombing.[32]

In the remainder of the 20th century, there were other instances in which chemical agents were used with devastating consequences (Table 8-2). In addition to the 1994 and 1995 sarin attacks in Japan, other attacks involved the following chemical agents[33]:

- Adamsite, diphenylchlorarsine, and mustard gas in Russia (1919)
- Bromomethyl ethyl ketone, chloropicrin, and mustard gas in Morocco (1923–1926)
- Chlorine, chloroacetophenone, mustard gas, phenyldichlorarsine, diphenylchlorarsine, and phosgene in Abyssinia (1935–1945)
- Chloroacetophenone, diphenylcyanoarsine, hydrogen cyanide, lewisite, mustard gas, and phosgene in Manchuria (1937–1945)
- Chloroacetophenone, mustard gas, and phosgene in Yemen (1963–1967)
- 2-Chlorobenzalmalononitrile in Vietnam (1965–1975)
- 2-Chlorobenzalmalononitrile in Iraq (1982–1988)
- Mustard gas, sarin, and tabun in Iran (1982–1988).

Table 8–2. A Timeline of Chemical Weapons History

1899, 1907: First and second peace conferences at The Hague. In 1899, European nations prohibited "the use of projectiles whose sole purpose is the release of asphyxiating or harmful gases." In 1907, the Conference added the use of poison or poisoned weapons to the prohibition.

1914–1918: The first large-scale attack with chemical weapons occurred on April 22, 1915, at Ieper in Belgium, during World War I.

1925: The Protocol for the Prohibition of the Use in War of Asphyxiating, Poisonous or Other Gases, and of Bacteriological Methods of Warfare was signed at Palais Wilson in Geneva.

1939–1945: Chemical weapons were deployed on a large scale in almost all theaters in World War II, leaving behind a legacy of old and abandoned chemical weapons.

1946–1991: During the Cold War, many nations produced and stockpiled chemical weapons, amounting to tens of thousands of tons, enough to kill much of human and animal life worldwide.

1988: Iraq used chemical weapons against Iran during the 1980-1988 conflict. Iraq also used mustard gas and nerve agents against Kurdish residents in northern Iraq.

1995: In Japan, the Aum Shinrikyo cult released the chemical agent sarin in a terrorist attack on the Tokyo subway. About 5,000 people became sick, and 12 died.

1997: With the entry into force of the Chemical Weapons Convention on April 29, 1997, The Organization for the Prohibition of Chemical Weapons immediately began its work to implement the Convention.

Source: Organization for the Prohibition of Chemical Weapons. Available at: http://www.opcw.org/29april/page02.html (accessed June 12, 2007).

Today, dozens of chemical agents are stockpiled in many countries, threatening combatants and noncombatants.

Chemical Agents and International Law

Since at least the early 1600s, international law has condemned what would today be regarded as chemical warfare. Subsequent development of such law can be seen in the Brussels Declaration of 1874 and at the Hague Peace Conference of 1899. Following the extensive use of chemical weapons during World War I, the international community strengthened the existing legislation restricting these weapons, leading to the Protocol for the Prohibition of the Use in War of Asphyxiating, Poisonous or Other Gases, and of Bacteriological Methods of Warfare. This treaty, known as the Geneva Protocol of 1925, entered into force in 1928.

As written, the Geneva Protocol prohibits "the use in war of asphyxiating, poisonous or other gases, and of all analogous liquids, materials or devices."

However, it does not prohibit possession of these weapons. In effect, the treaty was a "no-first-use" agreement. Additionally, some states parties (countries) reserved the right to use the weapons against states not party to the protocol. For these reasons, a more comprehensive prohibition of weapons was negotiated in the 1993 Chemical Weapons Convention (CWC). This agreement, which entered into force in 1997, is of "unlimited duration."

The CWC established the Organization for the Prohibition of Chemical Weapons (OPCW), a permanent international body whose membership consists of all states parties to the Convention, which oversees the implementation of the CWC. The CWC "reaffirms principles and objectives of and obligations assumed under the Geneva Protocol of 1925." Each state party to the CWC commits to never (1) develop, produce, otherwise acquire, stockpile, or retain chemical weapons or transfer, directly or indirectly, chemical weapons to anyone; (2) use chemical weapons; (3) engage in any military preparations to use chemical weapons; or (4) assist, encourage, or induce anyone, in any way, to engage in any activity prohibited to a state party under the Convention.

The CWC also commits each state party to "destroy chemical weapons it owns or possesses, or that are located in any place under its jurisdiction or control, in accordance with the provisions of this Convention" and "to destroy all chemical weapons it abandoned on the territory of another state party, in accordance with the provisions of this Convention." Any such destruction must ensure the safety of the population and the protection of the environment. The CWC incorporates an elaborate regimen to ensure compliance and specifies how its obligations are to be implemented. Although the CWC makes no direct reference to the concept of universality, the objective of universal adherence follows from the goal in its preamble to exclude the use of chemical weapons "for the sake of all mankind."

Despite the elaborate measures in the CWC, several challenges remain. First, not all countries have joined the treaty, challenging the concept of universality. Second, the CWC allows each country "to withdraw from this Convention if it decides that extraordinary events, related to the subject-matter of this Convention, have jeopardized the supreme interests of its country." Such discretion could potentially be exploited out of self-interest. Third, export/import controls remain underdeveloped. For example, some mustard and nerve agent precursors are not listed in the schedules of controlled chemicals. Fourth, the effectiveness of compliance monitoring systems has not truly been tested. Finally, prohibitions under the CWC are directed primarily to the actions of states and only marginally address the matter of individual responsibility. With the emergence of non-state actors with interest in these and other weapons, amendments to the existing CWC or a new treaty is needed to require a country to establish criminal jurisdiction applicable to foreign nationals who commit chemical weapons offenses either on its own territory or elsewhere, regardless of nationality.

Control of Chemical Weapons Proliferation

Despite the many attempts to limit the spread of chemical weapons, the ease with which certain classes can be developed and their sheer destructive potential make them attractive to any government or non-state entity that is seeking military advantage. Multilateral commitment is critical in controlling proliferation of such weapons. Critical also are intelligence gathering, challenge inspections, and monitoring of chemical transfers and technologies used in the development and manufacture of chemical weapons (Figure 8-4). When destroying existing chemical weapons, countries must exercise extreme caution so as to avoid adverse effects on local populations as well as the environment. To these ends, the CWC states that the following processes may not be used in the destruction of chemical weapons: "dumping in any body

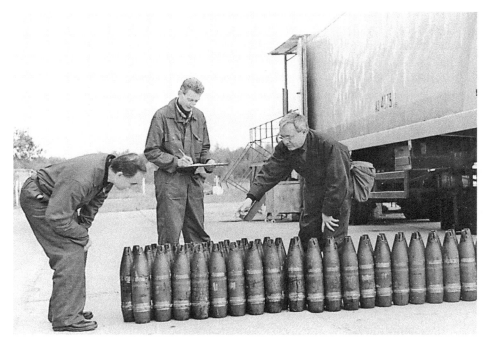

Figure 8-4. Organization for the Prohibition of Chemical Weapons (OPCW) inspectors inventory artillery munitions. (Source: Organization for the Prohibition of Chemical Weapons.)

of water, land burial, or open-pit burning." To augment the legal framework designed to control the spread of these weapons, national self-interest must not be underestimated in any multilateral agreement.

It is useful to remember that Napoléon Bonaparte once said, "Treaties are observed as long as they are in harmony with interests."

References

1. Lee EC. Clinical manifestations of sarin nerve gas exposure. JAMA 2003;290:659–662.
2. Okudera H, Morita H, Iwashita T, et al. Unexpected nerve gas exposure in the city of Matsumoto: Report of rescue activity in the first sarin gas terrorism. Am J Emerg Med 1997;15:527–528.
3. Kales SN, Christiani DC. Acute chemical emergencies. N Engl J Med 2004;350:800–808.
4. Department of Defense. The Medical NBC Battlebook. Aberdeen Proving Ground, MD: U.S. Army Center for Health Promotion and Preventive Medicine (USACHPPM), 2002.
5. Carlton FB Jr, Simpson WM Jr, Haddad LM. The organophosphates and other insecticides. In Haddad LM, Shannon MW, Winchester JF (eds.). Clinical Management of Poisoning and Drug Overdose, 3rd ed. Philadelphia: WB Saunders, 1998, pp. 836–845.
6. Sidell FR. Clinical effects of organophosphorus cholinesterase inhibitors. J Appl Toxicol 1994;14:111–113.
7. Sidell FR, Borak J. Chemical warfare agents: II. Nerve agents. Ann Emerg Med 1992;21:865–871.
8. Gunderson CH, Lehmann DR, Sidell FR, Jabbari B. Nerve agents: A review. Neurology 1992;42:946–950.
9. Sidell FR. What to do in case of an unthinkable chemical warfare attack or accident. Postgrad Med 1990;88:70–84.
10. Devereaux A, Amundson DE, Parrish JS, Lazarus AA. Vesicants and nerve agents in chemical warfare. Postgrad Med 2002;112:90–96.
11. Hall HI, Dhara VR, Price-Green PA, Kay WE, Surveillance for emergency events involving hazardous substances—United States, 1990–1992. MMWR CDC Surveill Summ 1994;43:1–6.
12. Kales SN, Castro M, Christiani DC. Epidemiology of hazardous materials responses by Massachusetts district HAZMAT teams. J Occup Environ Med 1996;38:394–400.
13. Burgess JL, Pappas GP, Robertson WO. Hazardous materials incidents: The Washington Poison Center experience and approach to exposure assessment. J Occup Environ Med 1997;39:760–766.
14. Nelson LS. Simple asphyxiants and pulmonary irritants. In Goldfrank LR, Flomenbaum NE, Lewin NA, et al. (eds.). Goldfrank's Toxicologic Emergencies, 7th ed. New York: McGraw-Hill, 2002, pp. 1453–1468.
15. Borak J, Sidell FR. Agents of chemical warfare: Sulfur mustard. Ann Emerg Med 1992;21:303–308.

16. Hurst CG, Smith WJ. Chronic effects of acute, low-level exposure to the chemical warfare agent sulfur mustard. In Somani SM, Romano JA Jr (eds.). Chemical Warfare Agents: Toxicity at Low Levels. Boca Raton, FL: CRC Press, 2001, pp. 245–260.

17. Davis KG, Aspera G. Exposure to liquid sulfur mustard. Ann Emerg Med 2001;37: 653–656.

18. Safarinejad MR, Moosavi SA, Montazeri B. Ocular injuries caused by mustard gas: Diagnosis, treatment, and medical defense. Mil Med 2001;166:67–70.

19. Ruhl CM, Park SJ, Danisa O, et al. A serious skin sulfur mustard burn from an artillery shell. J Emerg Med 1994;12:159–166.

20. Griffin D, Gabor K. eMedicine. CBRNE—Chemical detection equipment. Available at: http://www.emedicine.com/emerg/topic924.htm (accessed June 9, 2007).

21. Lynch EL, Thomas, TL. Pediatric considerations in chemical exposures: Are we prepared? Pediatr Emerg Care 2004;20:198–208.

22. Rotenberg JS, Newmark J. Nerve attacks on children: Diagnosis and management. Pediatrics 2003;112:648–658.

23. Kyle RR, Via DK, Lowy RJ, et al. A multidisciplinary approach to teach response to weapons of mass destruction and terrorism using combined simulation modalities. J Clin Anesth 2004;16:152–158.

24. Okumura T, Suzuki K, Fukuda A, et al. The Tokyo subway sarin attack: Disaster management. Part 2: Hospital response. Acad Emerg Med 1998;5:618–624.

25. Woodall J. Tokyo subway gas attack. Lancet 1997;350:296.

26. Sidell F. Proceedings of Seminar: Responding to the Consequences of Chemical and Biological Terrorism. USPHS/Office of Emergency Preparedness. Washington, DC: Government Printing Office, 1995, pp. 232–233.

27. Smart JK. History of Chemical and Biological Warfare Fact Sheets. (Special Study 50.) Aberdeen Proving Ground, MD: U.S. Army Chemical and Biological Defense Command, 1996.

28. Haber LF. The Poisonous Cloud: Chemical Warfare in the First World War. Oxford, England: Clarendon Press, 1986.

29. Prentiss AM. Chemicals in War: A Treatise on Chemical Warfare. New York: McGraw-Hill, 1937.

30. Hogg I. Bolimow and the first gas attack. In Fitzsimons B (ed.). Tanks and Weapons of World War I. New York: Beckman House, 1973.

31. Fries AA. Gas in attack. Chem Warfare 1919;2:3–8.

32. Infield GB. Disaster at Bari. New York: Macmillan Company, 1971.

33. World Health Organization. Public Health Response to Biological and Chemical Weapons: WHO Guidance, 2nd ed. Geneva: WHO, 2004.

9

Biological Weapons

Barry S. Levy and Victor W. Sidel

Biological weapons have been used in warfare, although infrequently, since ancient times. These agents are feared because they are generally invisible and easy to disseminate, some may spread easily from person to person, and some can cause horrific diseases. The public and health professionals have focused much attention on these agents since the dissemination of anthrax spores through the U.S. mail in September and October 2001. Five people died of inhalational anthrax, six more survived inhalational anthrax, and 11 others had confirmed or suspected cutaneous anthrax. (A laboratory worker later developed and survived cutaneous anthrax.) In addition, tens of thousands of postal, news-media, and other workers received prophylactic antibiotic treatment. And millions more feared that they too could be at risk of developing anthrax.

The biological agents in biological weapons are living organisms (usually microorganisms) or their toxic products. Although the main targets of these weapons are people, they can also be used against animals or plants to limit human food supplies or agricultural resources and thereby adversely affect human health and well-being indirectly.

Use of Biological Weapons

There is a long but sporadic history of the use of biological weapons since ancient times. Table 9-1 provides a summary of their use until World War II. During World War II, prisoners in German concentration camps were infected with various biological agents during tests of these weapons.[1] Great Britain and the United States, fearing the Germans would use biological weapons, developed their own: The British tested anthrax spores off the coast of Scotland on Gruinard Island, making it uninhabitable for decades; the United States developed anthrax spores, botulinum toxin, and other agents as biological weapons. Great Britain and the United States, however, never used these weapons.[1] Also during World War II, Japanese laboratories conducted extensive experiments on prisoners of war using many organisms, including those that cause anthrax, plague, gas gangrene, encephalitis, typhus, typhoid, hemorrhagic fever, cholera, smallpox, and tularemia.[2] The Soviet Union prosecuted some Japanese people for their involvement in these experiments, but the United States instead urged that other Japanese people who were involved be "spared embarrassment" so the United States could benefit from their knowledge.[3]

Development, production, and testing of biological weapons continued in several countries after World War II. Despite numerous allegations, however, no offensive use of these weapons has been substantiated or even fully investigated since World War II. In the 1950s and 1960s, the U.S. government conducted 239 top-secret, open-air disseminations of bacteria believed to be nonpathogenic, to test the efficiency of their dispersal. Bacteria were disseminated in the New York City subway system, Washington National Airport, the San Francisco Bay Area, and elsewhere. Some subsequent infections and deaths were attributed to one of these organisms. The University of Utah conducted secret, large-scale field tests at the U.S. Army Dugway Proving Ground of the agents that cause tularemia, Rocky Mountain spotted fever, plague, and Q fever.[4] The U.S. military developed a large biological weapons infrastructure of laboratories, test facilities, and production plants. By 1970, the United States had stockpiles of at least 10 different biological and toxin weapons.[3] Similar development of offensive biological weapons occurred in the Soviet Union.[5] (An accidental release of smallpox virus from the Soviet bioweapons program in 1971 in Aralsk, a small town on the shore of the Aral Sea, caused three deaths.[6])

In 1969, the Nixon administration, with the concurrence of the U.S. Department of Defense, which had previously declared that biological weapons lacked "military usefulness," announced that the United States would unilaterally dismantle its biological weapons program.[7] In 1972, the United

Table 9-1. Outline of History of Biological Warfare from Ancient Times to World War II

6th century B.C.E.	Persia, Greece, and Rome used diseased corpses to attempt to contaminate sources of drinking water.
400 B.C.E.	Scythian archers used arrows dipped in manure, blood, or decomposing bodies.
190 B.C.E.	Hannibal's forces threw poisonous snakes onto enemy ships.
1155 A.D.	Ottoman admiral Barbarossa poisoned enemy wells with the bodies of dead soldiers.
1346	Mongols besieging the Crimean seaport Kaffa placed cadavers of plague victims on hurling machines and threw them into Kaffa.
1495	The Spanish used wine infected with blood of leprosy patients against the French.
1650	A Polish general placed saliva of rabid dogs into hollow spheres and fired them against enemies.
1710	Russian troops used cadavers of plague victims to start an epidemic among enemy Swedish forces.
1754–1767	During the French and Indian War, British commander Sir Jeffrey Amherst sent smallpox-infected blankets to Native Americans.
1861	Union troops were affected by outbreaks of food poisoning during the U.S. Civil War.
1863	Confederate troops left dead animals in wells and ponds to deny fresh water to retreating Union forces.
1915–1916	Germans infected Romanian sheep bound for Russia with anthrax and *Pseudomonas* and infected horses of the French cavalry with bacteria that cause glanders.
1917	Germany was accused of poisoning wells with human corpses and dropping fruit, chocolate, and children's toys infected with lethal bacteria into Romanian cities.
World War I	Germany dropped bombs containing plague bacteria over British positions and used cholera in Italy.
1930s	Russian spies were arrested in China while carrying containers with agents of dysentery, cholera, and anthrax.
1930s	Japan fed infectious agents to prisoners and subjected them to anthrax bombs. Japan attacked at least 11 cities in China by contaminating food and water supplies or spraying the cities from aircraft with biological weapons.
1942	Anthrax bombs were tested at Gruinard Island by the British; all exposed sheep died within 3 days, and anthrax spores kept the island quarantined for five decades.

Adapted from: Metcalfe N. A short history of biological warfare. Medicine, Conflict and Survival 2002;18:271–282.

States, the Soviet Union, and other nations negotiated the Convention on the Prohibition of the Development, Prevention and Stockpiling of Bacteriological (Biological) and Toxin Weapons and on their Destruction (the Biological Weapons Convention, or BWC). The BWC prohibits, except for peaceful purposes, the development or acquisition of biological agents or toxins, as well as the weapons carrying them and the means of their production, stockpiling, transfer, or delivery. The U.S. Senate ratified the BWC in 1975, and it entered into force later that year.

The Soviet Union continued extensive development and testing of biological weapons after the BWC entered into force.[5,8,9] The Soviet bioweapons program employed 42,000 scientists, who weaponized anthrax, mounted smallpox on missiles, developed antibiotic-resistant plague and anthrax, and mass-produced hemorrhagic fever viruses.[10] As of August 2007, there were 174 nations that had signed or ratified the BWC. The BWC has been weakened by disagreements among its signatory nations on its future, by the lack of any system for compliance, by countries' performing research or other projects that are inconsistent with the treaty's objectives, and by the lack of consequences for countries accused of having violated the BWC. Of high priority is the need for establishing a system of verification.[11]

Two outbreaks related to biological weapons are worth noting. In 1979, an accidental release of anthrax spores from a Soviet biological weapons factory caused an outbreak of pulmonary anthrax with at least 79 cases, at least 68 of which were fatal.[7,10,12] In 1984, in Oregon, members of a cult intentionally contaminated salad bars with *Salmonella* bacteria at several restaurants; more than 700 people became ill, but no one died.[13]

During the 1980s, the Reagan administration initiated "defensive research" on biological weapons, which is permitted under the BWC. The budget for the U.S. Army Biological Defense Research Program (BDRP), which sponsored programs in a wide variety of academic, commercial, and government laboratories, increased dramatically. Much of this research was medical, including the development of immunizations and treatments against organisms that might be used as biological weapons.[14] Research and development of new biological weapons, which is outlawed by the BWC, may have also occurred.[7,8,15,16]

It is believed that 13 countries have offensive biological weapons programs.[17] Since the dissemination of anthrax spores in the United States in 2001, much attention in this country has been focused on preparedness for a potential terrorist attack with biological agents. (See Box 1-2.) The response to concerns about this threat has included plans for increased research on biological agents. Many people in the scientific community have voiced concerns about possible adverse effects of this research (Box 9-1).

Box 9-1 The Case Against Plans for a Biodefense Research Laboratory
David Ozonoff

I believe that biodefense constitutes a severe distortion of priorities in public health and a significant distortion of public health style, custom, etiquette, and culture. Biodefense research makes us less safe. It raises the specter of classified (secret) research. It has no true civilian oversight. And it creates an arms control problem.

Distortion of Priorities

People in the United States do not suffer much from tularemia, anthrax, plague, glanders, and other diseases associated with biological weapons. But we *do* suffer from tuberculosis, syphilis, gonorrhea, *Salmonella* infections, and whooping cough. We suffer from these preventable diseases, but we do not have public health infrastructure to adequately address them.

From 1996 to 2000, there were 33 grants awarded for research on prioritized bioweapons agents. From 2001 to January 2005, there were 497—a 15-fold increase! Meanwhile, there have been decreases in grants for research on microbial agents not related to biodefense: reductions of 41 percent and 27 percent in grants approved by the two main study sections at the National Institutes of Health (NIH) for diseases that people *do* acquire.

There has been a wholesale rearrangement of personnel assignments in state and local public health. We thought that biodefense money would be used to build our public health infrastructure, but this did not happen. What happened was much worse. Local and state governments started cutting taxes and cutting budgets for public health. When governments cut budgets for public health, they used biodefense money to pay staff members. But the biodefense money was earmarked for projects such as biodefense needs assessments and smallpox vaccination plans for hospitals. Public health workers who formerly operated programs addressing substance abuse, provided maternal and child health services, and performed all of the other routine and essential public health functions suddenly were making plans for smallpox vaccinations. They were taken off "bread-and-butter" public health work and assigned to projects of no general value to public health services and infrastructure.

Public Health Style

Public health has been organized categorically in areas such as substance abuse, maternal and child health, and vital statistics. Now, there is a military-like command structure, which does not work well in public health settings. We used to say that when public health works, nothing happens. Now

(continued)

Box 9-1 (*continued*)

everything is reversed: Nothing works until something happens. It makes us less safe.

Boston University is building a $178 million biodefense research laboratory adjacent to downtown Boston. While this laboratory will not make biological weapons, it may plausibly construct novel pathogens so that defenses can be developed against them, such as diagnostic kits and vaccines. Even with the best of safeguards, there will be risks that agents will escape from the laboratory or be stolen. We are now learning that laboratory-acquired infections and breaches of protocol in the nation's biodefense laboratories are more common than anyone suspected.[1] The proliferation of these laboratories increases the chances of a catastrophic incident.

Because of ease of access, guns and explosives are the weapons of choice for terrorists, not novel pathogens. An exception is when institutions develop novel pathogens, which can be stolen and used by terrorists.

Against this background, the construction of another high-containment biodefense laboratory at Boston University is an enterprise that will paradoxically make us less safe, not more safe. Despite strong concern among University faculty, medical center staff, and the surrounding community, construction has gone forward. A legal challenge is pending, but its chance of success is small. The biodefense research laboratory at Boston University and similar laboratories around the United States will bring classified and secret research to the medical community. There will likely be inadequate civilian involvement by nearby residents and laboratory workers who could possibly be affected. In addition, there will be no binding restriction that offensive, as opposed to defensive, biological-agent research would be performed at the Boston University laboratory or elsewhere. As the United States builds and operates these biodefense research laboratories, other countries will likely want to build and operate similar laboratories, stimulating a biological weapons arms race.

In sum, biodefense research laboratories, as planned, are likely to create more harm than benefit. They are not in the interest of public health.

Reference

1. The Sunshine Project: Biodefense. Available at: http://www.sunshineproject.org (accessed July 11, 2007).

Novel dangers lie in new genetic technologies, which permit the development of genetically altered organisms not known in nature. Stable, tailor-made organisms used as biological weapons could travel far and remain infectious, become resistant to antibiotic treatment, and rapidly infect a population, causing widespread illness and death.

**Table 9-2. Categories of Diseases and the Biological Agents
That Cause Them**

Category A

Anthrax *(Bacillus anthracis)*
Botulism *(Clostridium botulinum* toxin)
Plague *(Yersinia pestis)*
Smallpox (variola major)
Tularemia *(Francisella tularensis)*
Viral hemorrhagic fevers (filoviruses, such as Ebola and Marburg,
    and arenaviruses, such as Lassa and Machupo)

Category B

Brucellosis *(Brucella* species)
Epsilon toxin of *Clostridium perfringens*
Food safety threats (such as *Salmonella* species, *Escherichia
    coli* O157:H7, *Shigella)*
Glanders *(Burkholderia mallei)*
Melioidosis *(Burkholderia pseudomallei)*
Psittacosis *(Chlamydia psittaci)*
Q fever *(Coxiella burnetii)*
Ricin toxin from *Ricinus communis* (castor beans)
Staphylococcal enterotoxin B
Typhus fever *(Rickettsia prowazeki)*
Viral encephalitis (alphaviruses, such as Venezuelan equine encephalitis,
    eastern equine encephalitis, and western equine encephalitis)
Water safety threats (such as *Vibrio cholerae and Cryptosporidium parvum)*

Category C

Emerging infectious diseases, such as those caused
    by Nipah virus and hantavirus

Source: Centers for Disease Control and Prevention. Available at: http://www.bt.cdc
.gov/agent/agentlist-category.asp (accessed June 9, 2007).

Potential Biological Weapons and Their Adverse Health Effects

The many biological agents that might be used as weapons can produce both
physical and psychological effects.[18–20] Protocols for diagnosis, treatment,
and prevention are now widely available, with frequent updates from the
Centers for Disease Control and Prevention (CDC) and other sets of experts.
The CDC Web site on bioterrorism (http://www.bt.cdc.gov [accessed June 9,
2007]) is a useful source of information.

The CDC has developed three categories of biological agents, prioritized
according to the likelihood of their use and the severity of the diseases they
produce (Table 9-2):

- *Category A* (high-priority) agents pose a risk to national security because
  they can be easily disseminated or transmitted from person to person; can

cause high mortality and have major public health impact; might cause public panic and social disruption; and require special action for public health preparedness.

- *Category B* (second highest priority) agents are moderately easy to disseminate; cause moderate morbidity and low mortality; and require specific enhancements of diagnostic capacity and disease surveillance.
- *Category C* (third highest priority) agents include emerging pathogens that could be engineered for mass dissemination because of availability, ease of production and dissemination, and possible high morbidity and mortality and major health impact.

In 1999, the General Accounting Office, the investigative arm of Congress, analyzed the likelihood of a bioterrorist attack by several bacterial and viral agents (Table 9-3). (This table does not include botulinum toxin, one of the CDC Category A agents.)

The remainder of this chapter deals with the six CDC Category A agents: three bacteria (that cause anthrax, plague, and tularemia); a bacterial toxin (that causes botulism); and viruses that cause smallpox and the viral hemorrhagic fevers. Category B and Category C agents and the diseases that they cause are described in many sources, including the CDC Web site on bioterrorism (www .bt.cdc.gov [accessed June 9, 2007]); and Heymann DL (ed.), *Control of Communicable Diseases Manual,* 18th ed. (Washington, DC: American Public Health Association, 2004).

Anthrax

Anthrax is a highly virulent infectious disease of animals that can affect humans. It is not transmitted from person to person. The type of infection in humans is determined by the route of exposure. In the cutaneous form, anthrax spores or bacteria enter the body through breaks in the skin, causing itching, boils, and formation of a black scab, which can mimic a spider bite. Severe skin infections can lead to sepsis and microangiopathic hemolytic anemia. In the rare gastrointestinal form, eating infected meat or drinking water contaminated with anthrax spores or bacteria can result in nausea, vomiting, and diarrhea. In the most serious form, inhalational anthrax, symptoms include fever, chest pain, and difficulty breathing due to hemorrhagic mediastinitis, which is often fatal. Symptoms usually start within 2 to 7 days but may begin several weeks after exposure. Standard universal precautions should be used in the care of patients infected with anthrax; special isolation precautions are not required. All forms of the disease must be treated promptly with antibiotics.[21]

Preventive measures are indicated if an exposure has occurred. Spores can be washed off with soap and water. If contaminated, clothes should be changed.

Table 9-3. Characteristics of Selected Potential Bioterrorist Weapons

Agent	Ease of Manufacture	Stability	Lethal Effects	Likelihood of an Attack
Diseases Caused by Bacteria				
Anthrax	Virulent stock is hard to obtain and process	Spores are very stable; resistant to sunlight, heat, and some disinfectants	Very high for pulmonary anthrax	Possible, but requires sophistication to manufacture and disseminate.
Plague	Very difficult to acquire seed stock and to process	Can be long-lasting, but heat, disinfectants, and sunlight render it harmless	Very high	Possible, but not likely, because it is difficult to acquire suitable strain and to weaponize and disseminate it.
Glanders	Difficult to acquire seed stock; moderately difficult to process	Very stable	Moderate to high	Potential, but it is difficult to acquire, produce, and disseminate it.
Tularemia	Difficult to acquire correct strain; moderately difficult to process	Generally unstable in the environment; resists cold; killed by mild heat and disinfectants	Moderate if untreated; low if treated	Possible, but it is difficult to stabilize.
Brucellosis	Difficult to acquire seed stock; moderately difficult to process	Very stable; long persistence in wet soil or food	Very low	Not likely because of difficulty of getting stock, long incubation period, and low lethality.
Q Fever	Difficult to acquire seed stock; moderately difficult to process and weaponize	Stable; persists for months on wood and in sand.	Very low if treated	Not likely because of low lethality.

(continued)

Table 9-3. (*continued*)

Agent	Ease of Manufacture	Stability	Lethal Effects	Likelihood of an Attack
Diseases Caused by Viruses				
Hemorrhagic Fevers (Ebola and Marburg)	Very difficult to obtain and process; unsafe to handle	Relatively unstable	Depending on strain, can be very high	Unlikely because of difficulty of acquiring pathogen, safety considerations, and relative instability.
Smallpox	Difficult to obtain stock and to process; only confirmed sources are in the U.S. and Russia	Very stable	Moderate to high	Questionable because of limited availability, but consequences of an attack are deemed especially serious.

Source: General Accounting Office. Risk Assessments: The Biological Threat. As reported in the New York Times, November 1, 2001, p. B7.

Antibiotics should be given to everyone exposed. In the United States in the fall of 2001, fears of anthrax exposure fed demand for antibiotic prophylaxis, which was partially balanced by physicians' limiting unnecessary prescriptions for antibiotics in order to help prevent the development of antibiotic resistance. In such situations, physicians should counsel patients against overreacting and prescribe medications on the basis of sound clinical judgment. This is especially true because many hoaxes of anthrax dissemination have occurred since then.[22]

The anthrax vaccine is of uncertain efficacy against inhalation anthrax. Anthrax vaccine was developed during the 1950s, reformulated in the 1960s, and approved by the U.S. Food and Drug Administration (FDA) for general use in 1970. The Advisory Committee on Immunization Practices (ACIP) has recommended anthrax vaccination for groups that include the following[23]:

- People who work directly with the organism in the laboratory
- People who work with imported animal hides or furs in areas where standards are insufficient to prevent exposure to anthrax spores
- Military personnel deployed to areas with high risk for exposure to the organism
- People who handle potentially infected animal products in high-incidence areas (such as veterinarians who travel outside the United States to work in areas where the incidence is high).

Further complicating the question of efficacy is the possibility that new strains of anthrax may have been developed specifically to make the current vaccine ineffective.[24–27] Despite warnings by concerned groups,[28] the U.S. Department of Defense began an extensive immunization program in 1997.[29,30] Some military personnel, worried about adverse reactions to the vaccine, refused to be immunized and faced severe punishment.[31] The FDA inspected the sole facility producing the vaccine, found numerous deficiencies in the production process, and suspended immunizations for several years.[32–34] Production was resumed, and U.S. military personnel are again receiving mandated immunizations. In 2002, the Institute of Medicine reported that the current anthrax vaccine, although "far from optimal," is safe and likely to be effective. A number of analysts question the safety and efficacy of the current vaccine and its mandatory use for some U.S. soldiers.[35,35a]

Plague

Plague is caused by the bacterium, *Yersinia pestis,* which is found in rodents and fleas that infest rodents. Pneumonic plague, which occurs when *Y. pestis* infects the lungs, can spread from person to person via organisms suspended in respiratory droplets, but this usually requires close contact with the infected person. Used as a biological weapon, *Y. pestis* bacteria could be transmitted in an aerosolized form. Initial symptoms include fever, headache, weakness, shortness of breath, chest pain, cough, and sometimes bloody or watery sputum. Pneumonia may lead to respiratory failure, shock, and death. Antibiotics should be administered promptly.[23]

Bubonic plague, the most common form of this disease, occurs when an infected flea bites a person or when contaminated materials enter through a break in the skin. Symptoms include swollen, tender lymph nodes (buboes), fever, headache, chills, and weakness. This form of the disease is not transmitted from person to person.

Septicemic plague occurs when plague bacteria multiply in the blood—usually as a complication of another form of the disease. It too is not transmitted from person to person.[23]

Tularemia

Tularemia is caused by the highly infectious bacterium, *Francisella tularensis. F. tularensis* can enter the body via the skin, mucous membranes, gastrointestinal tract, or lungs. People can become infected by bites of infected arthropods; handling of infectious animal tissues or fluids; direct contact with or ingestion of contaminated food, water, or soil; and inhalation of infective aerosols. There is no person-to-person transmission. The case-fatality rate in the United States is about 1 percent. *F. tularensis* could be used as a biological weapon, most likely by aerosol release.[23] Symptoms include fever, headache, chills and rigors, generalized body aches, runny nose, sore throat, cough, shortness of breath, pleuritic pain, sputum production, nausea, vomiting, diarrhea, excessive sweating, progressive weakness, loss of appetite, weight loss, and skin ulcers. A vaccine against tularemia was used in the past to protect laboratory workers, but it is not currently available.[23]

Botulism

Botulinum toxin causes botulism. Botulism is caused by the potent neurotoxin produced by the bacterium, *Clostridium botulinum.* In the United States, an average of 110 cases are reported annually, about 72 percent of which are infant botulism (caused by spores germinating and producing toxin in the gastrointestinal tract) and about 25 percent are foodborne botulism. Foodborne botulism, usually caused by eating contaminated home-canned foods, is considered a public health emergency because there may be contaminated food remaining that could cause botulism in others.[23] Some additional cases are wound botulism (caused by spores germinating in wounds, including those of injection drug users).

Clinically, botulism is characterized by symmetric, descending flaccid paralysis of motor and autonomic nerves, most often starting with the cranial nerves. Symptoms include double vision, blurred vision, drooping eyelids, slurred speech, difficulty swallowing, dry mouth, and muscle weakness. Without treatment, botulism can cause descending paralysis of respiratory muscles and muscles of the arms and legs. Botulinum antitoxin, supplied by the CDC, can, if administered early, prevent progression of the disease and shorten symptoms in severe cases. About 5 percent of those affected die, often from respiratory failure. Survivors may suffer from fatigue and shortness of breath for many years afterward.[23]

Smallpox

Smallpox is a highly contagious and deadly viral disease in which human-to-human transmission occurs.[23,36,37] An extraordinary international effort eradicated the disease; it was last diagnosed in humans in 1981. The only remaining stockpiles of smallpox virus are being safeguarded by the United States and Russia until they are destroyed—a goal that has now been put on hold.[38,39] Allegations of weaponization of smallpox virus by Russia and possibly other countries have raised concerns that it might be used as a biological weapon, with potentially devastating consequences because vaccination programs have ceased.

Smallpox virus can be transmitted by inhalation, through mucous membrane contact with the fluid from the associated rash, and from touch contact with the clothing, bedding, or scabs of an affected person. The maculopapular rash of smallpox erupts quickly, rather than in stages as in chickenpox. It starts as small red macules, which become 2- to 3-mm papules within 1 to 2 days, then become 2- to 5-mm vesicles 1 to 2 days later. The rash starts in the mouth and throat, then occurs on the face and extremities, and then spreads to the rest of the body. Next, 4- to 6-mm pustules develop, remain present for 5 to 8 days, and are followed by crusting (Figure 9-1). All smallpox skin lesions are usually at the same stage of development. The following have been frequently confused with smallpox: drug eruptions, secondary syphilis, chickenpox, acne, insect bites, monkeypox, and generalized vaccinia and eczema vaccinatum. Symptoms usually start between 10 and 12 days after exposure, but they can begin as early as 7 days or as late as 17 days after exposure. High fever (often more than 40°C) occurs between 1 to 2 weeks after infection and is often accompanied by malaise, prostration, headache, and backache; abdominal pain and delirium may also develop.[40]

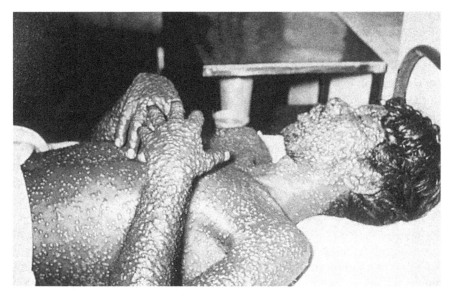

Figure 9-1. Adult male with smallpox lesions. (Public Health Image Library/Centers for Disease Control and Prevention).

Usually, smallpox is transmitted from person to person within families and among close contacts. The infected person is most contagious during the week after the rash appears. One person or a small number of people infected with smallpox would likely be cared for at home, with close contacts identified and quarantined. After infection with smallpox, antibiotics for secondary infections and supportive therapy are indicated. No antiviral agents have been effective against the disease, but smallpox vaccine can be given within 4 days after exposure to lessen the severity of or prevent illness.[40]

If smallpox virus were to be used as a biological weapon, hospitals would have to isolate entire wards and revaccinate hospital employees who previously had received vaccinations. Respiratory isolation (negative pressure ventilation) and contact precautions (using gloves, gowns, and masks) are necessary. Strict standard precautions must be followed in handling linen and clothing.

In late 2002, President George W. Bush announced a smallpox vaccination campaign to focus on vaccinating 500,000 military personnel, 500,000 health workers, and as many as 10 million emergency responders. Smallpox vaccination was implemented on a much smaller scale than planned and resulted in fewer than 40,000 health workers and emergency responders being vaccinated, with at least 145 serious adverse events and at least 3 deaths.[41] The diversion of resources for this campaign led to neglect of other urgent public health problems.[42]

Viral Hemorrhagic Fevers

Viral hemorrhagic fevers are divided into several categories, including those caused by filoviruses, such as Ebola and Marburg virus, and those caused by arenaviruses, such as Lassa virus. These viruses can be transmitted to people from reservoir hosts or vectors when their activities overlap. Viruses infecting reservoir rodents can be transmitted when people contact the rodents' urine, fecal matter, saliva, or other body excretions. Viruses associated with arthropod vectors are spread most often when the vector mosquito or tick bites a person, or when a person crushes a tick. Some vectors spread viruses to animals, with people becoming infected when they care for or slaughter these animals. Ebola, Marburg, Lassa, and other viruses can also spread person to person.[23]

Symptoms and signs include high fever, fatigue, dizziness, muscle aches, loss of strength, and exhaustion. In severe cases, there is bleeding under the skin, in internal organs, or from body orifices. Severe illness may lead to shock, nervous system malfunction, coma, delirium, and seizures.[23] There is no established cure. There are no protective vaccines available, except against yellow fever.[23]

Conclusion

Biological weapons have been used relatively infrequently in war, but they nevertheless represent a potential threat. Many public health professionals believe that this threat has been exaggerated, given the difficulty of developing or accessing, as well as using, these agents in warfare. Nevertheless, it is important for public health professionals to have an awareness of these potential weapons and what can be done to control them and prevent their use.

Acknowledgment: Hillel W. Cohen and Robert M. Gould have made important contributions to some of the policy analyses in this chapter.

References

1. Harris R, Paxman J. A Higher Form of Killing: The Secret Story of Chemical and Biological Warfare. New York: Hill and Wang, 1982.
2. Williams P, Wallace D. Unit 731: The Japanese Army's Secret of Secrets. London: Hodder & Stoughton, 1989.
3. Wright S. Evolution of biological warfare policy: 1945–1990. In Wright S (ed.). Preventing a Biological Arms Race. Cambridge, MA: MIT Press, 1990, pp. 26–68.
4. Cole LA. Clouds of Secrecy: The Army's Germ Warfare Tests over Populated Areas. Totowa, NJ: Rowman & Littlefield, 1988.

5. Alibek K with Handelman S. Biohazard. New York: Random House, 1999.
6. Broad WJ, Miller J. Report provides new details of Soviet smallpox accident. New York Times, June 15, 2002, p. A1.
7. Miller J, Engelberg S, Broad W. Germs: Biological Weapons and America's Secret War. New York: Simon and Schuster, 2001.
8. Wright S, Ketcham S. The Problem of Interpreting the U.S. Biological Defense Research Program. In Wright S (ed.). Preventing a Biological Arms Race. Cambridge, MA: MIT Press, 1990, pp. 243–266.
9. Preston R. The bioweaponeers. The New Yorker, March 9, 1998, pp. 52–65.
10. Garrett L. Betrayal of Trust: The Global Collapse of Public Health. New York: Hyperion, 2000.
11. Meier O. Verification of the Biological Weapons Convention: What is needed? Medicine, Conflict and Survival 2002;18:175–193.
12. Guillemin J. Anthrax: The Investigation of a Deadly Outbreak. Berkeley: University of California Press, 1999.
13. Török, TJ, Tauxe RV, Wise RP, et al. A large community outbreak of salmonellosis caused by intentional contamination of restaurant salad bars. JAMA 1997;278:389–395.
14. Piller C, Yamamoto KR. The U.S. Biological Defense Research Program in the 1980s: A Critique. In Wright S (ed.). Preventing a Biological Arms Race. Cambridge, MA: MIT Press, 1990, pp. 133–168.
15. King J, Strauss H. The hazards of defensive biological warfare research. In Wright S (ed.). Preventing a Biological Arms Race. Cambridge, MA: MIT Press, 1990, pp. 120–132.
16. Piller C, Yamamoto KR. Gene Wars: Military Control over the New Genetic Technologies. New York: William Morrow, 1988.
17. Leitenberg M. Biological weapons in the twentieth century: A review and analysis. Crit Rev Microbiol 2001;27:267–232.
18. DiGiovanni C Jr. Domestic terrorism with chemical or biological agents: Psychiatric aspects. Am J Psychiatry 1999;156:1500–1505.
19. Norwood AE, Holloway HC, Ursano RJ. Psychological effects of biological warfare. Mil Med 2001;166(Suppl 2):27–28.
20. Romano JA Jr, King JM. Psychological casualties resulting from chemical and biological weapons. Mil Med 2001;166(Suppl 2):21–22.
21. Swartz MN. Recognition and management of anthrax: An update. N Engl J Med 2001;345:1621–1626.
22. Cole LA. Anthrax hoaxes: Hot new hobby? Bull Atom Sci 1999;55:6–11.
23. Centers for Disease Control and Prevention. Anthrax: Vaccination. Available at: http://www.bt.cdc.gov (accessed June 9, 2007).
24. Stepanov AV, Marinin LI, Pomerantsev AP, Staritsin NA. Development of novel vaccines against anthrax in man. J Biotechnol 1996;44:155–160.
25. Wade N. Anthrax findings fuel worry on vaccine. New York Times, February 3, 1998, p. A6.
26. Broad WJ. Gene-engineered anthrax: Is it a weapon? New York Times, February 14, 1998.
27. Wade N. Tests with anthrax raise fears that American vaccine can be defeated. New York Times, March 26, 1998.
28. Sidel VW, Nass M, Ensign T. The anthrax dilemma. Med Global Survival 1998;5:97–104.

29. Graham B. Military chiefs back anthrax inoculations. Washington Post, October 2, 1996, p. A12.
30. Myers SL. U.S. armed forces to be vaccinated against anthrax. New York Times, December 16, 1997, pp. A1, A22.
31. American Public Health Association. Policy Statement Database: Anthrax Immunization (Policy Number 9930). Washington, DC: APHA, 1999. Available at http://www.apha.org/advocacy/policy/policysearch/default.htm?id=201 (accessed July 20, 2007).
32. Strong C. FDA cites 30 deficiencies in anthrax vaccine production. Associated Press, December 15, 1999.
33. Sciolino E. Shortage forces Pentagon to cut anthrax inoculations. New York Times, July 11, 2000, p. A14.
34. Sciolino E. Anthrax vaccination program is failing, Pentagon admits. New York Times, July 13, 2000.
35. Nass M. Anthrax vaccine not safe and effective. Emergency Medicine News 2002;24:44.
35a. Schumm WR, Webb FJ, Jurich AP, Bollman SR. Comments on the Institute of Medicine's 2002 report on the safety of anthrax vaccine. Psychological Reports 2002;91:187–191.
36. Tucker JB. Scourge: The Once and Future Threat of Smallpox. New York: Atlanta Monthly Press, 2001.
37. Henderson DA, Inglesby TV, Bartlett JG, et al. Smallpox as a biological weapon: Medical and public health management. JAMA 1999;281:2127–2137.
38. Miller J. U.S. set to retain smallpox stocks. New York Times, November 16, 2001.
39. W.H.O. delays end of smallpox virus. New York Times, May 19, 2002, p. A5.
40. Breman JG, Henderson DA. Diagnosis and management of smallpox. N Engl J Med 2002;346:1300–1308.
41. Centers for Disease Control and Prevention. Updated: Adverse events following civilian smallpox vaccination—United States, 2003. MMWR Morb Mortal Wkly Rep 2003;53:106–107.
42. Cohen HW, Gould RM, Sidel VW. The pitfalls of bioterrorism preparedness: The anthrax and smallpox experiences. Am J Public Health 2004;94:1667–1671.

10

Nuclear Weapons

Patrice M. Sutton and Robert M. Gould

> So long as any state has nuclear weapons, others will want them. So
> long as any such weapons remain, there is a risk that they will one day
> be used, by design or accident. And any such use would be cata-
> strophic.
> —Weapons of Mass Destruction Commission, June 2006.[1]

Nuclear weapons are the most destructive of all weapons. They were used
twice in World War II and have been detonated more than 2,000 times
in the course of their development. The acquisition, use, and possession of
nuclear weapons has had, for more than 60 years, profound impacts on
public health, military strategy, geopolitics, and the evolution of our global
society.

Nuclear weapons release vast quantities of energy suddenly by splitting the
nucleus of an atom (fission) and/or by fusing the nuclei of two atoms (fusion).
A nuclear explosion is fundamentally different from an explosion caused by a
conventional weapon. Nuclear weapons each have a potential explosive force
that is thousands or even millions of times greater than that of conventional
detonations, generate temperatures comparable to the interior of the sun
($27,000,000°F$), and release ionizing radiation into the environment.[2] Materials on the ground are transported up into a mushroom cloud, mix with
radioactive materials of the fireball, and return to Earth in minutes to weeks as
local fallout, and over longer periods as global fallout.[3]

Health Impacts of the Use of Nuclear Weapons

Hiroshima and Nagasaki, 1945

Nuclear weapons were used in warfare on August 6, 1945, when the U.S. military exploded a nuclear weapon over Hiroshima, Japan, and again 3 days later over Nagasaki (Figures 10-1 and 10-2). The use of these nuclear weapons caused approximately 210,000 deaths by the end of 1945.[4] These deaths were the result of exposure to heat, blast, and ionizing radiation (Table 10-1). As these forces acted synergistically, morbidity and mortality exceeded the sum of the effects caused by each of the these forces considered separately.[3] The instantaneous release of strong heat and light resulted in primary (flash) burns to directly exposed body parts and secondary burns from exposure to burning clothes or fires.[5]

The nuclear weapon used at Hiroshima had an explosive force equivalent to 15,000 tons of trinitrotoluene (TNT); the one used at Nagasaki, 21,000 tons of TNT.[4] People and objects in the path of the shock waves caused by the blast were crushed and/or blown far distances by high-velocity winds. The power of

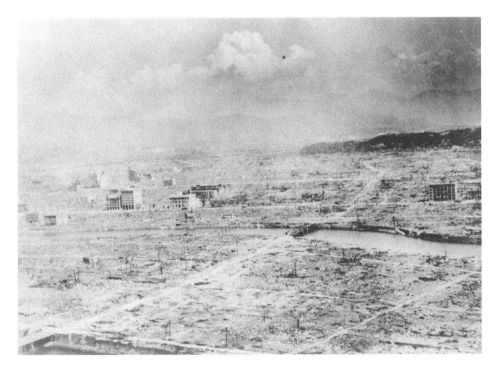

Figure 10-1.   General panoramic view of Hiroshima after atomic bomb was dropped on August 6, 1945. (Source: Library of Congress, Negative LC-USZ62-134192.)

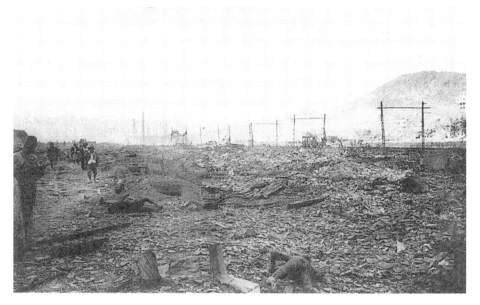

Figure 10-2. Nagasaki, August 10, 1945 (the day after the bombing), near the Matsuyan-Machi intersection close to the hypocenter. (Source: Photograph by Yosuke Yamahata; ©Shogo Yamahata.)

the explosion caused, first, primary injuries, such as ruptures of the abdominal wall and organs, and then secondary injuries, resulting from being pinned under and pressed by heavy objects and wounds caused by broken glass.[5]

Exposure to direct radiation from the explosions was intense. All victims within 1 km (0.62 miles) of the hypocenter died within 2 weeks.[5] The survivors had an increased incidence of malignancies, including leukemia, multiple myeloma, and cancers of the thyroid, breast, lung, colon, skin, and stomach.[4] Increased radiation dose was also associated with the development of cardiovascular and other nonmalignant diseases.[6] Among the 86,572 atomic bomb survivors with individual dose estimates, there were 440 solid cancer deaths and 250 noncancer deaths associated with exposure to radiation.[6a] Microcephaly with mental retardation was prevalent among children exposed in utero.[4] The use of nuclear weapons also had profound and persistent social and mental health impacts. Thousands of children were orphaned, and community life and social systems were devastated.

After World War II

The development of "hydrogen bombs" (thermonuclear weapons) after World War II exponentially increased the capacity of nuclear explosions to inflict

Table 10-1. Adverse Health Effects Associated with the Use of Nuclear Weapons

Burns	*Primary:* Flash burns to parts of the skin directly exposed to the heat rays. Flash burns result in severe keloids that begin to appear 1 to 5 months after the explosion. Infections and malnutrition complicate the healing of burns. *Secondary:* Scorch, contact, flame burns.
Wounds/Trauma	*Primary:* Injuries due to environmental pressure variations, hemorrhage, and rupture of abdominal and thoracic walls. *Secondary:* Injuries to individuals near the blast being blown far away, leading to instant or early death; injuries due to impact of penetrating and nonpenetrating flying objects on the body; burial, crushing, and fragments related to the destruction of dwellings and structures. In general, people are destroyed by the wind.
Acute radiation sickness	The three major forms in ascending order of severity are hematologic, gastrointestinal, and central nervous system-cardiovascular. *Dose level of 1–2 Sieverts (Sv)* = mild radiation sickness within a few hours, with vomiting, diarrhea, fatigue; reduction in resistance to infection; possible bone growth retardation in children. *Dose level >2 Sv* = virtually immediate nausea and vomiting with a loss of appetite and diarrhea in about a third of those exposed. *Dose level 2–4 Sv* = serious radiation sickness, bone marrow syndrome, hemorrhage; permanent sterility in women; death in several weeks as a result of bone marrow failure. *Dose level 4–12 Sv* = acute illness and early death; gastrointestinal syndrome produces progressive deterioration in days to weeks. *Dose level 10–50 Sv* = acute illness and death in days. *Dose level 20–150 Sv* = death in hours to days from neurological and cardiovascular breakdown.
Delayed effects of exposure to ionizing radiation	Cancer, chromosomal aberrations, birth defects (congenital malformations) and inheritable genetic damage, immunological disorders, sterility and impaired fertility, premature aging, and cataracts.
Infectious disease	Increased susceptibility to infection due to the direct effects of nuclear weapons and the subsequent hardships confronted.
Psychological/ stress-related disorders	Orphans, destruction of traditional society, devastation of community life and social systems, psychological effects.

harm (Figure 10-3). Whereas the bombs detonated at Hiroshima and Nagasaki were based on nuclear fission, thermonuclear weapons are based on nuclear fusion. Each has an explosive force of more than 1,000 Hiroshima bombs.

In 1962, the medical consequences of thermonuclear war—millions of deaths and no effective medical response—were described in a series of articles published in the *New England Journal of Medicine*.[7–9] During the Cold War era, U.S. government appraisals affirmed that a large-scale nuclear exchange was possible and that such a war would be "a calamity unprecedented in human history."[3] In 1986, the National Academy of Sciences projected tens

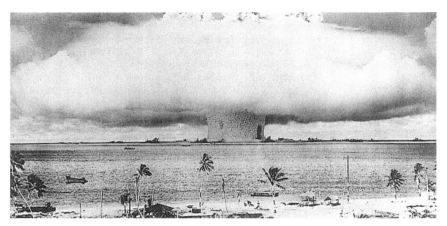

Figure 10-3. United States atomic-bomb test at Bikini atoll in the Pacific in 1946. (Source: Library of Congress, Negative LC-USZ62-66049.)

of millions deaths and severe injuries and illnesses occurring from a "limited" nuclear war—such as 1-megaton airbursts over the centers of the 100 largest U.S. urban areas.[10]

Although a deliberate, massive nuclear exchange between Russia and the United States is apparently no longer the daily danger that characterized life as recently as the early 1990s, the threat of nuclear war did not disappear with the collapse of the Soviet Union. The estimated magnitude of health consequences arising from the use of nuclear weapons under a variety of present-day scenarios are on the order of tens of thousands to millions of short-term fatalities (Table 10-2).[11–18] These scenarios include the following:

- The use of nuclear weapons against the Iranian nuclear facilities at Isfahan and the underground uranium enrichment plant at Natanz could cause at least 2.6 million immediate fatalities.[12,13] A nuclear attack on Iran could expose 10.5 million to more than 35 million people in the wider region to significant levels of ionizing radiation.[12,13]
- An attack on North Korea's nuclear facilities could result in more than 500,000 immediate deaths, 2 million other deaths and serious injuries, and extreme social and economic disruption in Japan and Korea as a result of people fleeing from the fallout plume.[12]
- Detonation by non-state actors of a 10- to 12.5-kiloton nuclear weapon in a large U.S. city could cause hundreds of thousands of immediate and delayed fatalities.[16,17]

Table 10-2. Estimated Magnitude of Casualties Related to the Detonation of Nuclear Weapons by States and Non-State Actors*

Projected Scenarios	Projected Magnitude of Casualties
Use by States	
Third World Urban Environment: Detonation of one 1-kiloton earth-penetrating "mininuke" in an urban environment	Tens of thousands of fatalities
Bombay (Mumbai): Detonation of one 15-kiloton or one 150–kiloton fission bomb	Between 160,000 to 866,000 deaths with a 15-kiloton explosion and between 736,000 and 8,660,000 deaths with a 150-kiloton weapon, depending on the population density in the part of the city that is targeted
North Korea (Yongbyon Nuclear Weapons and Power Facilities): Detonation of 1.2-megaton explosion using a B83 "Robust Nuclear Earth Penetrating Weapon"	More than 500,000 people killed immediately, with 2 million other serious injuries and deaths
Iran: Detonation of three B61-11 earth-penetrating nuclear weapons, each with a yield of 340 kilotons, OR detonation of a 1.2 megaton explosion using a B83 "Robust Nuclear Earth Penetrating Weapon" at Iranian nuclear facilities	An estimated 2.6 to 3 million fatalities within 48 hours; in the wider region, 10.5 to more than 35 million people would incur significant radiation exposure
India-Pakistan War: Detonation of twenty-five 15-kiloton warheads on Pakistani targets and nine 15-kiloton warheads on Indian targets	Millions of short-term fatalities; potentially greater numbers of deaths secondary to famine and disease epidemics resulting from the disruption of food production and distribution systems and destruction of water and sewage systems
Eight U.S. Cities: Launch of a single Russian submarine's missiles bearing nuclear weapons as a consequence of current U.S. and Russian reliance on a strategy of "launch on warning" of strategic missiles (that is, after a missile attack has been detected but before the missiles arrive)	More than 7 million deaths, with millions of other people exposed to potentially lethal doses of radiation in fallout
Use by Non-State Actors	
New York City or Washington, DC: Detonation of one 10- to 12.5-kiloton nuclear weapon by a terrorist	Approximately 230,000 to 250,000 prompt and delayed fatalities

*The results of the scenarios are highly dependent on the initial assumptions. Wind speed, direction, altitude, time of day, day of week, season, height of burst, population density, and assumptions concerning the health consequences of exposure to ionizing radiation are among the factors that influence the outcome of the detonation of a nuclear weapon. These estimates do not include the mental health, environmental, social, economic, and other consequences of the detonation of a nuclear weapon.

Other present-day scenarios include the following:

- The inadvertent launch of nuclear weapons that remain on high alert[11]
- The use of nuclear weapons in India[14] or Pakistan[15]
- The explosion of a 1-kiloton earth-penetrating "mininuke" in an urban population center.[18]

In all scenarios, the projected number of acute deaths underestimates the scope of the devastation. Deaths, injuries, and illnesses resulting from the environmental, social, and economic disruption that accompany the use of nuclear weapons defy calculation but are thought to equal or exceed the estimated combined impacts of blast, heat, and radiation.[3]

Health Impacts of the Acquisition and Possession of Nuclear Weapons

Testing of Nuclear Weapons

During the 60 years since the U.S. bombing of Hiroshima and Nagasaki, more than 2,000 nuclear weapons have been detonated in the atmosphere, in the oceans, in space, and underground as part of nuclear weapons testing programs. These programs have been conducted by the United States, by the former Soviet Union, and, to a much lesser degree, by the other nuclear weapons states

Table 10-3. Worldwide Nuclear Weapons Testing Involving Nuclear Explosions

	Atmospheric	Underground	Total
United States	215	815	1,030
Soviet Union	219	496	715
France	50	160	210
United Kingdom	21	24	45
China	23	22	45
India	0	4	4
Pakistan	0	2	2
North Korea	0	1	1
Total	**528**	**1,524**	**2,052**

Sources: National Resources Defense Council. Archive of Nuclear Data. Known Nuclear Tests Worldwide, 1945–1996, and 1975–2002 [India and Pakistan]; International Physicians for the Prevention of Nuclear War. Radioactive Heaven and Earth: The Health and Environmental Effects of Nuclear Weapons Testing In, On and Above the Earth. New York: Apex Press, 1991; Onishi N and Sanger DE. U.S. holds direct talks in North Korea. New York Times. June 21, 2007.

(Table 10-3). Between 1951 and 1965, U.S. atmospheric nuclear explosions at the Nevada Test Site alone released more than 12 billion curies of radioactive material into the atmosphere. Approximately half of the radioactive fallout from atmospheric testing returned to Earth near the test locations and in downwind areas within a few hundred kilometers of the test locations; the remainder of the fallout was distributed in a non-uniform manner across the world.[19]

Local populations downwind of atmospheric nuclear explosions received large doses of radiation from fallout.[19,20] Indigenous, colonized, and minority populations disproportionately incurred hazardous environmental impacts and detrimental social, economic, and cultural impacts of testing because their lands served as the main sites for testing of nuclear weapons by each of the declared nuclear powers.[21–24] The directly impacted population also included 210,000 U.S. military personnel who participated in 200 nuclear tests conducted after 1945 (Figure 10-4).[25] Additional unidentified populations living in areas where weather, topography, and other local conditions led to

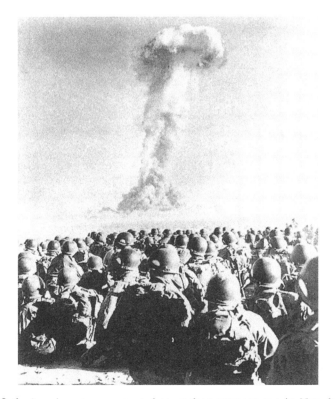

Figure 10-4. American troops exposed to nuclear weapons test in Nevada in 1951. (Source: Library of Congress, Negative LC-USZ62-47325.)

"hot spots" of fallout were likely to have received doses three to six orders of magnitude larger than average exposures.[19] Radioactive isotopes in fallout also concentrated in the food chain; for example, children drinking fresh milk from backyard cows and goats in the era of atmospheric testing were at high risk for exposure to radioactive iodine-131.[26]

The primary human health impacts of exposure to fallout are cancer and other delayed effects of exposure to ionizing radiation. Any exposure to ionizing radiation can be harmful, and the risks of developing cancer are proportional to the dose: the higher the exposure, the greater the risk.[27] Females exposed to ionizing radiation are at greater risk than males, and children are at greater risk than adults.[27] In addition to cancer, exposure to ionizing radiation can cause (1) somatic mutations that might lead to birth defects and ocular disorders and (2) heritable mutations that might increase disease risks in future generations.[28] (See Box 5-1 in Chapter 5.)

The National Cancer Institute estimates that 11,300 to 212,000 additional cases of thyroid cancer will ultimately occur among the U.S. population due to iodine-131 exposure from nuclear weapons testing.[26] It is estimated that the global dissemination of radioactive fallout will have produced 430,000 fatal cancers by the year 2000.[19] Because some portions of radioactive fallout are long-lived, human exposure will persist and related adverse health effects will continue to occur for thousands of years among future generations.

Beginning in 1963, nuclear explosions were conducted underground, which greatly reduced the quantity of radioactive fallout that entered the atmosphere in the short term and transferred the longer-term hazards to future generations. As a result, as of 1989, almost 14 million curies of radioactive materials had been deposited in more than 60 locations around the world.[19] Containment of these radionuclides for the tens of thousands of years during which they will release high levels of radiation is not assured.[19]

Production of Nuclear Weapons

Development of the U.S. nuclear weapons arsenal involved an expansive industrial complex of facilities that was owned by the government and operated by contractors. It employed more than 600,000 individuals and produced approximately 70,000 nuclear weapons over 45 years. At least 365 facilities participated in U.S. nuclear weapons activities as subcontractors, suppliers, or service providers, including scores of private companies used to process and transport huge volumes of highly radioactive material.

Uranium miners, primarily inhabitants of tribal and minority lands, incurred some of the most hazardous exposures in the production process. Workers in the nuclear weapons complex were exposed to radioactive and toxic materials, including heavy metals, silica, acids, organic solvents, and other occupational hazards.[29–31] Routine and sporadic operational releases of hazardous radioactive and toxic materials caused widespread contamination of surrounding communities and ecosystems.[32] By the mid-1990s, the radioactive and other hazardous waste products of the U.S. nuclear weapons complex had accumulated at more than 91 sites in 28 states and territories, with remediation complicated by thousands of areas contaminated with large quantities and exotic mixtures of hazardous and radioactive contaminants. U.S. government estimates of the legacy of radioactive and/or hazardous weapons waste is about 24 million cubic meters (6.3 billion gallons), containing 900 million curies.[33] The production of nuclear weapons also led to extensive contamination of soil (approximately 73 million cubic meters) and groundwater (1.5 billion cubic meters).[33] Contaminated surface and subsurface groundwater throughout the U.S. nuclear weapons complex is leaching, migrating, and moving offsite, posing a threat to major rivers and aquifers, which, in some cases, feed municipal water supplies.[34]

In 2000, the U.S. Department of Energy (DOE) estimated that the cost to remediate contaminated soil and groundwater, manage nuclear and hazardous wastes, stabilize nuclear materials, and decontaminate and decommission nuclear facilities throughout the nuclear weapons complex will be in the range of $200 to $250 billion. The National Academy of Sciences has stated: "At many sites, radiological and non-radiological hazardous wastes will remain, posing risks to humans and the environment for tens or even hundreds of thousands of years. . . . Complete elimination of unacceptable risks to humans and the environment will not be achieved, now or in the foreseeable future."[35]

In land that was part of the Soviet Union, widespread waste discharges have left even larger areas of contamination. As much radiation as 1.7 billion curies was poured into rivers and lakes or injected deep underground into rock formations.[36] Approximately 120 million curies of high-level waste remain in Lake Karachai, a 50-acre lake in the Chelyabinsk region of Siberia. A person standing at some points on the lake's shore would receive a fatal dose of radiation in a few hours. The dumping of radioactive liquids into rivers and reservoirs at the Siberian sites of plutonium production sites, Tomsk-7 on the Tom River and Krasnoyarsk-26 on the Yeni-sey River, has left these rivers contaminated for hundreds of miles downstream.[36] Workers in the Soviet nuclear weapons program were routinely exposed to excessive radiation, with consequent health risks.[37]

Threats to public health throughout the nuclear weapons complex were not widely recognized until the mid-1980s, when the safety of U.S. nuclear weapons–related reactors was scrutinized after the explosion and meltdown of the Chernobyl nuclear reactor in Ukraine in April 1986.[30] Numerous hearings, reports, and investigations by governmental agencies, the U.S. Congress, and the news media ensued, and many critical health and safety issues were identified. During the next two decades, there were an increasing number of reports of sick workers, communities, and ecosystems throughout the U.S. and Soviet Union nuclear weapons complexes (Box 10-1).[30–37]

Subsequently, two U.S. government programs were established to provide partial restitution to certain impacted populations.[38,39] The Radiation Exposure Compensation Program provides fixed payments, ranging from $50,000 to $100,000, to uranium miners, mill workers, ore transporters, onsite participants in atmospheric testing, and individuals living or working "downwind" of the Nevada Test site. Claimants must be diagnosed with specified cancers and chronic diseases that could have resulted from exposure to radiation released during above-ground nuclear weapons tests or in the course of uranium mining and processing. In 2001, the Energy Employees Occupational Illness Compensation Program extended recognition of the occupational health impacts of weapons production to other groups of exposed workers with radiation-induced cancers, beryllium diseases, or silicosis. Program benefits include a lump-sum payment of $50,000 to $150,000, medical expenses, and medical monitoring for workers diagnosed with beryllium sensitivity. However, these programs do not cover all impacted populations. For example, individuals exposed to iodine-131 in fallout in childhood during the 1950s would qualify for compensation and medical care if the Radiation Compensation Act program were extended to the public.[40]

The Role of Secrecy

Conducting what is an inherently dangerous industrial operation behind a wall of secrecy exacerbated the health impacts of building and maintaining nuclear weapons, a legacy that has been characterized as "... a kind of secret, low-intensity radioactive warfare ... waged against unsuspecting populations."[41]

Specifically, efforts to identify and prevent the adverse health effects from nuclear weapons development and production have been impeded by government policies, allegedly justified by national security considerations, that:

1. Gave the responsible parties a virtual monopoly on the collection and analysis of human and environmental exposure and health outcome data related to the nuclear weapons complex
2. Failed to initiate research adequate to establish the effect of exposures on public health and environmental health
3. Shielded nuclear weapons operations from independent federal and state regulation and oversight
4. Fostered a system where information relevant to public health was either not publicly available or available only in sanitized form in order to avoid adverse public reactions.[30]

Box 10-1 Human Health Effects of Weapons Production
Tim K. Takaro and Laurence J. Fuortes

An often hidden cost of war to the public is the price paid by workers who are injured or killed in weapons production. Throughout the ages, the most obvious hazard has been accidental discharge of explosives. However, more insidious hazards associated with chronic diseases may be more significant.

Whereas little is known of the impacts of nuclear weapons production in other states with nuclear weapons, mortality and morbidity in the former Soviet Union, the United Kingdom, and the United States has been substantial. Thousands of workers were exposed to chemical, physical, and radiological hazards during nuclear weapons development, testing, production, and clean-up, including many soldiers and sailors who were intentionally exposed (and monitored) during early atmospheric nuclear weapons tests.

In the United States, a program was begun in 1996 to screen U.S. Department of Energy (DOE) nuclear weapons workers and compensate those who became ill as a result of their work.[1] Each of the 12 largest DOE sites was found to have increased mortality for one or more radiation-related cancers when compared with the general population. (Radiation doses were even higher in the former Soviet facilities, although mortality and morbidity data are lacking.[2]) The program detected hundreds of cases of occupationally related illnesses. DOE has begun compensating victims of radiation-related cancer, as well as chronic lung disease induced by beryllium, asbestos, and silica. More than 70,000 claims have been filed, and costs of the program already exceed $1 billion.[3] During the first 5 years of the surveillance program, more than 11,600 examinations were performed on the more than 250,000 workers thought to have had significant exposures during their work for DOE. Among those examined, 72 percent had significant noise-induced hearing loss, 21 percent had evidence for asbestos-related or other lung disease, and 1.4 percent were found to have been sensitized to beryllium.[4]

Workers in the munitions industry are also likely to be exposed to various toxic substances, including energetic organonitrogen compounds, solvents, unstable metallic primers, depleted uranium (DU), beryllium-alloy tools, and radiation. Occupational exposure to trinitrotoluene (TNT) has been associated with dose-dependent discoloration and irritation of the skin, acute and chronic liver toxicity, low-grade anemia, aplastic anemia, DNA mutations, cataracts, and sperm abnormalities.[5–8] One study of munitions workers found a two-fold increase in sudden heart attacks associated with occupational nitrate exposure.[9] Another study found a four-fold increase in hepatobiliary cancers among workers exposed to nitrates in the munitions industry.[10]

Toxic metals are another hazard of the industry. Chronic beryllium disease, a cause of often-fatal pulmonary fibrosis, has been diagnosed in hundreds of nuclear weapons workers. Conventional munitions workers and military

(continued)

Box 10-1 (*continued*)

aircraft mechanics are also exposed to beryllium from the grinding and sanding of beryllium-alloy parts and tools. Because bushings, chisels, punches, screwdrivers, hammers, wrenches, and other tools made of beryllium alloys are generally softer than steel, they deform and may need periodic reshaping; sanders or grinders are used to reshape the tools, resulting in potential exposure to beryllium-containing dust. Plutonium-induced lung fibrosis has been reported in nuclear weapons workers.[11] DU, used in making armor-piercing weapons because of its density and exothermic properties, can expose workers via inhalation, ingestion, or contamination of wounds and can cause kidney damage. Because DU emits alpha particles that can be inhaled, there is also the potential for pulmonary fibrosis and lung cancer.

Thousands of other workers in private companies have also been involved in dangerous weapons production work,[12] and residents of communities around such facilities have been adversely affected as well.[13] As in the former Soviet republics, the full extent of past and existing health impacts from these and other, more clandestine biological and chemical weapons production is still unknown. Investigations have not yet begun for some populations.

References

1. Silver K, Wilson B. The Energy Employees Occupational Illness Compensation Program Act. Federal Facilities Environmental Journal 2005;16(3):89–104.
2. Shilnikova NS, Preston DL, Ron E, et al. Cancer mortality risk among workers at the Mayak nuclear complex. Radiat Res 2003;159:787–798.
3. Davis J. Energy Employees Occupational Illness Compensation Program. Health Physics 2004;86:210–211.
4. Available at: http://www.cdc.gov/niosh/sbw/osh_prof/takaro2.html (accessed June 28, 2007).
5. Hathaway JA. Trinitrotoluene: A review of reported dose-related effects providing documentation for a workplace standard. In Minutes of the Seventeenth Explosives Safety Seminar, Vol. 1. Denver, CO: September 14–16, 1976, pp. 693–705.
6. Ahlborg G Jr, Einistö P, Sorsa M. Mutagenic activity and metabolites in the urine of workers exposed to trinitrotoluene (TNT). Br J Indus Med 1988;45:353–358.
7. Harkonen H, Karki M, Lahti A, Savolainen H. Early equatorial cataracts in workers exposed to trinitrotoluene. Am J Ophthalmol 1983;95:807–810.
8. Liu HX, Qin WH, Wang GR, et al. Some altered concentrations of elements in semen of workers exposed to trinitrotoluene. Occup Environ Med 1995;52:842–845.
9. Stayner L, Dannenberg A, Thun M, et al. Cardiovascular mortality among munitions workers exposed to nitroglycerin and dinitrotoluene. Scand J Work Environ Health 1992;18:34–43.
10. Stayner L, Dannenberg A, Bloom T, Thun M. Excess hepatobiliary cancer mortality among munitions workers exposed to dinitrotoluene. J Occup Med 1993; 35:291–296.
11. Newman LS, Mroz MM, Ruttenber AJ. Lung fibrosis in plutonium workers. Radiat Res 2005;164:123–131.
12. U.S. Department of Energy Federal Register notice, January 17, 2001, pp. 4003–4009.
13. Clines FX. Disaster zone is urged after Soviet nuclear blast. New York Times, September 29, 1990, p. 7.

Secrecy permeated weapons operations and the conduct of radiation-related science. The U.S. government sponsored several thousand human radiation experiments between 1944 and 1974—many without informed consent, including secret intentional releases of radiation into the environment.[42]

Other Costs to Public Health: Resource Diversion

Between 1940 and 1996, the United States spent $5.5 trillion (in constant 1996 dollars) on nuclear weapons and related programs.[43] Nuclear weapons spending exceeded all other categories of government spending except for non-nuclear national defense and Social Security during this period.[43] Annual U.S. spending for DOE nuclear weapons activities during the Cold War (1948–1991) was, on average, $4.2 billion (in 2004 dollars).[44] Current and planned spending on comparable activities has steadily risen from a post–Cold War low of $3.4 billion in fiscal year (FY) 1995, to more than $6.9 billion in FY 2006.[44]

The allocation of vast resources for nuclear weapons activities continues. In 2004, an estimated 51,000 persons were employed at main laboratories, factories, and offices related to these activities in the United States.[45] In April 2006, the Bush administration unveiled the most sweeping realignment and modernization of the nation's massive system of laboratories and factories for nuclear bombs since the end of the Cold War. The U.S. plan is for a revitalized research, development, and production complex that can ensure a "responsive" nuclear weapons infrastructure. "Complex 2030" will have the capacity to design, develop, certify, and produce refurbished and new warheads in quantity and sustain underground nuclear-test readiness.[46]

International Control of Nuclear Weapons

Over the past 50 years, nuclear weapons have proliferated in both the vertical dimension (expanded arsenals of existing nuclear weapon states) and the horizontal dimension (acquisition of nuclear weapons by countries that did not possess them before). The early U.S. monopoly on nuclear weapons lasted only until 1949, when the Soviet Union acquired them. Until the 1960s, the United States maintained a vast superiority over the Soviet Union in nuclear weapons and delivery systems. During this period, development of nuclear weapons was influenced by a strategic doctrine that targeted highly populated cities. This doctrine came to be known as "mutually assured destruction."

Partial Test Ban Treaty

Initially, design and development of nuclear weapons relied on extensive atmospheric testing (see Table 10-3). The Partial Test Ban Treaty of

1963—which was developed, in part, as a response to health concerns about radioactive fallout from atmospheric testing—banned nuclear tests in the atmosphere, under water, and in outer space. Subsequently, proliferation of nuclear weapons accelerated with underground detonations, almost tripling the number of prior tests over the next three decades.

In the 1960s, with the Soviet Union achieving virtual nuclear weapons parity with the United States, the strategies of both nations shifted from targeting of cities to "counterforce"—targeting of strategic weapons. Counterforce strategies employed weapons with redundant warheads deployed through aircraft and land- and sea-based missile systems. This change, aimed at crippling an adversary's capacity to retaliate to a nuclear strike with devastating effects on the attacker, lowered the threshold for considering a "first-strike" use of nuclear weapons. As such, this transition may have heightened the potential for apocalyptic health consequences, given the number of targets located close to major population centers. Worldwide production of nuclear weapons also increased markedly, with the U.S. stockpile reaching an historic high of approximately 32,000 warheads in 1967.

Nuclear Nonproliferation Treaty

In 1968, international agreement to stem the proliferation of nuclear weapons was formalized in the Nuclear Nonproliferation Treaty (NPT). The NPT prohibits the acquisition of nuclear weapons by non-nuclear weapon states—in exchange for protection of the states that eschew acquisition by the nuclear weapon states and a commitment to nuclear and general disarmament by the nuclear weapon states. As of 2006, a total of 188 nations had agreed to the NPT. It was only four nations short of universal membership; Israel, India, and Pakistan have never agreed to it, and, in 2003, North Korea withdrew.

The NPT permits all nations to have full access to nuclear energy for peaceful purposes, with inspections conducted by the International Atomic Energy Agency (IAEA) to verify compliance with the Treaty's nonproliferation goals. The IAEA has thus been charged with the contradictory roles of discouraging active proliferation while encouraging "latent" proliferation—because nuclear power reactors account for a supply of raw materials and intellectual know-how that provides capability for producing nuclear weapons. Civilian nuclear power and nuclear research programs have been integrally involved with the nuclear weapons programs of South Africa, India, and North Korea and underlie current concerns about the potential acquisition of nuclear weapons by Iran.[47]

The NPT obligation of the nuclear weapons states to pursue nuclear and general disarmament is firmly established in international law (see Chapter 21). In 1996, the International Court of Justice, the judicial branch of the United

Nations and the highest court in the world on general questions of international law, ruled that (1) the threat or use of nuclear weapons is generally illegal, and (2) states have an obligation to pursue in good faith and to conclude negotiations on the elimination of nuclear weapons.[48]

Nuclear-Weapons-Free Zones

One demonstrated pathway toward nations' meeting their NPT nonproliferation obligations has included the establishment of regional nuclear-weapons-free zones (NWFZs). In general, NWFZs prohibit the manufacture, production, possession, testing, acquisition, receipt, and deployment of nuclear weapons within them.[49] Regional NWFZs have been established in Latin America and the Caribbean, the South Pacific, Southeast Asia, and Central Asia. A treaty establishing an NWFZ has been negotiated for Africa, but, as of early 2007, it had not yet entered into force.

Limitations on the Deployment of Strategic Nuclear Weapons

Beginning in the 1970s, the United States and the Soviet Union concluded a series of agreements aimed at setting limits on the deployment of strategic offensive weapons systems. These were known as the Strategic Arms Limitation Talks (SALT I and II); the Strategic Arms Reductions Treaties (START I and II); and the Strategic Offensive Reductions Treaty (SORT, or the Moscow Treaty). The United States and Russia agreed in the Moscow Treaty to reduce their strategic nuclear warheads such that the aggregate number of warheads would not exceed 1,700 to 2,200 for each country by the end of 2012. However, they may retain as many warheads as they desire, because nuclear weapons are not required to be destroyed—only taken out of operation, with launchers left intact.

Limitations on offensive deployments were negotiated in the context of signing the 1972 Anti-Ballistic Missile (ABM) Treaty. This treaty set limits on defensive systems recognized as being integral to enhancing offensive nuclear capabilities. In 2002, the United States withdrew from the ABM Treaty so that it could remove the legal barrier to its attempts to develop its National Missile Defense (NMD) program, which is potentially capable of enhancing both space-based and land-based offensive operations.

Comprehensive Test Ban Treaty

The achievement of control measures that move beyond limiting weapons deployment to undermining weapons development has proved elusive. After decades of concerted public pressure, a Comprehensive Nuclear Test Ban

Treaty (CTBT) banning nuclear explosions for either military or civilian purposes was signed in 1996. The CTBT has yet to be ratified by 10 of the 44 designated "nuclear-capable states" necessary for its entry into force, although a moratorium on the underground explosive testing of nuclear weapons has held. However, the United States and Russia are currently conducting nuclear tests by other means, such as by exploding weapons-grade plutonium and high explosives underground. Because these explosions do not involve a self-sustaining nuclear reaction they are called "subcritical."

Control of Fissile Material

The world's plutonium stockpile is currently estimated to be 1,855 metric tons—enough for more than 225,000 nuclear weapons.[50] In May 2006, the United States proposed the Fissile Material Cut-off Treaty to the 65-nation Conference on Disarmament, which would ban production of weapons-grade fissile material. However, the treaty contained no verification measures, and large stockpiles of fissile material held by current nuclear weapons states would not be affected.

Post–Cold War Proliferation of Nuclear Weapons

With the collapse of the Soviet Union in 1991, the United States reaffirmed the centrality of nuclear weapons as an integral component of "credible" U.S. offensive posture. U.S. "counterproliferation" policy sees nuclear weapons as tools to impede the proliferation of chemical, biological, and nuclear or radiological weapons.[51]

In 2001, the U.S. Nuclear Posture Review (NPR) asserted a military role for nuclear weapons far into the future—in stark conflict with the NPT obligation of the United States to work toward the elimination of nuclear weapons. Moreover, the 2002 National Security Strategy of the United States discounted most nonproliferation treaties in favor of a doctrine of "preemptive" war, including the possible use of nuclear weapons, against countries and organizations perceived to be hostile to the United States.[52]

Commensurate with these policies, the United States in the mid-1990s, under its Stockpile Stewardship Program, began advancing nuclear weapons research at DOE weapons facilities through computer simulation, enhanced laser technologies, subcritical testing, and other programs. The United States continues to modernize its nuclear warhead and delivery systems and the industrial capacity for designing, testing, and deploying strategic nuclear weapons.[53] In 2005, the United States proposed a new program for developing "reliable replacement warheads" which could ultimately cost billions of dollars and lead to the construction of thousands of new nuclear warheads.

Recommended Future Restrictions on Nuclear Weapons

Today, nine nations possess approximately 27,000 nuclear weapons (Table 10-4), and nuclear materials and technologies are widely distributed throughout the world. Current nuclear weapons and related capabilities remain inextricably linked to catastrophic public health consequences (see Table 10-2). Preventive measures include strengthening disarmament and nonproliferation measures, phasing out nuclear power, and abolishing nuclear weapons.

Strengthening Disarmament and Nonproliferation Measures

The existence and proliferation of nuclear weapons continues to be fueled by the view of more than 50 years that nuclear weapons are strategically desirable and, if in "the right hands," can be safely possessed. However, national security strategies that rely on possession of nuclear weapons serve as a constant stimulus for other nations to acquire them.[54]

Table 10-4. Global Nuclear Weapons Stockpile

Country	Strategic Nuclear Warheads[*]	Total Nuclear Warheads[†]
Russia	~3,500	~16,000
United States	~5,235	~10,000
China	~20	~200
France	~288	~350
United Kingdom	~200	~200
Israel	N/A	~100
India	N/A	~70-110
Pakistan	N/A	50-110
North Korea	N/A	<10
Total	~10,000	~27,000

[*]The number of nuclear warheads deployed on ballistic missiles or bombers with a range greater than 5,500 km.
[†]The sum of deployed strategic warheads, tactical weapons, and weapons held in reserve.
N/A: not available.

Sources: Carnegie Endowment for International Peace. Worldwide nuclear stockpiles. Washington, DC, 2006; Norris RS, Kristensen HK, U.S. nuclear forces, 2006. Bull Atom Scientists 2006;62:68–71; Norris RS, Kristensen HK. Russian nuclear forces, 2006. Bull Atom Scientists 2006;62:64-67; Norris RS, Kristensen HK. Chinese nuclear forces, 2006. Bull Atom Scientists 2006;62:60–63; Bull Atomic Scientists. The Bulletin Online. Five minutes to midnight. Last modified January 15, 2007. http://www.thebulletin.org/minutes-to-midnight/nuclear.html (accessed July 4, 2007); Yardley J. North Korea to close reactor in exchange for raft of aid. New York Times. February 13, 2007.

Strong international support remains for the two basic ideas at the heart of the NPT: (1) that more fingers on more nuclear triggers makes the world more dangerous, and (2) that nonproliferation by the "have-nots" accompanying disarmament by the "haves" will lead to a safer world.[1] The Weapons of Mass Destruction (WMD) Commission, chaired by former IAEA Director General Hans Blix and including former U.S. Secretary of Defense William Perry, is the most recent international effort to propose a practical framework to achieve nuclear disarmament. In June 2006, the Commission concluded that "a nuclear disarmament treaty is achievable and can be reached through careful, sensible and practical measures."[1]

Many of the WMD Commission's recommendations flow from existing international controls. They include the following:[1]

- Measures to strengthen and enhance the effectiveness of the existing NPT commitments
- Expanding nuclear-weapons-free zones
- Ratifying the CTBT and entering it into force
- Effectively controlling all stocks of fissile material and ceasing production of fissile material for weapon purposes
- Taking U.S. and Russian nuclear weapons off "hair-trigger" alert
- Reducing strategic arms, including a legally binding commitment to irreversibly dismantle these weapons
- Having every nuclear weapons state commit to not deploy nuclear weapons on foreign soil
- Refraining from developing nuclear weapons with new military capabilities
- Eschewing new missions, systems, or doctrines that blur the distinction between nuclear and conventional weapons or lower the threshold for the use of nuclear weapons.

Phasing Out Nuclear Power

Although these recommendations would strengthen safeguards against weapons proliferation, the "latent" proliferation threats posed by the civilian nuclear power industry were not addressed in the WMD Commission report. There are 443 commercial nuclear reactors in 30 countries, providing an expanding source of nuclear materials and know-how useful for weapons programs. Although vigorous control measures to secure existing facilities and materials remain essential, truly effective primary prevention of nuclear proliferation requires phasing out of nuclear power. Although nuclear power has increasingly been promoted as a path for reducing global greenhouse-gas emissions while meeting the world's increasing energy requirements, recent studies have demonstrated that the weapons proliferation potential of nuclear power, coupled with the intractable problems of nuclear waste disposal, safety, and cost, make it a very risky and unsustainable option.[55]

Abolition of Nuclear Weapons

The final conclusion of the 2006 WMD Commission report regarding nuclear weapons was that "All states possessing nuclear weapons should commence planning for security without nuclear weapons [and] start preparing for the outlawing of nuclear weapons."[1] Nuclear abolition has been supported by numerous global military and political leaders, including the mayors of more than 1,400 cities in 120 countries and regions.

Advocacy for nuclear abolition was sparked at the dawn of the nuclear age and remains essential to preventing nuclear catastrophe. In 1944, on learning that there was no German bomb to deter, one Manhattan Project scientist, Sir Józef Rotblat, left the Project rather than contribute to the development of a weapon with such catastrophic potential. In doing so, he performed what has been described as "one of most principled acts of the 20th century."[56] In 1995, he received the Nobel Peace Prize, along with the Pugwash Conferences on Science and World Affairs for their efforts to eliminate nuclear weapons. In 2002, while advising an audience of physicians and public health professionals regarding the urgent need for abolition of nuclear weapons, Dr. Rotblat observed, "A colossal effort will be required, . . . the courage and the will to embark on this great task, to restore sanity in our policies, humanity in our actions, and a sense of belonging to the human race."[57]

Physicians, public health professionals, and students in the health sciences have a unique role to play in the abolition of nuclear weapons. Nuclear abolition has been endorsed by leading medical and public health organizations, including the American Medical Association, the American College of Physicians, the American Public Health Association, and the International Physicians for the Prevention of Nuclear War (IPPNW) and its U.S. affiliate, Physicians for Social Responsibility.

In 1985, IPPNW was awarded the Nobel Peace Prize in recognition of the essential role of health professionals in the spread of authoritative information to awaken public opinion as to the catastrophic consequences of atomic warfare. Today, IPPNW and its affiliates in 58 countries unite tens of thousands of health professionals and students in the still urgent goal of creating a more peaceful and secure world, freed from the threat of nuclear annihilation.

Proposal for a Nuclear Weapons Convention

In 1997, the United Nations General Assembly called for negotiations leading to the conclusion of a Nuclear Weapons Convention. IPPNW and other organizations drafted the Model Nuclear Weapons Convention (MNWC) as part of the international campaign to stimulate negotiations on an international treaty to abolish nuclear weapons. Costa Rica introduced the MNWC into the General Assembly, and the United Nations distributed it to all of its member states. The MNWC would prohibit the development, testing, production, stockpiling, transfer, use, and threat of use of nuclear weapons. Nations possessing nuclear weapons would be required to destroy their arsenals in phases over 15 years. The Convention would also prohibit the production of weapons-usable fissile material and require delivery vehicles to be destroyed or converted to make them not capable of delivering nuclear weapons. The Convention outlines a series of phases for the elimination of nuclear weapons: taking nuclear weapons off alert, removing weapons from deployment, removing nuclear warheads from their delivery vehicles, disabling the warheads, removing and disfiguring the "pits," and placing the fissile material under international control. In the initial phases, the United States and Russia are required to make the deepest cuts in their nuclear arsenals. The United Nations has not taken any further action on the MNWC, but IPPNW and other organizations are campaigning for its adoption.

References

1. Weapons of Mass Destruction Commission. Weapons of Terror: Freeing the World of Nuclear, Biological, and Chemical Arms. Final report. Stockholm, Sweden: WMD Commission, 2006.
2. Glasstone S, Dolan PJ. The Effects of Nuclear Weapons, 3rd ed. Washington, DC: U.S. Government Printing Office, 1977.
3. Office of Technology Assessment. The Effects of Nuclear War. Washington, DC: U.S. Government Printing Office, 1979.
4. Yokoro K, Kamada N. The public health effects of the use of nuclear weapons. In Levy BS, Sidel VW (eds.). War and Public Health (updated edition). Washington DC: American Public Health Association, 2000, pp. 65–83.
5. Kusano N. Atomic Bomb Injuries (revised edition). Tokyo: Tsukiji Shokan, 1995.
6. Yamada M, Wong FL, Fujiwara S, et al. Noncancer disease incidence in atomic bomb survivors, 1958–1998. Radiat Res 2004;161:622–632.
6a. Preston DL, Shimizu Y, Pierce DA, et al. Studies of mortality of atomic bomb survivors. Report 13: Solid cancer and noncancer disease mortality, 1950–1997. Radiat Res 2003;160:381–407.
7. Nathan DG, Geiger HJ, Sidel VW, Lown B. The medical consequences of thermonuclear war: Introduction. N Engl J Med 1962;266:1127.

8. Ervin FR, Glazier JB, Aronow S, et al. The medical consequences of thermonuclear war: I. Human and ecological effects in Massachusetts of an assumed nuclear attack on the United States. N Engl J Med 1962;266:1127–1136.

9. Sidel VW, Geiger HJ, Lown B. The medical consequences of thermonuclear war: II. The physician's role in the postattack period. N Engl J Med 1962;266:1137–1145.

10. Daugherty W, Levi B, von Hippel F. Casualties due to the blast, heat and radioactive fallout from various hypothetical nuclear attacks on the United States. In Solomon F, Marsten RQ (eds.). The Medical Implications of Nuclear War. Washington, DC: National Academy of Sciences, National Academy Press, 1986. Available at: http://books.nap.edu/openbook.php?record_id=940&page=207 (accessed June 9, 2007).

11. Forrow L, Blair B, Helfand I, et al. Accidental nuclear war: A post-cold war assessment. N Engl J Med 1998;338:1326–1331.

12. Wilk P, Stanlick S, Butcher M, et al. Projected Casualties among U.S. Military Personnel and Civilian Populations from the Use of Nuclear Weapons Against Hard and Deeply Buried Targets. Washington DC: Physicians for Social Responsibility, 2005.

13. Physicians for Social Responsibility. Medical Consequences of a Nuclear Attack on Iran. Washington, DC: Physicians for Social Responsibility, May 2006. Available at: http://www.psr.org/site/PageServer?pagename=security_main_iranfactsheet (accessed June 9, 2007).

14. Ramana MV. Bombing Bombay? Effects of nuclear weapons and a case study of a hypothetical explosion. (IPPNW Global Health Watch Report no. 3.) Cambridge, MA: International Physicians for the Prevention of Nuclear War, 1999.

15. Wilson N. Regional war in South Asia: Effects on surrounding countries. Med Global Survival 1999;6:24–27.

16. Helfand I, Forrow L, Tiwari J. Nuclear terrorism attack. BMJ 2002;324:356–359.

17. U.S. Homeland Security Council and U.S. Department of Homeland Security. National Planning Scenarios. Created for Use in National, Federal, State, and Local Homeland Security Planning Activities. Washington DC: April 2005. Available at: http://media.washingtonpost.com/wp-srv/nation/nationalsecurity/earlywarning/NationalPlanningScenariosApril2005.pdf (accessed July 4, 2007).

18. Sidel VW, Geiger HJ, Abrams HL, et al. The threat of low-yield earth-penetrating nuclear weapons to civilian populations: Nuclear "bunker busters" and their medical consequences. Cambridge, MA: International Physicians for the Prevention of Nuclear War, 2003.

19. International Physicians for the Prevention of Nuclear War, Inc., Institute for Energy and Environmental Research. Radioactive Heaven and Earth: The Health and Environmental Effects of Nuclear Weapons Testing In, On and Above the Earth. New York: Apex Press, 1991.

20. Simon SL, Bouville A. Radiation doses to local populations near nuclear weapons test sites worldwide. Health Phys 2002;82:706–725.

21. Makhijani A. A readiness to harm. In Makhijani A, Hu H, Yih K (eds.). Nuclear Wastelands: A Global Guide to Nuclear Weapons Production and Its Health and Environmental Effects, by a Special Commission of International Physicians for the Prevention of Nuclear War and the Institute for Energy and Environmental Research. Cambridge, MA: The MIT Press, 1995.

22. Guyer RL. Radioactivity and rights: Clashes at Bikini Atoll. Am J Pub Health 2001;91:1371–1376.

23. Bauer S, Gusev BI, Pivina LM, et al. Radiation exposure due to local fallout from Soviet atmospheric nuclear weapons testing in Kazakhstan: Solid cancer mortality in the Semipalatinsk historical cohort, 1960–1999. Radiat Res 2005;164:409–419.

24. Kawano N, Hirabayashi K, Matsuo M, et al. Human suffering effects of nuclear tests at Semipalatinsk, Kazakhstan: Established on the basis of questionnaire surveys. J Radiat Res (Tokyo) 2006;47(Suppl A):A209–A217.

25. Hansen D, Schriner C. Unanswered questions: The legacy of atomic veterans. Health Physics 2005;89:155–163.

26. Institute of Medicine. Exposure to the American people to Iodine-131 from Nevada Nuclear-Bomb Tests: Review of the National Cancer Institute Report and Public Health Implications. Washington, DC: National Academy Press, 1999.

27. National Academy of Sciences, National Research Council Committee to Assess Health Risks from Exposure to Low Levels of Ionizing Radiation. Health Risks from Exposure to Low Levels of Ionizing Radiation: BEIR VII, Phase 2. Washington, DC: National Academies Press, 2006.

28. Sowa M, Arthurs BJ, Estes BJ, Morgan WF. Effects of ionizing radiation on cellular structures, induced instability and carcinogenesis. EXS 2006;(96):293–301.

29. Sumner D, Hu H, Woodward A. Health hazards of nuclear weapons production. In Makhijani A, Hu H, Yih K (eds.). Nuclear Wastelands: A Global Guide to Nuclear Weapons Production and Its Health and Environmental Effects, by a Special Commission of International Physicians for the Prevention of Nuclear War and the Institute for Energy and Environmental Research. Cambridge, MA: The MIT Press, 1995, pp. 65–104.

30. Geiger HJ, Rush D, Michaels D. Dead Reckoning: A Critical Review of the Department of Energy's Epidemiologic Research. A report by the Physicians Task Force on the Health Risks of Nuclear Weapons Production. Washington, DC: Physicians for Social Responsibility, 1992.

31. Thomas S, Frank L. Special report: An investigation into illnesses around the nation's nuclear weapons sites. Tennessean, Beginning February 9, 1997. Available at: http://www.tennessean.com/special/oakridge/part1/frame.shtml (accessed July 4, 2007).

32. Makhijani A, Schwartz SI. Victims of the bomb. In Schwartz SI (ed.). Atomic Audit: The Costs and Consequences of U.S. Nuclear Weapons Since 1940. Washington, DC: Brookings Institution Press, 1998, pp. 395–431.

33. U.S. Department of Energy, Office of Environmental Management. Linking Legacies: Connecting the Cold War Nuclear Weapons Production Processes to Their Environmental Consequences. (DOE/EM-0319.) January 1997.

34. Radioactive Waste Management Associates. Danger Lurks Below: The Threat to Major Water Supplies from U.S. Department of Energy Nuclear Weapons Plants. Washington, DC: Alliance for Nuclear Accountability, April 2004. Available at: http://www.ananuclear.org/Issues/EnvironmentalCleanup/tabid/76/Default.aspx (accessed June 9, 2007).

35. Wald M. Nuclear sites may be toxic in perpetuity, report finds. New York Times, August 8, 2000.

36. U.S. Department of Energy, Office of Environmental Management. Closing the Circle on the Splitting of the Atom: The Environmental Legacy of Nuclear Weapons Production in the United States and What the Department of Energy Is Doing About It. Washington, DC: U.S. Department of Energy, January 1996.

37. Donnay A, Cherniack M, Makhijani A, Hopkins A. Russia and the Territories of the Former Soviet Union. In Makhijani A, Hu H, Yih K (eds.). Nuclear Wastelands. A

Global Guide to Nuclear Weapons Production and Its Health and Environmental Effects, by a Special Commission of International Physicians for the Prevention of Nuclear War and the Institute for Energy and Environmental Research. Cambridge, MA: The MIT Press, 1995, pp. 285–392.

38. U.S. Department of Justice. Radiation Exposure Compensation Program. Available at: http://www.usdoj.gov/civil/torts/const/reca/about.htm (accessed June 9, 2007).

39. U.S. Department of Labor. Energy Employees Occupational Illness Compensation Program. Available at: http://www.dol.gov/esa/regs/compliance/owcp/ca_eeoic.htm (accessed June 9, 2007).

40. Hoffman FO, Apostoaei AI, Thomas BA. A perspective on public concerns about exposure to fallout from the production and testing of nuclear weapons. Health Phys 2002;82:736–748.

41. Lown B. Foreword. In Makhijani A, Hu H, Yih K (eds.). Nuclear Wastelands: A Global Guide to Nuclear Weapons Production and Its Health and Environmental Effects, by a Special Commission of International Physicians for the Prevention of Nuclear War and the Institute for Energy and Environmental Research. Cambridge, MA: The MIT Press, 1995, p. xiii.

42. U.S. Department of Energy. Final Report of the Advisory Committee on Human Radiation Experiments. Washington, DC: U.S. Government Printing Office, 1995. Available at: http://www.hss.energy.gov/healthsafety/ohre/roadmap/achre/report.html (accessed July 4, 2007).

43. Schwartz SI (ed.). Atomic Audit: The Costs and Consequences of U.S. Nuclear Weapons Since 1940. Washington, DC: Brookings Institution Press, 1998, pp. 3–5.

44. Paine CE. Weaponeers of Waste: A Critical Look at the Bush Administration Energy Department's Nuclear Weapons Complex and the First Decade of Science-Based Stockpile Stewardship. Washington DC: Natural Resources Defense Council, April 2004, pp. 5–6,45. Available at: http://www.nrdc.org/nuclear/weaponeers/weaponeers.pdf (accessed June 9, 2007).

45. Los Alamos Study Group. Sites within the U.S. Nuclear Weapons Complex. Available at: http://www.lasg.org/sites-index.htm (accessed June 9, 2007).

46. National Nuclear Security Administration. Statement of Thomas P. D'Agostino, Deputy Administrator for Defense Programs, National Nuclear Security Administration, Before the House Armed Services Committee Subcommittee on Strategic Forces, April 5, 2006. Available at: http://www.nnsa.doe.gov/docs/congressional/2006/2006-04-05_HASC_Transformation_Hearing_Statement_(DAgostino).pdf (accessed June 9, 2007).

47. Hersh SM. The Iran plans: Would President Bush go to war to stop Tehran from getting the bomb? The New Yorker, April 17, 2006.

48. Burroughs J. The (Il)legality of Threat or Use of Nuclear Weapons: A Guide to the Historic Opinion of the International Court of Justice. Münster, Germany: International Association of Lawyers Against Nuclear Arms, 1997.

49. Burroughs J. The Legal Framework for Non-use and Elimination of Nuclear Weapons. Briefing paper for Greenpeace International. New York: Lawyers' Committee on Nuclear Policy, February 2006.

50. Albright D, Kramer K. Plutonium Watch: Tracking Plutonium Inventories. Washington DC: Institute for Science and International Security, June 2004. Available at: http://www.isis-online.org/global_stocks/plutonium_watch2004.html (accessed June 9, 2007).

51. Kristensen HM. Nuclear Futures: Proliferation of Weapons of Mass Destruction and US Nuclear Strategy. British American Security Information Council, March 1998.

Available at: http://www.basicint.org/pubs/Research/1998nuclearfutures(2).pdf (accessed June 9, 2007).

52. Bush GW. The National Security Strategy of the United States. September 2002. http://www.whitehouse.gov/nsc/nss.html (Accessed June 9, 2007).

53. Lichterman A, Cabasso J. War Is Peace, Arms Racing Is Disarmament: The Non-Proliferation Treaty and the U.S. Quest for Global Nuclear Dominance. Oakland, CA: Western States Legal Foundation, May 2005. Available at: http://wslfweb.org/docs/warispeace.pdf (accessed June 9, 2007).

54. El Baradei M. Rethinking Nuclear Safeguards. Washington Post, June 14, 2006, p. A23.

55. Smith B. Insurmountable Risks: The Dangers of Using Nuclear Power to Combat Global Climate Change. Tacoma Park, MD: Institute for Energy and Environmental Research Press, May 2006.

56. Watkins M. Tribute to Joseph Rotblat. Pugwash Online, September 5, 2005. Available at: http://www.pugwash.org/publication/obits/obit-rotblat-press-canada.htm (accessed June 9, 2007).

57. Rotblat J. The Nuclear Issue: Where Do We Go From Here? Keynote speech to the International Physicians for the Prevention of Nuclear War 15th World Congress, The Summit for Survival. Washington, DC, May 4, 2002.

IV

VULNERABLE POPULATIONS

11

The Impact of War on Children

Joanna Santa Barbara

The focus of this chapter is on children affected directly or indirectly by war. Children who live in war zones may be killed or injured physically or psychologically. They may be internally displaced by the violence or flee to another country. They may be forced or drawn into military service. Many other children are affected by war, including children of serving soldiers, children of war veterans, children of victims of warfare and genocide, children whose lives are affected by the amounts of public resources spent on the war system, and children whose lives are overshadowed by the arsenals of nuclear weapons that have the potential to destroy civilization.

Children are particularly vulnerable to the impacts of war in several ways. Children affected by war are likely to suffer multiple, cumulative adverse effects over many years or decades. They are dependent for their proper development on an intact family and attentive family members who can adequately address their physical and emotional needs. War may impair both the physical and emotional resources that parents can provide for their children. War completely deprives some children of parents and other caregivers. Orphaned children and children with absent, depressed, or highly stressed parents suffer in ways different from the ways adults suffer.

Children are more vulnerable to some of the physical risks in war, such as death from diarrheal illness due to contaminated water. Unprotected children in war are at particular risk of rape and abduction. Children who are abducted into, or who voluntarily join, militias are vulnerable to the destruction of their formerly socialized moral system. Child soldiers are especially vulnerable to developing dysfunctional attachments and adopting violent and exploitative behavior after armed conflict has ended.

Life Trajectory

Adverse impacts of war on children affect the quality of life for many more years in their life trajectory than would be true for older people. Consider a child who has lost a leg to a landmine explosion. Some societies keep disabled family members at home, depriving them of normal social relations and of education. The whole life of this child will be lived in the shadow of a war injury, because she or he is less likely to be employed and to marry. Consider also the lives of millions of children growing up in refugee camps—displaced by war, their opportunities in life are markedly distorted by political events. Many will never resume a normal life trajectory.

> She will never marry with this condition. My husband has died, my two sons have died. My hope is lost for myself and my daughter. She is always depressed. When she is home she just sits and does nothing. She has no friends any more as she is ashamed of going anywhere in public. What are we going to do?
> —Mother of 17-year-old Adela, who lost both of her legs in a landmine incident 2 years previously.[1]

Physical Impacts

Death

Methods are poor for collecting information on child deaths during war. Hundreds of thousands of children die from direct violence in war each year.[2] The primary causes of death among 15- to 29-year-olds worldwide are unintentional injuries and infectious diseases, followed closely by war and homicide.[3] Children are often deliberately killed in war. They may be a part of fighting forces or part of the civilian population affected by conflict, and they may be specifically targeted by fighting forces. Ethnic cleansing often targets children in order to wipe out the next generation.

Injury

Children may sustain serious injuries and or lifelong disabilities, losing limbs, vision, hearing, or other neurological functions. They suffer injuries from sexual assaults.

Children are more vulnerable than adults to some kinds of injury in war. Landmines kill and mutilate 8,000 to 10,000 children each year[4] (see Chapter 7). Compared with adult landmine victims, children have higher fatality rates and experience more serious physical damage and permanent disabilities from their injuries. A child who survives a landmine blast is likely to be seriously injured and permanently disabled. Avulsion of one or both feet or lower limbs, shrapnel fragmentation wounds to the pelvis and abdomen, and blinding in one or both eyes are common. Conductive deafness is almost inevitable.[5] Facial disfigurement may occur.[6]

Disability

Millions of children are disabled by war, many of whom have grossly inadequate access to rehabilitation services. In one sample of war-injured children nearly 40 percent remained permanently disabled.[7]

Illness

Healthy living conditions and access to health services deteriorate in war. Many more children succumb to illnesses from these causes than from the direct violence of war. Many children become malnourished and contract infectious diseases from overcrowding in camps for refugees and internally displaced persons. They may develop parasitic infestations from a variety of sources, waterborne diseases from poor water and sewage systems, and sexually transmitted infections from rape. Children are more vulnerable than adults to many of these circumstances, especially to death by dehydration from diarrheal illness.

Malnutrition and Growth Retardation

Malnutrition and starvation may result from disruption of agriculture, blocked trade of food supplies, displacement from home, and limited supplies in camps for refugees and internally displaced persons. The most vulnerable group of children are those younger than 5 years of age. Some children are already malnourished due to poverty, which may have contributed to the onset of war. For example, in Somalia during 1993 and Liberia in 1995, more than 50 percent of children in some regions suffered from moderate or severe malnutrition.[8] Starvation and malnutrition contribute substantially to the mortality of war-affected children, especially by increasing vulnerability to infectious illness. Long-term malnutrition and protein-energy undernutrition result in cognitive and social-emotional impairment, with little improvement on nutritional recovery.[9] Malnutrition of children, inadequate medical supplies and medication, and inadequate water treatment—all largely due to economic sanctions—contributed to the deaths of an estimated 350,000 to 500,000 children in Iraq[10] (see Chapter 15).

Destruction of Health Services

Health care services are sometimes deliberately targeted for destruction in war and typically become difficult or impossible to access. One of the most dangerous aspects of war for children is the disruption of rural immunization programs.

> By 1973, in Uganda, immunization coverage had reached an all-time high of 73 percent. After the fighting started in that country, coverage declined steadily until, by 1990, fewer than 10 percent of eligible children were being immunized with antituberculosis vaccine, and fewer than 5 percent against diphtheria, pertussis, and tetanus, measles, and poliomyelitis.[2]

Psychological Impact

The events of war expose children to experiences that cause acute terror or horror, prolonged fear, grief over loss, anger about their adverse experiences, and chronic frustration of their needs and wishes. The exposure of children to events of war has been studied with the use of the Child War Trauma Questionnaire and various modifications of this instrument.[11–13] Psychological symptoms in war-affected children have been researched using a variety of instruments, usually focusing on posttraumatic stress disorder (PTSD), anxiety, grief, and depression[14] (see Chapter 4). In addition, levels of a broader range of disorders have been examined, including attention-deficit hyperactivity disorder (ADHD) and aggressive behavior.[15]

Children experience varying degrees of fear and terror related to the direct violence of bombing, shelling, sniper fire, and landmines; exposure to dead, burned, or injured bodies; and the experience of their own injuries. They may live in states of prolonged anxiety with fear of further attack, concern about lost family members, and worry about finding enough food for themselves or siblings. Children in flight from a war zone, unprotected children, and those attached to militias may be especially subject to prolonged fear. Exposure to horrifying experiences, in which they perceive threats to life, may leave memories that cannot be assimilated and recur intrusively, interrupting their lives.

Children grieve losses of parents, siblings, peers, and community; of home, school, pets, and agricultural animals; and of a limb, eye, or unscarred face. Their grief may be prolonged as depression. They feel anger to possibly unknown perpetrators of their suffering or to a vividly remembered attacker or rapist. Those who are old enough are aware of the difference between earlier times and their hard, constrained life in a refugee camp or as head of an unparented family, and they feel sad, resentful, and frustrated about the circumstances of their lives.

Symptoms of anxiety, intrusive memories, depression, and anger may be fleeting or may last long after the events that caused them. Age, gender, severity of exposure, and cumulative exposure to multiple events are factors that determine mental health outcomes.[14] Many affected children suffer several or all of these debilitating states together.[16]

Children under the most trying circumstances may also find capacity for joy, determination to overcome the difficulties of their lives, and commitment to work on behalf of their people for a better life.

Symptoms of PTSD include recurrent intrusive memories or nightmares of the horrifying event, avoidance of reminders, and an attitude of vigilance for possible recurrence. Although some children manage to function well despite such symptoms, others may be seriously debilitated. Appearance of symptoms after exposure to extremely adverse events differs greatly in various populations, from 22 to 94 percent in one series of studies.[9] The prevalence of symptoms decreases after the adverse events cease but may persist in some young people for up to 12 years.[17] Children aged 5 to 11 years may be more vulnerable.[15,18] Preschoolers may not understand the full meaning of the experience and therefore have some protection, whereas schoolchildren understand the reality of threats while remaining extremely vulnerable to their impacts. Adolescents, who generally show somewhat fewer symptoms than younger children, may be able to summon various psychological coping mechanisms.

Anxiety symptoms, such as worrying and showing behaviors that parents and teachers describe as fearful, nervous, high-strung, and tense, are prominent in war-affected children. In a study of Palestinian children, parents and teachers of about half the survey population described these behaviors, as did about half of 12- to 18-year-olds.[15]

Depression, which affects many children who have suffered losses and deprivations in war, is characterized by feeling unhappy, crying more than usual, and failing to derive pleasure from usual activities. In the study of Palestinian children, about half of the children, in both the 6-to-11-years and 12-to-18-years age groups, had these symptoms.[15] In the same study, high rates of conduct disorder, which includes aggressive and rule-breaking behavior such as lying and stealing, were demonstrated in Palestinian children, especially in boys.

Abnormal attachment might also be considered among the psychological problems of war-affected children. This issue has been little studied. Children who lose their parents in war may be adopted into other families, in which they may be treated as equal to other siblings or as unwanted underlings. In the latter case, they will lack opportunity for development-enhancing attachment to adults. Even worse is the case of children abducted into militias. The only adults available for attachment are likely to be deficient in nurturant capacity, offering very poor models of adult behavior to these children.

Spiritual and Moral Impacts

Systems of meaning enable children to make sense of their place in the world, feel like worthwhile persons, possess a set of values to apply to their behavior, and have hope for the future. These systems may derive elements from religious teachings, but religion is only one of several sources for such constructs. Each of these systems may be disrupted by the experience of war.

The cruel events of war and the indifference or malice of others may cause children to feel meaningless as individuals. Previously protected by benign adults who are now absent or helpless, the child may experience terror and feel insignificant and worthless.

In order to resocialize children to become merciless fighters as child soldiers, their socialized values are broken down. For other children in desperate circumstances (such as children in refugee camps or street children), the only means of survival may be stealing, extortion, and prostitution. Such experiences may override previous values and may create a negative sense of self-worth. Children may perceive "the enemy" as less than "human," as adults do frequently. Children who have known no other way of life may lose hope for the future, especially in intractable conflicts. For example, in one survey, 25 percent of Palestinian youths indicated that they were "thinking of becoming a martyr"—sacrificing their lives for their people's cause.[19]

Social and Cultural Impacts

> I feel miserable. I can't play football with my friends anymore or help my mother bring up water from the well. Why has this happened to me? I am so disappointed with my life. I don't understand why this has happened.
>> —Ali, age 10 years, who lost one leg and severely injured the other and lost part of one hand as a result of a landmine explosion that occurred while he was collecting scrap metal 200 meters from his house. He dropped out of school because it was too difficult for him to get there and back.[1]

Children are highly dependent for their optimal development on relationships with their peers and members of their families and communities, as well as social institutions. In war, each of these relationships may be adversely affected or ended. Family members may die or leave. A village may be burned and its residents scattered. Children's education may cease because their schools have been destroyed, their families have had to flee, or they have been severely injured. Children who are displaced during war may not participate in various rituals, festive days, and folk songs and dances, depriving them of their culture and its meaning to them.

Resilience

Children are remarkably resilient. Even those who have been wounded and those who are physically or mentally ill, disabled, or malnourished have areas of good function. They continue to fetch water, help with the cooking, care for younger siblings, and, if they have access to a school, attend classes and do their homework. And, given the most limited opportunities, they are often able to play, laugh, and create. Their resilience in the face of great adversity is promoted by the presence of family and community.[9]

Resilience of moral values in the face of attempts to resocialize children to be child soldiers, as discussed in the next section, bears some relation to length of exposure to negative models. In Mozambique, for example, children who stayed less than 6 months in the militia camps displayed, after their liberation, aggressive behavior and distrust of adults, reactions that quickly subsided as the children came to define themselves as victims of PTSD. In contrast, the self-concepts of children who had remained in the camps for longer than 1 year became strongly intertwined with those of their captors. The use of violence as a principal means of exerting social control and influence over others continued. Some even joined another armed group in another country as mercenaries.[9]

Child Soldiers

During the past two decades, there has been serious erosion of the norm of excluding children from combat roles. There are probably more than 300,000 child soldiers worldwide participating in more than 40 percent of the world's armed organizations.[20] With the increased availability of small arms and light weapons (see Chapter 6), children are actively recruited or abducted by military groups and forced to fight in war—in contravention of international law. This is a deliberate strategy, not just resorted to when an army runs out of

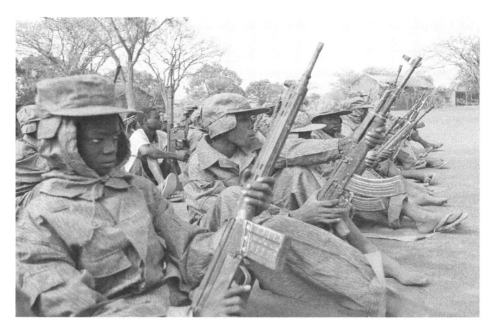

Figure 11-1. Child soldiers of the rebel Sudan People's Liberation Army (SPLA) wait for their commander at a demobilization ceremony at their barracks in Malou, southern Sudan, in February 2001. Under an agreement with the United Nations Children's Fund (UNICEF), the SPLA has demobilized 2,500 child soldiers between 8 and 18 years of age. (Source: Associated Press Photo/Sayyid Azim.)

adults. Children are available for abduction or persuasion, especially when orphaned or living as street children, or when aggregated in schools or camps for refugees or internally displaced persons. In some cases, children comprise the majority of soldiers in a militia (Figure 11-1).

Some children may join military groups voluntarily to avenge the death of a family member; others have very few options because of political, economic, and societal pressures or because of domestic abuse. Joining militia groups may provide children with the assurance that their basic needs will be met—which is often difficult in times of war.

Children are exposed to horrific acts of violence to desensitize them and make them more able to commit violent acts, during both war and its aftermath. Child soldiers also perform tasks such as hunting, spying, carrying and guarding goods, and relaying messages in addition to participating in violent combat. Girls may also cook, clean, and care for the sick, and they are often forced to provide sexual services.

They would eat and drink, then they would call for you. They were so many. It was so painful.... If you refused, they used sticks to whip you.... They all had sex with me.... A man would come, then another and another. I wasn't even the youngest. Some girls were even younger than me. Even the commanders called for you.... They said they'd kill you if you ran away.
>   —A girl abducted at the age of 13 by an armed
>   group in Burundi.[21]

Child soldiers may live dominated by fear of pain or death at the hands of their commanders if they transgress; they long to escape and sometimes succeed. Or they may assimilate to the group behavior and norms of the militia and enjoy the rewards of looting and killing. Some child soldiers are forced to use drugs and alcohol to disinhibit them and to blunt their fear of battle. Child soldiers are used as layers and clearers of landmines, shields for adult soldiers, suicide bombers, and participants in human waves of onslaught. They often commit atrocities, even against their own families and villages. They are unlikely to be aware of international laws constraining behavior in war.

The use of child soldiers greatly worsens life for noncombatant children in an area. They may be killed because of erroneous misidentification with child soldiers. They may lose access to education because of the risk of abduction from school and lose health services because of targeting of clinics.

At the end of a war, child soldiers may continue to be a dangerous group in the population. They may retain their arms and use them in criminal activities. They may join militias of neighboring countries. Efforts to help former child soldiers usually include the elements of disarmament, demobilization, rehabilitation, and reintegration into their home communities. Resources for such programs are generally sparse. Very few programs have been evaluated for effectiveness.

Former child soldiers need considerable physical care. They may have serious wounds or may suffer from loss of hearing, vision, or limbs. Rates of human immunodeficiency virus (HIV) and sexually transmitted infections are high. Many girls are pregnant. Drug addiction is a significant problem. Children's needs for psychological rehabilitation are especially great. Possibly a majority suffer from PTSD—97 percent in one study.[22]

Reintegration of these children into their former communities can be very difficult. Finding their families in the chaos of a war zone is the first problem. Families fear and reject children who have committed atrocities against their people. There is also the problem of orphaned ex-soldiers whose family members have been killed in the war.

"Night Commuters"

Among the many adverse impacts on noncombatant children in war zones involving child soldiers are the adaptations children must make to avoid abduction into militias. In the Gulu area in northern Uganda, thousands of "night commuter" children, who fear being abducted at night from their rural homes by marauders from the Lord's Resistance Army, trekked long distances to towns, where they slept in makeshift shelters in poor conditions, before returning at daybreak. With progress in the peace process in 2007, this has ended.

Torture

Torture is the deliberate infliction of pain or suffering in order to punish, induce submission, or extract information from the victim or a third person (see Chapter 14). Occasionally, children are tortured during war. Torture is also a way to inflict deliberate pain and suffering in the course of pursuit of other purposes, such as rape or arrest and imprisonment of children.[23]

> According to the United Nations Special Rapporteur on Torture, 7-month-old Muhammad Ardiansyah was reportedly suspended by his legs and left hanging in the sun for several hours in Aceh, Indonesia, in 1998. The Indonesian security forces reportedly wanted his mother to reveal the whereabouts of her husband, suspected of separatist activity. Both mother and child were later released.

Rape and Prostitution

Rape of children in war is especially destructive to their development. It may be associated with physical injuries. It may include torture. Family members may be forced to watch or participate. Psychological sequelae may occur, including profound shame and self-blame. Victims may be unable to access health care or other forms of assistance. Pregnancy and sexually transmitted infections may occur. Victims may be expelled from their families and may be considered not marriageable.

Wherever there are aggregations of military men and desperate poverty, prostitution increases, as girls resort to exchanging sex for having their and their families' survival needs met.

What Can Be Done

Listed below are 11 measures that can reduce or end the impact of war on children.

1. *End war.* Any degree of immersion in war will negatively impact children. Conflict between and within countries must be addressed by nonviolent means.

2. *Incorporate education for a "culture of peace" in assistance to war-affected children.* A country ending war by ceasefire has a 44 percent probability of re-entering a war during the next 5 years.[24] One measure to reduce this probability is peace education that is designed to prevent the polarization and dehumanization that are part of war and the lead-up to war. This education can increase awareness of human rights and nonviolent modes of addressing conflict.[2] Such education oriented to children can increase ethnic tolerance.[25]

3. *Implement international humanitarian law regarding protection of children in war.* International law addresses the protection and care of children affected by armed conflict, including the Geneva Conventions and their additional protocols (developed between 1949 and 1977); the Convention on the Rights of the Child (1989); and a series of United Nations Security Council resolutions.[26] The Machel Report of 1996 drew international attention to the suffering of children in war, delivered an agenda for action, and resulted in the appointment of a special representative of the United Nations Secretary-General to act on behalf of war-affected children.[2] Since 1999, there have been annual sessions on this issue in the Security Council, which has mandated the inclusion of child protection advisors in each United Nations peacekeeping mission.

These instruments deal with special protection of war-affected children with regard to food, clothing, medicine, education, and family reunion. In addition, they are intended to protect children from ethnic cleansing and recruitment into armed forces. However, compliance with these instruments is poor, especially on recruiting children to be soldiers.[26] The International Criminal Court and the ad hoc Criminal Tribunals for Yugoslavia and Rwanda cover child-related crimes in war.[26] It is not clear what actions they will take.

4. *Prevent the use of child soldiers.* Prevention of the use of child soldiers must begin with efforts to prevent war. There has been much emphasis on buttressing global ethical norms against the use of child soldiers. These are embodied in many documents, preeminently the Declaration on the Rights of the Child (1959). However, groups who use child soldiers are not characterized by adherence to high ethical standards; they repeatedly break promises to demobilize their child soldiers and to refrain from recruiting them. P. W. Singer, a senior fellow in foreign policy studies at The Brookings Institution, suggested that the focus should be more on disincentives to groups using child soldiers.[20] One form of disincentive would be the clear criminalization of leaders of such groups and assertive prosecution of them in war crimes tribunals and in the International Criminal Court. Another form of disincentive

would be curbs to trade in the commodities of the criminal economies often involved in conflicts engaging child soldiers.

5. *Ensure that general economic sanctions against a country are never used again.* Children and poor adults suffer most from economic sanctions. Use of economic sanctions should become a war crime, just as is laying siege to a city to starve its population.

6. *Ensure special consideration for children who are in flight from war zones and who live in camps for refugees and internally displaced persons, especially children who are unaccompanied by adults.* Special considerations need to be given for family reunion, systems of distribution of resources (to women rather than to men), internal layout of camps (to prevent attacks on girls), the provision of facilities for education and play, and special help for child-headed families.

7. *Institute measures to reduce sexual exploitation and gender-based violence against women and girls in war.* These measures include training of soldiers, including peacekeeping forces; inclusion of relevant interventions in humanitarian responses to population emergencies in war; reporting and support systems for victims of rape in camps for refuges and internally displaced persons; the prosecution of rape as a war crime; and making organized rape a crime against humanity.

8. *Facilitate humanitarian assistance to ensure that the health infrastructure of children's lives is not destroyed.* Perpetrators should be prosecuted for actions such as destroying clinics, schools, and hospitals—all of which are protected by international law. Where access to health services, such as immunization, is hindered by the violent conflict, there should be humanitarian ceasefires to enable access.[27]

9. *Include children's interests in peace agreements.* Since 1999, several peace agreements have specifically referred to children in the post-violent conflict arrangements for disarmament, demobilization, and reintegration.[26] Children have been recognized as both victims and perpetrators of violence in several truth-and-reconciliation commissions, but children have played little role in these systems.

10. *Extend healing and rehabilitation programs for war-affected children.* These programs should include physical healing, especially rehabilitation from disabilities, psychological healing, access to education, and access to the arts, play, and sports.

Important principles of such work include the following:

- Building on support systems in the community of the child
- Ensuring cultural sensitivity and the use of culturally appropriate meanings in assisting children
- Planning with much community participation

- Working with children in groups and settings that do not involve stigmatization
- Working not only at an expressive level, but also at a level of reconstructing meaning—helping the child deal with dysfunctional meanings emerging from adverse experiences (such as "What has happened is my fault.")
- Evaluating effectiveness of programs.

Special programs for child soldiers are necessary and should be aimed at reuniting them with members of their families and communities whenever possible.

Although many such programs have been instituted, little evaluation has been done. Two programs that have been evaluated have shown modest improvements.[25,28]

11. *Involve children in reconciling and reconstructing war-torn societies, and consider children's interests in restoring institutions.* Involvement may include reconstructing schools, establishing systems for child protection, and including children with disabilities. In Northern Ireland, for example, children have been involved in reconciliation of a war-divided society through schools and in community groups.[29]

References

1. Save the Children. Fragile Footsteps: Children and Landmines. 2003. Available at: http://www.savethechildren.org/publications/landmines.pdf (accessed June 12, 2007).
2. Machel G. The Impact of Armed Conflict on Children: Report of the Expert of the Secretary General of the United Nations. New York: United Nations, 1996. Available at: http://www.unicef.org/graca/a51-306_en.pdf (accessed June 12, 2007).
3. Blum RW, Nelson-Mmari K. The health of young people in a global context. J Adol Health 2004;35:402–418.
4. United Nations Children's Fund. Key Facts about Children and Landmines: Profile of UNICEF. Available at: http://www.maic.jmu.edu/journal/3.3/profiles/unicef.htm (accessed June 12, 2007).
5. Pearn J. Children and war. J Paediatr Child Health 2003;39:166.
6. Scheper E. On the Brink: Prevention of Violent Conflict and Protection of Children in Deeply Divided Societies. UNICEF Conference on Religious Women, Children and Armed Conflict at the University of Cordoba, 2002.
7. Terzic J, Mestrovic J, Dogas Z, Furlan D, Biocic M. Children war casualties during the 1991–1995 wars in Croatia, Bosnia and Herzegovina. Croat Med J 2001; 42: 156–60.
8. Djeddah C, Shah PM. Report of the Study on the Nutritional Impact of Armed Conflict on Children. Geneva: Food and Agriculture Organization, 1996.
9. Barenbaum J, Ruchkin V, Schwab-Stone M. The psychosocial aspects of children exposed to war: Practice and policy alternatives. J Child Psychol Psychiatr 2004; 45:41–62.

10. Lennon S. Sanctions, Genocide, and War Crimes. Paper presented to the International Law Association on Feb 29, 2000. Available at: http://www.zmag.org/CrisesCurEvts/Iraq/sanctions.htm (accessed June 12, 2007).

11. Macksoud M, Aber LJ. The war experiences and psychosocial development of children in Lebanon. Child Dev 1996;67:70–88.

12. Macksoud M. Assessing war trauma in children: A case study of Lebanese children. J Refugee Stud 1992;5:1–15.

13. Macksoud M. Helping children cope with the stresses of war: A manual for parents and teachers. New York: United Nations Children's Fund, 1993.

14. Meier E. Effects of trauma and war on children. Pediatr Nurs 2002;28:626–629.

15. Miller T. Health of Children in War Zones: Gaza Child Health Survey. Hamilton, Canada: McMaster University, 2000.

16. Thabet AAM, Abed T, Vostanis P. Comorbidity of PTSD and depression among refugee children during war conflict. J Child Psychol Psychiat 2004;45:533–542.

17. Kinzie JD, Sack W, Angell R, et al. A three-year follow up of Cambodian young people traumatized as children. J Am Acad Child Adolesc Psychiatry 1989;28:501–504.

18. Garbarino J, Kostelny K. The effects of political violence on Palestinian children's behavior problems: A risk accumulation model. Child Dev 1996;67:33–45.

19. Macintyre D. Children of the Revolution. Independent (UK), October 18, 2004. Available at: http://pamolson.org/ArtChildRev.htm (accessed June 12, 2007).

20. Singer PW. Children at War. Berkeley and Los Angeles: University of California Press, 2006.

21. Amnesty International. Burundi: Poverty, Isolation and Ill-treatment—Juvenile Justice in Burundi. London: Amnesty International, 2002. Available at: http://web.amnesty.org/library/Index/engAFR160112002?OpenDocument&of=COUNTRIES%5CBURUNDI (accessed June 12, 2007).

22. Derluyn I, Broekaert E, Schuyten G, De Temmerman E. Post-traumatic stress in former Ugandan child soldiers. Lancet 2004;363:861–863.

23. Amnesty International. Hidden scandal, secret shame: Torture and ill-treatment of children, 2000. Available at: http://web.amnesty.org/library/pdf/ACT400382000 ENGLISH/$FILE/ACT4003800.pdf (accessed April 28, 2006).

24. Collier P, Elliott VL, Hegre H, et al. Breaking the Conflict Trap: Civil War and Development Policy. A World Bank Policy Research Report. Washington, DC: World Bank and Oxford University Press, 2003.

25. Woodside D. Psychological trauma and social healing in Croatia. Med Conf Surviv 1999;15:355–367.

26. Harvey R. Children and Armed Conflict: A Guide to International Humanitarian and Human Rights Law. The Children and Armed Conflict Unit of the International Bureau for Children's Rights, 2003. Available at: http://www.essex.ac.uk/armedcon/story_id/000044.pdf (accessed June 12, 2007).

27. Peters MA. A Health-to-Peace Handbook: Ideas and Experiences of How Health Initiatives Can Work for Peace. Hamilton, Canada: McMaster University, 1996.

28. Dybdahl R. Children and mothers in war: An outcome study of a psychosocial intervention program. Child Development 2001; 72: 1214–1230.

29. Department of Education, Northern Ireland. Report of a Survey of Provision of Education for Mutual Understanding in Post-Primary School, 1999–2000. Available at: http://www2.deni.gov.uk/inspection_services/publications/EMUPPS.pdf (accessed April 2, 2006).

12

The Impact of War on Women

Mary-Wynne Ashford

The health effects of war spread far from the battlefield and endure long after the last shot is fired. Men and women, boys and girls suffer different injuries and die in different ways in war. Reports that are gender-blind miss the specific ways that women are targeted and the long-lasting impact of their injuries.

Population of Women Affected by War

Women in the following groups suffer gender-specific effects of war:

- Single and unaccompanied women
- Voluntary and involuntary combatants or support workers at the front
- Direct victims of an enemy attack
- Victims of sanctions
- Civilians living in a zone of conflict
- Captives
- Refugees and internally displaced persons
- Partners and families of returned combatants
- Widows
- Immediate and late victims of landmines
- Survivors in postconflict zones.

Although this chapter focuses on the adverse effects of war on women, women should not be characterized as helpless victims. Women's contributions to sustaining their families and communities are essential to the survival of society. Women in crisis situations rise to the challenges of reconstructing their communities, caring for children and injured people, and reestablishing social traditions that reduce tensions among groups of people. Furthermore, war may paradoxically affect some women positively, because the disruption of society may provide opportunities for them to assume new roles in their communities.[1]

More men than women are killed in battle, but battle deaths are only part of the story of war. Women's deaths that result from sanctions, the destruction of civil infrastructure, landmines, and suicide may be omitted in calculating the human cost of a war because they occur after the end of the conflict. Many injuries leave permanent physical and mental disabilities that render the victim dependent on others for survival. And many of these disabilities result from gender-based violence, such as rape and mutilation.

Factors That Make Women Vulnerable in War

Physical Factors

Because they generally are smaller and weaker than men, women must rely on social bonds, traditions, and risk avoidance to protect themselves against assault. These strategies are unreliable in wartime.

Systematic mass rape is used as a deliberate tool of ethnic cleansing and humiliation of the enemy. In addition, women are more susceptible to human immunodeficiency virus (HIV) infection than men. One young Eritrean soldier stated, "I have seen so many of my friends die at the front and I know that I might die. Why should I worry about a disease that would take years to kill me when I might die tomorrow?"[2]

According to the Joint United Nations Programme on HIV/AIDS (UNAIDS), rates of sexually transmitted infections among military populations during peacetime are generally 2 to 5 times higher than in civilian populations; during war, they can be 50 or more times higher.[3] In 1994, the prevalence of HIV infection among Rwandan soldiers was estimated to be 65 percent.[4]

Traditions of female genital mutilation contribute to the adverse sequelae of rape during war. Where women and girls have undergone extreme forms of genital mutilation, they may suffer extensive injuries if their genitalia are reopened by a sharp instrument or by the force of sexual penetration.[5] If these injuries lead to incontinence of urine or feces, the women may be abandoned by their families and excluded from their communities. Other forms of gender-based violence are forced pregnancy, forced miscarriage, sexual enslavement, and mutilation.

Pregnant women and those with small children are especially vulnerable because they cannot move quickly and quietly to escape the enemy. In areas of armed conflict, obstetrical care is poor; more spontaneous abortions and miscarriages occur; and maternal and infant mortality rates are high. In Bosnia and Iraq, physicians had to perform some cesarean sections without anesthesia.[6,7]

Cultural Factors

Inferior Social Status of Women

Women are vulnerable in societies where they do not have basic rights of autonomy, including the following rights:

- To own property
- To choose whom to marry
- To divorce
- To have access to family planning
- To refuse sexual intercourse
- To be protected against physical assault and mutilation
- To be equal before the law
- To vote and to be elected to office
- To have employment.

The absence of these rights makes women dependent on men for their security and support and leaves them vulnerable during wartime when the men are gone. In addition, where women have been restricted from educational opportunities and therefore are unable to read, write, or use numbers, their health and their opportunities to generate significant income are adversely affected. If women do not have the right to refuse sexual intercourse with their HIV-infected husbands, they are susceptible to acquiring infection with HIV. Women who do not have property rights may turn to prostitution in order to survive on their own and may thus contribute to the spread of HIV.

Women's Roles and Responsibilities

Women are the caregivers in most societies, with responsibilities not only for children but also for elderly, ill, and disabled people (Figure 12-1). Because of their responsibility for cooking, they are often responsible for collecting firewood. In war zones and refugee camps, this task is fraught with danger,

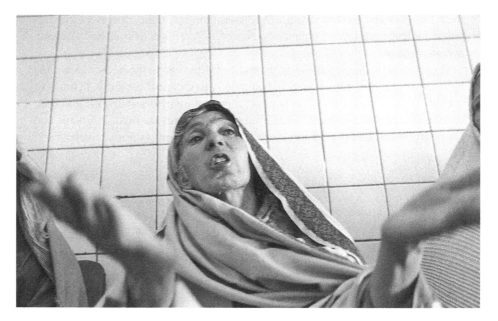

Figure 12-1. A 45-year-old woman who had two sons killed during war and a daughter injured by a bomb at their home cries during her therapy session at a mental health hospital in Kabul, Afghanistan. Due to the tragedies suffered by the women, many have developed mental health problems, including anxiety, depression, and other related disorders. (Source: Associated Press Photo/Silvia Izquierdo.)

because women must leave relative safety to walk long distances seeking wood. These are the times when they are most likely to be raped, injured, or killed by snipers.[7] Their responsibility for others reduces their mobility and forces them to make compromises to protect people who are even more vulnerable.

Exploitation of Women to Humiliate Male Enemies

In the genocides in Rwanda and in Darfur, male combatants were convinced that the best way to humiliate the enemy was to torture and rape enemy women. The belief that women are part of the legitimate booty of war is widespread. From ancient times, historians have recorded that victorious warriors returned home from battle with women captured as slaves.

Systematic rape in war is part of ethnic cleansing, because the forced impregnation of women dilutes the ethnic purity of the enemy, and "defiled" women are stigmatized and often cast out of their communities along with their offspring. As a result, they suffer the health consequences of deprivation and exclusion for many years after a war. Systematic rape in some countries has included the deliberate spreading of HIV/AIDS through rape.[3]

Mass rape in war has been documented in Bosnia, Cambodia, Liberia, Peru, Somalia, and Uganda. In Sierra Leone, 94 percent of displaced households surveyed reported incidents of sexual assault, including rape, torture, and sexual slavery. At least 250,000—and perhaps as many as 500,000—women were raped during the 1994 genocide in Rwanda.[8]

During World War II, 100,000 to 200,000 "comfort women" were captured by the Japanese and subjected to years of brutal sexual exploitation. Most of the women were Korean; others were Chinese, Filipina, Indonesian, Burmese, and Dutch. In army documents, women were described as war supplies. The goal appears to have been to provide the Japanese troops with many virgin women who would not transmit sexually transmitted infections. Fewer than 10 percent of comfort women survived to the end of the war:

> In some military outfits, the comfort women were ordered to commit suicide along with the Japanese soldiers. In other locations, they were killed in the caves or trenches or even locked in submarines to be sunk in a deep sea.[9]

Destruction of Civil Infrastructure

The targeting of water purification systems, electricity grids, sewage disposal plants, food distribution systems, hospitals, and communication lines amounts to war on public health.[7] This ruthless assault on basic survival needs for the population is especially devastating for women. In war zones, women continue to be responsible for procuring and preparing food and caring for their dependents. Faced with food and fuel shortages, lack of electricity, shortages of medicines, and lack of safe water, women face issues of survival daily.

Women in Refugee Camps

Women refugees are vulnerable to violence, rape and extortion in camps, where, often, warlords control food distribution and protection. In camps, women are also vulnerable if they become pregnant and deliver babies without trained birth attendants.

Female Combatants

Women may join armed forces during a war, or they may be captured and forced to join militias as combatants, cooks, or sex slaves. Although some women are forced to become combatants, others join armed forces voluntarily out of a sense of patriotism and a desire to take advantage of education and training opportunities they could otherwise not afford.

In recent years, more women in the U.S. armed forces have pressed charges of sexual harassment, rape, and assault against men in their units.[10] Many others do not press charges because they fear that they will not be believed, that the charges will not be taken seriously, and that they will suffer reprisals for making complaints. Official military policy provides "zero tolerance" for gender-based violence, but enforcement lags behind policy.

Examples of the Impact of War on Women

Prewar Period

Women suffer increased oppression in the period before war. Gendered social changes are sensitive indicators that provide early warning of impending armed conflict. They include[11]

- Propaganda emphasizing hypermasculinity
- Gender-specific unemployment
- Gender-specific refugee migrations
- Growth of fundamentalism
- Increase in households headed by single women
- Increased barriers to women's access to health and education
- Perception of women as property
- Violation of women's human rights
- Trafficking of women, the sex trade, and prostitution
- Increased incidence of domestic violence
- Increased sale of valuables.

Microlevel changes in women's daily lives warn of impending conflict. For example, in Sierra Leone as the war was brewing, women would rise very early and go to the market to get all their business done as quickly as possible; markets closed early because people were afraid. In Burundi, women would normally come down from the mountains in the morning; if they did not, people anticipated danger, because the men had probably sent them back for a reason.

War Period

Noeleen Heyzer, Executive Director of the United Nations Development Fund for Women (UNIFEM), visited women in desperate circumstances in war and postwar settings. (UNIFEM had an annual core budget of $45 million in 2004, compared to the annual budget in that year for the United Nations Children's Fund [UNICEF] of approximately $2 billion.) She visited the "Valley of Widows" in Colombia, where women had lost their husbands and their land to civil war and drug lords. She visited Bosnia, where women described abductions, rape camps, and forced impregnation. And she visited Rwanda, where women had been gang-raped and purposely infected with HIV. These stories were repeated in East Timor, the Democratic Republic of Congo, and Guatemala.

> Only the horror and pain were the same. Clearly the nature of war has changed. It is being fought in homes and communities—and on women's bodies—in a battle for resources and in the name of religion and ethnicity. Violence against women is used to break and humiliate women, men, families, communities, no matter which side they are on.[3]

A 2002 report documented the failure of the international community to protect women in conflict zones and to provide opportunities for women to participate meaningfully in prevention of armed conflict and in peace-building.[3] However, the report also provided positive examples of women taking charge of their communities after conflict, rebuilding and restoring hope, generally with few resources and little outside support[3]:

> Violence against women in conflict is one of history's great silences. We were completely unprepared for the searing magnitude of what we saw and heard in the conflict and post-conflict areas we visited. We knew the data . . . but knowing all this did not prepare us for the horrors women described. Wombs punctured with guns. Women raped and tortured in front of their husbands and children. Rifles forced into vaginas. Pregnant women beaten to induce miscarriages. Fetuses ripped from wombs. Women kidnapped, blindfolded and beaten on their way to work or school. We saw the scars, the pain and the humiliation. We heard accounts of gang rapes, rape camps and mutilation. Of murder and sexual slavery. We saw the scars of brutality so extreme that survival seemed for some a worse fate than death.

Soldiers have long regarded rape and pillage as privileges earned in battle. A U.S. Marine Corps drill instructor once said:

> This is the reality of war. We Marines like war. We like killing. We like raping females. This is what we do.[10]

Brigadier General Janis Karpinski, who was the highest-ranking official to lose a job because of the Abu Ghraib prison scandal, testified at the Commission of Inquiry for Crimes against Humanity Committed by the Bush Administration. She reported that a surgeon for the Coalition's joint task force had said in a briefing that several women in the U.S. armed forces in Iraq had died of dehydration in the extreme heat because they stopped drinking fluids in the late afternoon, despite temperatures up to 120°F. The women were afraid that if they needed to use the latrine in the night, they would be assaulted and raped. Karpinski alleged that on the death certificates the cause of death was altered to remove dehydration as a possible factor. These charges have been neither corroborated nor disproven. Kathy Gilberd, co-chair of the National Lawyers Guild's Military Law Task Force, stated that "people who report assaults still face command disbelief, illegal efforts to protect the assaulters, [and] informal harassment from assaulters, their friends or the command itself."[12]

Refugees

Women and children comprise almost three-fourths of refugees worldwide.[13] Women who have been forced to flee are usually separated from their husbands and often from their source of income and protection. Living conditions in camps are often inadequate. Gender-based violence poses risks of injury and disease.

Postwar Period

Violence against women does not stop with a ceasefire. Domestic violence increases in the aftermath of war, even in the countries that have been victorious.[14] The tolerance of brutality, torture, and killing that develops during a war is slow to change; weapons are widely available; unemployment and scarcity cause high levels of frustration; ex-combatants may be suffering psychological trauma including posttraumatic stress disorder; and women who have been sexually assaulted may not be easily reintegrated into their communities. The rule of law is not reestablished immediately after war, and gender-based violence continues with impunity.

Military families are at high risk for spousal abuse. In 2001, there were more than 18,000 incidents of spousal abuse reported to the Family Advocacy Program of the U.S. Department of Defense, 84 percent of which involved physical abuse. Between 1995 and 2001, there were 267 domestic-violence homicides in the military community.[15] A U.S. Army survey of 55,000 soldiers at 47 bases found that one third of families suffered some kind of domestic violence, from slapping to murder—twice the rate found in groups of civilians. The Pentagon has disclosed that, on average, one child or spouse dies each week at the hands of a relative in the U.S. military.[16]

Widows in many societies are unable to claim property after war because the property is transferred to male relatives of their husbands. A widow in such a situation may be plunged into poverty unless she has a son to defend her rights to land.[17]

During and after war, trafficking in women and children flourishes. From 1995 to 2000, human trafficking worldwide grew almost 50 percent.[18]

What Can Be Done to Limit or End the Vulnerability of Women Due to War?

Prevent War

The most effective way to end the vulnerability of women due to war would be to stop leaders from using armed violence to resolve conflicts. This may no longer be a utopian dream if trends reported in the 2005 Human Security Report continue[19]:

> Over the past dozen years, the global security climate has changed in dramatic, positive, but largely unheralded ways. Civil wars, genocides and international crises have all declined sharply. International wars, now only a small minority of conflicts, have been in steady decline for a much longer period, as have military coups and the average number of people killed per conflict per year.

Since 1986, when Ferdinand Marcos was toppled as president of the Philippines in a "velvet revolution," 60 dictators have been expelled and their governments replaced by fledgling democracies. The collapse of the Berlin Wall in 1989 led to the expulsion of communist dictators in Central and Eastern Europe. In South America, Chile and Argentina succeeded in ousting their military dictators, and recently the Rose Revolution in (Soviet) Georgia and the Orange Revolution in Ukraine brought democracy to those countries. All of these revolutions were nonviolent, except in Romania.

The 2005 Human Security Report did not disaggregate data to expose the effects of war on women. In addition, it did not address morbidity and mortality caused by sanctions, destruction of civil infrastructure, forced flight, torture, or indirect health effects of war, such as the spread of HIV infection. The authors attributed the changing security climate to the United Nations, the increasing influence of international law, and the upsurge of international activism by civil society.

Ensure Women's Human Rights

The more equal the society, the less likely it is to use military force.[20] The fertility rate, the percentage of women in the labor force, and the percentage of women in the national legislature can be used as indicators of the degree of gender equity. Fertility is a variable related to women's status, education, empowerment, and employment. Nations with high fertility rates are almost twice as likely to experience internal conflict as those with low fertility rates. Nations with 10 percent of women in the labor force are almost 30 times more likely to experience internal conflict than are nations with 40 percent women in the labor force.

> States (nations) characterized by gender discrimination and structural hierarchy are permeated with norms of violence that make internal conflict more likely.[21]

As women participate more in governance, a nation becomes more likely to resolve disputes without military violence. A nation that has twice the number of years of female suffrage as another is almost five times as likely to use nonviolent means to resolve conflict; in addition, a 5 percent decrease in the proportion of women in the national legislature correlates with an almost five times greater likelihood of the use of military force.[20]

Ratify and Implement Existing Agreements

The second most effective action to protect women would be to implement the legal instruments that address equal human rights for women, including the following:

- The Charter of the United Nations
- The Universal Declaration of Human Rights
- The Convention on the Elimination of All Forms of Discrimination Against Women
- The Covenant on Economic, Social and Cultural Rights
- The Covenant on Political and Civil Rights
- The Beijing Declaration and Platform for Action
- Security Council Resolution 1325.

The health of women depends on enforcement of national and international political decisions relating to equality and human rights.

Fast-track Implementation of U.N. Security Council Resolution 1325

In 2000, the Security Council of the United Nations unanimously adopted Resolution 1325, which commits nations to fully integrate women in all stages of conflict prevention, conflict resolution, and postconflict reconstruction and peace-building.[22] This far-reaching resolution, which has the power of international law, recognizes the strength and special expertise of women. It should result in greater influence of women on policy decisions and infusion of protection of women's rights into all decisions made by negotiating teams in peace talks. It should engage women in planning humanitarian aid and in rehabilitation of societies after war. The progress of implementing this resolution is slow, but some countries have come forward as "friends of 1325" and have committed to advancing its principles.

In 2000, the Department of Peace-Keeping Operations stated: "[W]omen's presence in peacekeeping missions improves access and support for local women; it makes male peacekeepers more reflective and responsible and it broadens the repertoire of skills and styles available within the missions, often with the effect of reducing conflict and confrontation."[3]

Address the Role of Women in *Responsibility to Protect*

Responsibility to Protect (R2P), a report of the International Commission on Intervention and State Sovereignty, calls for international intervention if a nation is unwilling or unable to protect all of its citizens. Various nonmilitary interventions, such as targeted economic and political sanctions, are recommended before any consideration of military action is considered. Women must be part of plans to implement R2P in order to expose the likely impact on women of any proposed intervention. The criterion considered for intervention under R2P is the same as those for medical interventions: "Above all, do no harm."

Address Women's Needs When Planning Peacekeeping and Humanitarian Operations

Gender training is necessary for peacekeeping troops and humanitarian aid workers to prevent recurrence of rape and exploitation of women and girls by men who have power and money. Greater efforts must be made to ensure that humanitarian aid reaches women and is not first diverted to men. It is important to do the following:[23]

- Make safety of women and children the central concern when establishing refugee camps
- Provide adequate cooking fuel to avoid the necessity for women to leave the relative security of the camp to collect firewood
- Provide efficient cooking stoves to conserve fuel.

Increase the Numbers of Women in Decision-making Bodies

Increasing the numbers of women in governance at all levels improves the likelihood that a nation will use nonviolent means to resolve conflict.[20] The Fourth World Conference on Women, which was held in Beijing in 1995, called for a 30 percent minimum representation of women in decision-making bodies. Setting quotas for women's participation can be one step toward this goal. So can mandating that half of the nominations to an elected body must be women.

Establish or Restore Justice Systems, Education, Health Care, and Economic Opportunities for Women Immediately after War

It is important to restore the rule of law and women's access to justice. Women in postwar communities should be able to claim land that is rightfully theirs. Peace and reconciliation commissions are part of the rehabilitation process and must address gender-based violence.

Other important activities include the following:

- Providing antiretroviral drugs for women and children infected with HIV
- Providing literacy and numeracy education, information technology training, and computers so that the advancement of women can parallel that of men
- Providing aid targeted to income-generating opportunities for women, both microloans and loans for larger enterprises similar to the loans given to men
- Providing psychosocial support and reproductive health services for women in need of emergency assistance and during postconflict reconstruction. The special health problems arising from female genital mutilation require surgical, medical, and psychological care.
- Providing international support for community-based education initiatives, such as those in Kenya and Senegal, to end female genital mutilation. Since 1997, more than 1,000 villages in Senegal and Burkina Faso have publicly declared an end to harmful traditional practices, including forced genital mutilation and forced marriages.[24]
- Enforcing prosecution of rape and gender-based violence as war crimes and crimes against humanity.

Conclusion

The empowerment of women is slow, but, where it is advancing, the trend away from the use of armed violence is clear. Ensuring equal rights for women in every country would not only increase stability but would also fulfill the mandate of the United Nations and the dictates of international law. Global civil society is demanding that nations end war and atrocities against all people. Action to protect women is a first step in this direction.

References

1. Mertus JA. War's offensive on women: The humanitarian challenge in Bosnia, Kosovo, and Afghanistan. Bloomfield: Kumarian Press, 2000.
2. Garfield R. The impact of economic embargoes on the health of women and children. J Am Med Women's Assoc 1997;52:181–184.
3. Rehn E, Sirleaf EJ. Women, war, peace: The independent experts' assessment on the impact of armed conflict on women and women's role in peace-building. New York: United Nations Development Fund for Women (UNIFEM), 2002.
4. Roseberry W. AIDS prevention and mitigation in Sub-Saharan Africa. Washington, DC: World Bank, 1996.
5. Human Rights Watch. Sexual violence in the context of refugees. New York: Human Rights Watch, 1993.
6. Bhatia B, Kawar M, Shahin M. Women's survey: The impact of the Gulf crisis on the women in Iraq. Health and welfare in Iraq after the Gulf crisis: An in-depth assessment. Cambridge: Harvard International Study Team, 1991.
7. Mann J, Drucker E, Tarantola D, McCabe MP. Bosnia: The war against public health. Med Global Survival 1994;1:130–146.
8. United Nations High Commissioner for Refugees. Sexual violence against refugees: Guidelines on prevention and response. Geneva: UNHCR, 1995.
9. Chung CS. Testimonies of the global tribunal on violations of women's human rights. In Reilly N (ed.). United Nations World Conference on Human Rights. Vienna: Center for Women's Global Leadership, 1993.
10. Allison A. An excellent reason not to join the military. May 5, 2006. Available at: http://www.AlterNet.org/stories/35792 (accessed June 12, 2007).
11. McPhedran M, Sherret L, Bond J. R2P Missing women—Canada's responsibility to perceive. Fragile, Dangerous and Failed States: Implementing Canada's International Policy Statement. Fragile States Conference, 2005. Available at: http://www.iwrp .org/pdf/R2P_mcphedran.pdf (accessed July 19, 2007).
12. Cohn M. Military hides cause of women soldiers' deaths. January 30, 2006. Available at: http://www.Truthout.org (accessed June 12, 2007).
13. 2005 Global Refugee Trends: Statistical Overview of Populations of Refugees, Asylum-Seekers, Internally Displaced Persons, Stateless Persons, and Other Persons of Concern to the United Nations High Commissioner for Refugees, June 9, 2006. Available at: http://www.unhcr.org/statistics.html (accessed June 12, 2007).
14. Meintjes S, Pillay A, Turshen M. (eds.) The Aftermath: Women in Post-conflict Transformation. New York: Zed Books, 2001.
15. National Coalition Against Domestic Violence. Available at: http://www.ncadv.org/ files/Military_.pdf (accessed June 12, 2007).
16. Schmitt E. Military struggling to stem an increase in family violence. New York Times, May 23, 1994, A1, A12.
17. Berger L. Conflict prevention, gender and early warning: A work in progress. Third Expert Consultative Meeting on Gender and Early Warning, London, 2002.
18. EU toughens line on human trafficking. Financial Times, London, 2001. March 17, 2001, p6.
19. Mack A, Nielsen Z. (eds.). Human Security Report: War and Peace in the 21st Century. New York: Oxford University Press, 2005.

20. Caprioli M. Gendered conflict. J Peace Res 2000;37:51–68.
21. Caprioli M. Primed for violence: The role of gender inequality in predicting internal conflict. Int Stud Q 2005;49:161–178.
22. United Nations Security Council Resolution 1325 on Women, Peace and Security. Women's International League for Peace and Freedom, 2000.
23. Patrick E. Beyond firewood: Fuel alternatives and protection strategies for displaced women and girls. New York: Women's Commission for Refugee Women and Girls, 2006.
24. Female Genital Mutilation. Tostan: Women's Health and Human Rights, 2005.

13

Displaced Persons and War

Michael J. Toole

The cycle of war, intimidation, hunger, migration, and death that has affected millions of civilians in several continents during the past three decades poses one of the greatest contemporary public health challenges. Refugee camps have become the modern-day international public health equivalent of the clinical medicine emergency department (Figure 13-1). The indirect public health consequences of war have been mediated by mass population displacements, food shortages, hunger, and the destruction of health services and have been especially severe in low-income countries, where basic services and food reserves are already inadequate. In some situations, especially in sub-Saharan Africa and in Asia, the public health impact of population displacements induced by war has been relatively more severe than the direct impact of the violence.

Refugees who have crossed international borders fleeing war or persecution for reasons of race, religion, nationality, or membership in particular social and political groups are protected by the United Nations Convention Relating to the Status of Refugees (1951) and the Additional Protocol (1967).[1] During the two decades following the end of World War II, the most dramatic refugee emergencies took place in South Asia—first when 10 million people were displaced after the partition of India and Pakistan, and later when Bangladesh seceded from Pakistan. The number of dependent refugees under the protection and

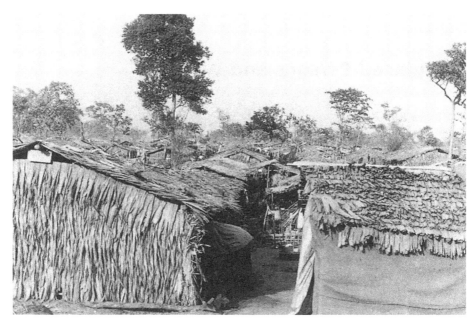

Figure 13-1. Huts made of thatch and burlap at Khao-I-Dang camp for Cambodians in Thailand in 1980. (Photograph by Barry S. Levy.)

care of the United Nations High Commissioner for Refugees (UNHCR) has steadily increased, from approximately 6 million in 38 countries in 1980, to almost 20 million in 97 countries in 1990 (see Table 13-1). By the end of 2005, the number of refugees had declined to about 12 million due to several large repatriations of refugees to their homelands (such as Angola, Afghanistan, and Rwanda) and a general downward trend in the global number of armed conflicts[2] (Figure 13-2).

Most refugees are still in Africa, the Middle East, and Central Asia. However, during the 1990s, there was a rapid increase in the number of refugees in Europe, following the collapse of the Soviet Union. Almost 2 million refugees were displaced within or fled from the republics of the former Yugoslavia between 1992 and 1995.[3] Almost 1 million refugees fled the Kosovo region of Serbia in 1999 as a result of widespread human rights abuses. Nevertheless, the reasons for the flight of refugees generally remain the same: war, civil strife, and persecution.

The term "complex humanitarian emergency" came into popular use after the Kurdish refugee exodus in 1991. The Centers for Disease Control and Prevention (CDC) has defined it as "a situation affecting large civilian populations which usually involves a combination of factors including war or civil

Table 13-1. Source of the 12 Largest Refugee Populations, 2005

Source	Number
Former Palestine	2,972,000
Afghanistan	2,192,000
Iraq	889,000
Myanmar (formerly Burma)	727,000
Sudan	671,000
Democratic Republic of Congo (DRC)	451,000
Burundi	438,000
Somalia	328,000
Vietnam	305,000
Colombia	258,000
Liberia	219,000
Eritrea	215,000

Source: United States Committee for Refugees and Immigrants. World Refugee Survey, 2006. Washington, DC, 2006.

strife, food shortages, and population displacement, resulting in significant excess mortality."[4] Jonathan Goodhand and David Hulme from the University of Manchester's Institute for Development Policy and Management have defined a "complex political emergency" as a conflict that combines a number of features[5]:

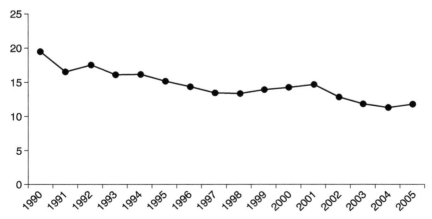

Figure 13-2. Millions of refugees worldwide, by year, 1990–2005. (Source: United States Committee for Refugees and Immigrants. World Refugee Survey, 2006. Washington, DC, 2006.)

Box 13-1 Darfur
Susannah Sirkin

Sudan, Africa's largest country geographically, is also ethnically diverse, with more than 300 tribes and 100 languages. An Arab minority (representing about 39 percent of the population), located mainly in the North, rules a non-Arab, "black African" majority of Christians, Muslims, and Animists (representing about 52 percent of the population). The British ruled Sudan from 1899 to 1953 as Anglo-Egyptian Sudan, administering the country as two separate entities, the North and the South.

Sudan has largely been at war with itself since it declared independence from Great Britain in 1956. During decades of onslaughts by the North related to access to oil reserves in the South and the regime's attempts to Islamize this region, 2 million non-Arabs were killed; untold numbers of civilians were abducted, enslaved, and raped; and 4–5 million people were displaced. Rebel forces arose to defend their turf and people, with rebel factions also committing war crimes. The conflict ended in 2004, with the signing of the Comprehensive Peace Agreement.

Just as that war ended, another bloody conflict erupted in Darfur, Sudan's far-western region. Home to almost 7 million people—most of them non-Arab Muslim agriculturalists who also owned livestock, as well as many Arab Muslim nomadic pastoralists, Darfur had been long neglected by the government in Khartoum. Tensions between various tribes have been exacerbated by desertification and shrinking grazing lands. Fighting broke out in 2003 when non-Arab villagers in north Darfur who had organized into militias attacked Sudanese military outposts in protest over long-ignored grievances. The Sudanese military used the attacks as a pretext to launch an all-out assault on the people of Darfur, destroying lives and livelihoods. The government also began to arm Arab nomads, sponsoring militia groups known as the Janjaweed (literally, "bandits on horseback"). The Janjaweed, in concert with the Sudanese military, have waged a campaign of destruction and terror— entering villages, killing men, raping women, burning houses and crops, and looting livestock and household possessions.[1]

Since the intense violence in Darfur erupted, the genocidal campaign[2] has totally destroyed hundreds of villages, caused the deaths of between 200,000 and 400,000 people, and displaced more than 2 million people within Darfur and more than 200,000 into neighboring Chad, where the war is expanding.

We at Physicians for Human Rights (PHR) began to examine the crisis in 2004, sending three teams of experts into the region to investigate human rights violations and destruction of villages and livelihoods. We interviewed refugees in Chad who told us horrific stories about the violence that drove them from their villages. We saw the harsh environment into which they had

(*continued*)

fled and documented the threat to survival imposed on them by forced migration. At the time of our first team visit, humanitarian relief was virtually absent on the Chad–Sudan border; one of our medical investigators said that this was the most difficult region for delivering aid that she had ever seen.

Dozens of interviews corroborated widespread attacks on villages. Sudanese aircraft circled villages and dropped bombs during predawn raids. Janjaweed militias then entered the villages in the early morning, shooting men, raping women,[3] and burning houses to the ground, pillaging and plundering as they went. There was strong evidence of genocide, an intent to destroy a population in whole or in part: Men, women and children were pursued and frequently shot in the back. Livestock were stolen or killed. Wells were poisoned. Hundreds of thousands of people were forced to flee into an environment with extreme heat, strong winds and dust storms, no water, no shelter, and almost no roads. Survival was difficult, if not impossible, without outside assistance.[4] Compounding the crisis were the Sudanese Government's overt efforts to obstruct both humanitarian assistance and the international protection force authorized by the United Nations.

In interviews with residents of three former villages, all respondents described a complete evacuation of their villages, 39 percent observed or were subjected to sexual assault, and 59 percent said they had heard racial epithets as they fled. Of the women our team interviewed, 52 percent had been widowed in the attacks.

The challenges now entail ending the conflict with a just and sustainable peace agreement, protecting the survivors and arranging for reparations, including compensation, as international law requires. Refugees and internally displaced persons will not be able to return and rebuild their lives without security. As of July 2007, the United Nations-African Union mission in Darfur (UNAMID) is expected to stabilize the situation with a long-awaited peacekeeping force of up to 26,000 troops and police, mainly drawn from African nations. This will augment the African Union force, which had not been capable of protecting the population in this vast terrain. The global response to this situation has been spotty, hampered by the lost credibility and diminished influence of the United States and the indifference of so many nations. But our common humanity dictates that we must respond to this most heinous human rights crime and act to protect the people of Darfur.

References

1. Report of the International Commission of Inquiry on Darfur to the United Nations Secretary-General. Geneva, January 25, 2005.
2. Convention on the Prevention and Punishment of the Crime of Genocide. Adopted by Resolution 260 (III) A of the United Nations General Assembly on December 9, 1948.

(continued)

Box 13-1 (*continued*)

3. The Use of Rape as a Weapon of War in the Conflict in Darfur, Sudan. A paper prepared for the U.S. Agency for International Development/Office of Transition Initiative by the Harvard School of Public Health/Physicians for Human Rights. October 2004.

4. Darfur—Assault on Survival: A Call for Security, Justice, and Restitution. Physicians for Human Rights. Cambridge, MA, February 2006. Available at: http://www.physicians forhumanrights.org/library/report-sudan-2006.html (accessed June 12, 2007)

- It often occurs within, but also across, national boundaries.
- It has political antecedents, often relating to competition for power and resources.
- It is protracted in duration.
- It is embedded in, and is an expression of, existing social, political, economic, and cultural structures and cleavages.
- It is often characterized by predatory social formations.

The most dramatic example of mass population displacement in the 1990s occurred in Rwanda as a result of attempted genocide of the Tutsi minority by extremist elements of the Hutu majority between April and June 1994. In July, when the Rwandan Patriotic Front militarily defeated the Rwandan government and took over the country, 1 million ethnic Hutus abruptly fled to the former Zaire (now the Democratic Republic of Congo [DRC]), provoking an unprecedented refugee crisis.

The most recent crisis to cause major population displacement was the ethnic conflict in West Darfur, Sudan. By mid-2007, this bitter conflict, which has directly targeted civilians, had led to internal displacement of more than 2 million people, with more than 200,000 people fleeing to the refugee camps in neighboring Chad[2] (Box 13-1 and Figure 13-3).

Although the number of refugees has steadily declined worldwide, the number of internally displaced persons remains high. Approximately 21 million people have fled their homes to escape war and persecution and to search for food and shelter, often in remote locations, without crossing international boundaries (Figure 13-4).[2] Therefore, they do not qualify for the protection and assistance provided to refugees by the international community (Table 13-2). An estimated 10 million of these internally displaced persons live in three African countries: Sudan, the DRC, and Uganda. In addition, almost 3 million people have been displaced by armed conflict within Colombia.

Those who are internally displaced are in an especially precarious situation because they remain within or close to zones of conflict, and international relief agencies experience extreme difficulty in providing them with relief aid.

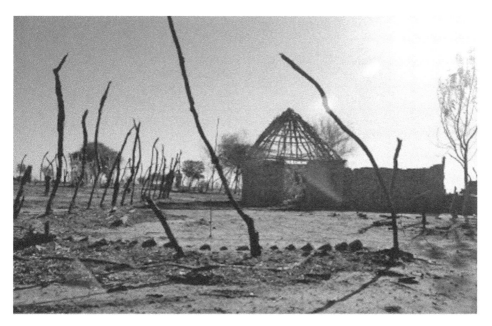

Figure 13–3. Remains of village destroyed by Janjaweed militia, Darfur, Sudan. (Photograph by Michael Wadleigh [www.gritty.org] for Physicians for Human Rights.)

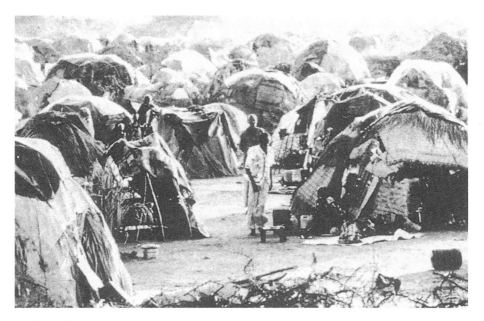

Figure 13-4. Tent city housing internally displaced Somalis in Baidoa in 1992. (Photograph by Michael J. Toole.)

213

Table 13-2. The Largest Internally Displaced Populations, 2005

Country	Number
Sudan	5,335,000
Colombia	2,900,000
Uganda	1,740,000
Democratic Republic of Congo (DRC)	1,664,000
Iraq	1,300,000
India	600,000
Zimbabwe	569,000
Azerbaijan	558,000
Myanmar (formerly Burma)	540,000
Côte d'Ivoire (Ivory Coast)	500,000
Algeria	500,000
Somalia	382,000

Source: United States Committee for Refugees and Immigrants. World Refugee Survey, 2006. Washington, DC, 2006.

Although the Geneva Conventions guarantee the basic human rights of civilian victims of war, the International Committee of the Red Cross, which is mandated with implementing the Conventions, is often denied access to these populations by governments or rival political organizations.

Public Health Consequences

The critical health problems affecting refugees and internally displaced persons are similar in nature, but their severity may be greater among internally displaced populations because assistance is often delayed and inadequate in quantity. Internally displaced persons may suffer more injuries because they are located close to zones of conflict. Refugees and internally displaced persons are often victims of landmines, especially as they travel between zones controlled by rival armed factions (see Chapter 7).

Mortality Rates

A community cannot be "healthy" if its death rate remains high. The most specific indicator of health status among refugee populations is the crude mortality rate (CMR). CMRs have been estimated from hospital and burial records, community-based surveys, and 24-hour burial site surveillance. Among the many problems in estimating mortality under emergency conditions are:

- Inadequate access to information
- Recall bias in surveys
- Families' failure to report perinatal deaths
- Inaccurate estimates of population size
- Lack of standard reporting procedures.

In general, however, bias tends to underestimate CMRs, because deaths are usually undercounted and population size is often exaggerated.[6]

Most reports of mortality related to complex emergencies have come from displaced populations. Comparisons of mortality between displaced and non-displaced populations that are affected by conflict and famine are problematic, because displacement itself may reflect a more serious baseline situation. Nonetheless, comparisons between displaced and nondisplaced populations, and between refugees and local host-country populations, show that in almost all cases the displaced and refugee populations experience significantly higher CMRs.[4]

During the early phase of an emergency, it is useful to express the CMR as deaths per 10,000 people per day. The median annual CMR in low-income countries is approximately 9 per 1,000 people, corresponding to a daily rate of approximately 0.25 per 10,000.[7] In emergencies, a daily rate of 1.0 per 10,000 has been commonly used as a threshold to indicate an elevated CMR.[6] Between March and May 1991, the average daily CMR among 400,000 Kurdish refugees on the Turkey–Iraq border was 4.2 per 10,000—a death rate 18 times higher than the normal rate in Iraq.[8] After the massive influx of Rwandan refugees into the North Kivu region of the DRC in July 1994, daily CMRs ranged between 25 and 50 per 10,000 per day,[9] among the highest ever documented among refugees (Figure 13-5).

Recently, complex emergencies have occurred without excess mortality being reported among displaced populations. For example, although mortality rates among Kosovar refugees in Albania and Macedonia in 1999 remained lower than 1 per 10,000 per day, significant threats to the health of the affected populations were present. In East Timor, after a referendum on independence in 1999, more than 1,000 civilians were massacred by militia cadres opposed to independence from Indonesia, and three-fourths of the population was displaced. In the months after the massacre, the death rate in East Timor did not exceed 1 per 10,000 per day; however, in the squalid refugee camps in West Timor, the CMR reached 2.1 per 10,000 per day and remained greater than 1 per 10,000 for several months.

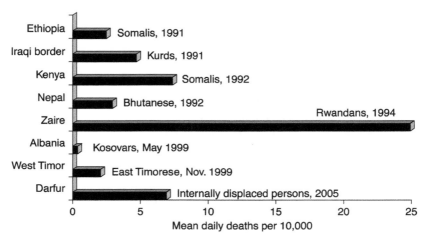

Figure 13–5. Crude mortality rates, selected refugee and displaced populations, 1991–2004.

Demographic Risk Groups

Most deaths in refugee populations have occurred among children younger than 5 years of age. For example, 65 percent of deaths among Kurdish refugees on the Turkish border occurred in the 17 percent of the population aged 0 to 5 years.[8] However, this is not always the case. For example, in Goma in the DRC, during the first month after the refugee exodus from Rwanda in 1994, mortality rates were comparable in all age groups because the major cause of death was cholera, which is equally lethal at any age.

Mortality data disaggregated by gender are frequently not available. However, during 1992, in the Gundhum II camp for Burmese refugees in Bangladesh, the death rate among Muslim Rohingya female infants (less than 1 year of age) was almost twice the rate among male infants; among refugees older than 5 years of age, the death rate among females was 3.5 times that for males. This was attributed to lesser access to health services for girls than for boys in the context of a conservative social environment. Among Kurdish refugees on the Turkey–Iraq border in 1991, however, the death rates among male and female children were approximately equal.[10]

Causes of Death

The most commonly reported causes of death among refugees during the early influx phase are diarrheal diseases, measles, acute respiratory infections, and other infectious diseases.[11] Epidemics of severe diarrheal disease have been increasingly common; cholera epidemics have occurred in refugee camps in Malawi, Zimbabwe, Swaziland, Nepal, Bangladesh, Turkey, Afghanistan, Burundi, and the DRC. Case-fatality rates (CFRs) for cholera in refugee camps have ranged between 3 and 30 percent. In addition, outbreaks of dysentery caused by *Shigella dysenteriae* type 1 have been reported in Malawi, Nepal, Kenya, Bangladesh, Burundi, Rwanda, Tanzania, and the DRC. Dysentery CRFs have been as high as 10 percent in young children and the elderly. In the Goma area of eastern Zaire, between 40,000 and 45,000 Rwandan refugees may have died from cholera or dysentery (accounting for 80 to 90 percent of all deaths) during the month after their arrival in mid-July 1994.[9]

Measles epidemics have caused high death rates among refugees. For example, during a 3-month period in 1985, more than 2,000 measles-associated deaths were documented in the Ethiopian refugee camp of Wad Kowli in eastern Sudan.[12] Since 1990, measles outbreaks have been reported among new refugees in camps in Nepal, Zimbabwe, and Malawi, contributing to high death rates in those camps. Large refugee camps for Somalis in Ethiopia, Iraqis in Turkey, and Rwandans in Tanzania and the DRC have been spared measles epidemics, probably because measles vaccination coverage rates in the refugees' countries of origin were relatively high. However, during the civil conflict and famine in Somalia in 1992–1993, widespread outbreaks of measles occurred, most likely because the country's health system had collapsed and most children were not immunized against measles and other childhood vaccine-preventable diseases.

Malaria has been reported as a major cause of death in camps in Thailand (1979), Malawi (1988–1993), eastern Sudan (1988), western Ethiopia (1991), Kenya (1992), and the DRC (1994). High malaria-specific death rates among refugees have been associated with movements from areas of low malaria endemicity through, or into, areas of high endemicity and with the development of chloroquine resistance.

Refugees in camps in Somalia, Ethiopia, Kenya, Sudan, and Chad have experienced outbreaks of hepatitis E virus infection, with attack rates between 6 and 8 percent and CFRs among pregnant women between 8 and 17 percent.[13] In 2004, an epidemic of hepatitis E affected thousands of displaced persons in West Darfur and in the refugee camps of neighboring Chad.[14] Investigation of the epidemic was aided by the use of a newly licensed rapid diagnostic kit. In addition, outbreaks of meningococcal meningitis have been reported in refugee camps in Thailand (1980), Sudan (1985), Ethiopia (1988), Malawi (1991), Burundi (1994), the DRC (1994), and Sudan (2005).

Although there is significant overlap between those countries affected by war and population displacement and those where the prevalence of HIV infection is high, it is not clear that population displacement increases vulnerability to HIV transmission. Until recently, few data have been available on the prevalence of HIV in refugee populations. It has been postulated that refugees and other conflict-affected populations might be at greater risk of acquiring HIV because of sexual exploitation, the breakdown of traditional societies and values, and the disruption of programs for treatment of sexually-transmitted infections and promotion of condoms.

Nevertheless, there is some evidence that conflict might actually inhibit the spread of HIV. When the 20-year conflict in Angola ended in 2002, the country had a significantly lower HIV prevalence (5 to 10 percent in Luanda and 1 to 3 percent in rural areas) than that in all other Southern African countries (15 to 40 percent). Between 2001 and 2003, UNHCR surveys of pregnant women in 20 refugee camps in Kenya, Rwanda, Sudan, and Tanzania found lower prevalence of HIV infection among refugees than in the surrounding population in each of the four countries, except Sudan. The studies noted that (1) most refugees moved from low to high HIV prevalence countries; (2) most refugees lived in remote rural areas with restricted freedom of movement; and (3) nongovernmental organizations (NGOs) have often mounted HIV prevention programs targeted at "captive" camp populations.[15]

In armed conflicts in Eastern Europe, a high proportion of mortality among civilians has been caused by trauma associated with the violence. Nevertheless, there has also been increased mortality in these conflicts due to the collapse of the public health system. Chronic conditions, such as cardiovascular diseases, cancer, and kidney disorders, have been inadequately treated because the medical care system has focused on the management of war-related injuries. Medical services in most parts of Bosnia and Herzegovina were overwhelmed by the demands of war casualties. Preventive health services, including childhood immunization and prenatal care, ceased in many areas. Hospitals were systematically targeted by the military in some areas; in Sarajevo, 38 of the original 42 ambulances were destroyed.[16] The collapse of health services in Bosnia and Herzegovina had significant public health effects. For example, the perinatal mortality rate increased in Sarajevo from 16 deaths per 1,000 live births in 1991 to 27 per 1,000 during the first 4 months of 1993.[17]

Nutritional Deficiencies

In the emergency phase of a refugee crisis, acute energy depletion is a life-threatening condition and leads to excess mortality. A critical factor is the synergy between malnutrition and infection. The prevalence of malnutrition may be increased by high rates of infectious diseases, such as measles, diarrhea, and dysentery. Infections lead to decreased appetite, increase the metabolic rate, and exacerbate acute malnutrition. These factors may differentially affect certain demographic groups within the population. The most vulnerable groups include children younger than 5 years of age and unaccompanied children, pregnant and lactating women, elderly people, disabled people, those who are chronically ill (including people with tuberculosis and HIV infection), people in households without an adult male, and people in disadvantaged ethnic or religious groups.

Because weight is more sensitive than height to sudden changes in food availability, nutritional assessments during emergencies focus on measuring weight-for-height. Moderate to severe acute malnutrition is defined as a weight-for-height ratio more than two standard deviations below the mean of the CDC/National Center for Health Statistics/World Health Organization (WHO) reference population.[18] All children with edema are classified as having severe acute malnutrition. As a screening measurement, the mid-upper arm circumference (MUAC) may also be used to assess acute undernutrition, although there is not complete agreement on which cut-off values should be used as indicators.

In some settings, refugee children who were adequately nourished on arrival in camps develop acute malnutrition due to inadequate food rations or severe epidemics of diarrheal disease. For example, in early 1991, the prevalence of acute malnutrition among Kurdish refugee children 12 to 23 months of age increased after a severe outbreak of diarrheal disease, from less than 5 percent to 13 percent during a 2-month period.[19]

As a result of an armed conflict in Darfur, Sudan, which began in early 2003, approximately 100,000 refugees fled to Chad during that year. By May 2004, the camps were overcrowded, water and sanitation were inadequate, and an outbreak of hepatitis E, a waterborne viral disease, had occurred in some camps. In June, a joint agency survey found the overall acute malnutrition prevalence among children to be 36 percent, with 5.5 percent severely malnourished. Blanket supplementary feeding was introduced for all children younger than 5 years of age and all pregnant or lactating women. According to food basket monitoring, the average energy content of the food ration reached 1,967 kilocalories per person per day by October 2004 (which approximated the official ration). A September survey found that the prevalence of acute malnutrition had decreased to 20 percent; although this represented an improvement, the rate remained very high by international standards (Figure 13-6 and Box 13-1).

In addition, high incidence rates of several micronutrient deficiency diseases have been reported in many refugee camps, especially in Africa. Refugee and displaced children are at high risk of developing vitamin A deficiency, because food rations usually contain inadequate vitamin A. In addition, common infectious diseases, such as measles and diarrheal disease, may deplete their body stores of vitamin A. In 1990, more than 18,000 cases of pellagra, caused by food rations deficient in niacin, were reported among Mozambican

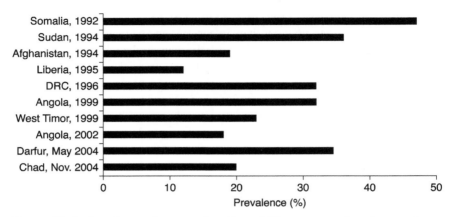

Figure 13–6. Prevalence of acute malnutrition, children younger than 5 years of age, selected refugee and displaced populations, 1992–2004.

refugees in Malawi.[20] Numerous outbreaks of scurvy (vitamin C deficiency) were documented in refugee camps in Somalia, Ethiopia, and Sudan between 1982 and 1991.[21]

Internally Displaced Persons

Although reliable data on the internally displaced are difficult to gather, very high death rates have been documented in some populations. In 1993, in Southern Sudan, civil war resulted in mass population displacement, hunger, and death rates up to 15 times those reported in nonconflict times.[22] In 2005, cross-sectional surveys in two conflict-affected African countries, Sudan and the DRC, found high mortality rates among civilian populations. In West Darfur, the survey sampled 215,000 internally displaced persons in four sites. The CMRs ranged between 6.0 and 9.3 per 10,000 per day; between 68 and 93 percent of deaths were associated with violence, and most were deaths of adult men.[23] The DRC survey sampled 19,500 households throughout the country and found the mortality rate to be 40 percent higher than the preconflict rate, amounting to 38,000 excess deaths per month, and 3.9 million excess deaths since the conflict began in 1998.[24] Death rates were highest in the eastern zones of the country, where the conflict had been most intense. Unlike West Darfur, the survey in the DRC found that most excess deaths were due to nonviolent causes, such as communicable diseases. (See also Chapter 17.)

Among internally displaced persons in countries affected by severe famine, high adult mortality rates have been reported. For example, in the Somali town of Baidoa, 59 percent of 15,105 deaths reported between August 1992 and February 1993 were among adults.[25] Although the main causes of death among internally displaced persons are similar to those among refugee populations, the prevalence of acute malnutrition among internally displaced persons has tended to be extremely high. In southern Somalia during 1992, the prevalence of acute malnutrition among children younger than 5 years of age in displaced persons camps in Marka and Qorioley was 75 percent, compared with 43 percent among town residents.[26]

Refugees and internally displaced persons in Bosnia and other parts of the former Yugoslavia suffered from intentional injuries inflicted during the course of bitter interethnic fighting. An estimated 200,000 civilians died during the last 3 years of the conflict (1992 to 1995)—more than 15,000 in Sarajevo alone.[16] Population surveys in southern and central Somalia found that between 4 and 11 percent of deaths from April 1992 to January 1993 were caused by war-related trauma.[27]

Sexual assault of displaced women has been increasingly common; for example, reports from the former Yugoslavia estimated that at least 20,000 Bosnian, Serbian, and Croatian displaced women had been raped.[28] The UNHCR documented 192 cases of rape of Somali refugee women in Kenyan camps during a 7-month period in 1993; in addition, several thousand unreported rapes were estimated to have occurred.[3] In West Darfur, the systematic rape of women and girls by the Janjaweed militia has been documented by human rights organizations, such as Amnesty International, and humanitarian aid agencies, such as Médecins Sans Frontières. Members of the Janjaweed militia are drawn from Darfurian and Chadian Arab-speaking tribes that have been fighting the sedentary non-Arab Muslim Sudanese population of the West Darfur region of Sudan in a battle over resource and land allocation. (See also Chapter 12.)

Response to Population Displacement Emergencies

Epidemiological data have documented those health problems that consistently cause most deaths and severe illnesses among refugees and internally displaced populations and have identified women and young children as being at highest risk. Most deaths are preventable with the use of currently available and affordable measures. Relief programs, therefore, must channel all available resources toward identifying, treating, and preventing cases of measles, diarrheal disease, malnutrition, acute respiratory infection, and, where prevalent, malaria—especially among women and young children.

Initially, refugees may suffer severe anxiety or depression, compounded by complete dependence on the generosity of others for survival. If refugee camps are located near borders or close to areas of continuing armed conflict, the desire for security is an overriding concern. Because most refugees (up to 80 percent) and internally displaced persons are women and children, the first priority of any relief operation is to ensure adequate protection of these vulnerable people.

In order to diminish the sense of helplessness and dependency, refugees should be given an active role in the planning and implementation of relief programs. Nevertheless, giving total control of the distribution of relief items to so-called "refugee leaders" may be dangerous. For example, leaders of the former, Hutu-controlled Rwandan government took control of the distribution system in DRC refugee camps in July 1994, resulting in diversion of relief supplies to young male members of the former Rwandan Army. Surveys indicated that households headed by single women had diminished access to food and shelter material, which led to increased malnutrition rates among children in those households.[9]

The critical elements of a relief program in response to sudden population displacement are clean water, food, sanitation, and shelter. UNHCR recommends that at least 15 to 20 liters of potable water be provided daily to each person. Although there is a consensus on the minimum quantity and quality of food required by these populations for survival, the timely provision of adequate food supplies remains a critical issue in many parts of the world, especially in Africa. In addition to the minimum caloric requirement of 2,100 kilocalories per person per day, adequate micronutrients need to be provided in ration foods, through fortification of ration cereals or routine supplementation, especially with vitamin A. General rations should consist of familiar and culturally acceptable foods, and adequate cereal grinding mills, cooking utensils, and cooking fuel must be provided. Food should be distributed, preferably by women—who have been shown to be fairer than men—to family units, with special care taken to ensure that socially vulnerable groups in the community receive their fair share. Minimum standards for humanitarian assistance have now been codified by the Sphere Project, and a Code of Conduct for humanitarian agencies has been developed and adopted by most agencies.[29]

Beyond the provision of the these basic needs, the following elements of a public health program should be established as soon as possible:

1. *A health information system:* Including surveillance of mortality, nutritional status, and morbidity from diseases of public health importance
2. *Diarrheal disease control:* Including oral rehydration therapy (ORT) in a supervised setting, appropriate treatment of dysentery, community hygiene education, and cholera preparedness
3. *Immunization:* Including immediate measles immunization for children 6 months to 12 years of age; provision, when the emergency subsides, of

other WHO Expanded Program on Immunization antigens (diphtheria-pertussis-tetanus, oral polio vaccine, and BCG [bacille Calmette-Guérin]); and identification of sources for meningitis vaccine (Figure 13-7)

4. *Basic curative care:* Including an emphasis on maternal and child health; establishment of a referral system; development of a list of essential drugs; preparation of standard treatment guidelines (at least for diarrhea, malaria, and acute respiratory infection); and selection, training, and deployment of community health workers

5. *Selective feeding programs:* Including supplementary feeding for vulnerable groups, such as young children, pregnant and lactating women, and the elderly; therapeutic feeding for severely malnourished children; and the provision of micronutrient supplements to vulnerable groups.

6. *Endemic disease control and epidemic preparedness:* Endemic disease control and epidemic preparations include the following:
   - Establishing surveillance, including standard case definitions
   - Developing standard case management protocols
   - Agreeing on policies for prevention (including vaccination and prophylaxis)

(continued)

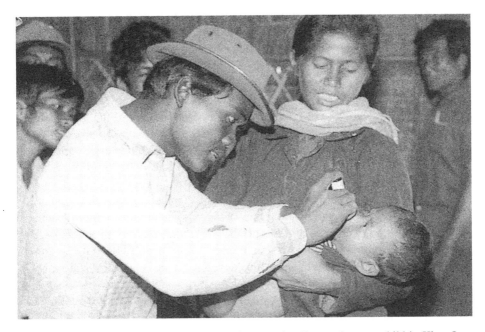

Figure 13-7. Public health worker administers oral polio vaccine to a child in Khao-I-Dang camp for Cambodians in Thailand. (Photograph by Barry S. Levy.)

- Identifying a laboratory to confirm index cases of epidemic diseases
- Identifying sources of relevant vaccines
- Establishing reserves of essential medical supplies (such as ORT, intravenous solutions, and antibiotics)
- Identifying treatment sites, triage systems, and training needs
- Identifying expert assistance for epidemic investigation
- Developing environmental management plans
- Implementing community education and prevention programs.

Innovative and culturally appropriate programs of counseling, support, and rehabilitation are often necessary to address the needs of people who have experienced the violence of shelling, landmines, and sexual assault. In addition, there is a need to develop specialized approaches to caring for unaccompanied children, such as those Rwandan children in the camps of the DRC and Tanzania in 1994. A reproductive health program should be established that provides a basic minimum set of services, including prevention of HIV infection.

Once the emergency relief phase is over, new challenges arise. Public health programs need to be community-based and integrated with other development programs that aim to minimize dependency on the outside world, restore dignity to stressed communities, and prepare for eventual repatriation of displaced persons to their homelands. Training of community health workers, particularly women, should be the cornerstone of these longer-term programs. New and sometimes sensitive issues, such as family spacing and the prevention of HIV infection, need to be addressed through community development processes.

Relief management decisions need to be based on sound technical information, coordinated action, information sharing, and careful evaluation of the impact and effectiveness of interventions. Responsibilities for the implementation of relief programs should increasingly be shared with proven, competent, and experienced indigenous and foreign NGOs (see Chapters 22 and 23). However, the core group of international relief agencies with appropriate experience and technical competence in emergency management remains small and overstretched. The public health needs of displaced populations cannot be adequately addressed by traditional, Western-style curative care in expensive, difficult-to-manage hospital settings. Therefore, there is an urgent need for relevant training programs in emergency public health for NGO personnel and limited operational research to develop effective and innovative approaches to emergency health problems.

Recent emergencies have followed a predictable pattern of political unrest, civil war, human rights abuses, food shortages, and, finally, mass population displacement. There has been almost no preparedness for these emergencies within the public health community. Agencies involved in health development projects should integrate preparedness planning into all aspects of public health programs. Health information systems should incorporate plans to simplify and focus on major health problems in the event of emergencies. Immunization, diarrheal disease control, and community health worker training programs should likewise incorporate emergency contingency plans.

Finally, greater attention needs to be given to the early prevention of conflict situations that give rise to mass population displacement. Early warning systems have been in place in disaster-prone regions for the past decade. However, their warnings have often been ignored. Determined diplomacy applied to warring parties early in a conflict might preclude the need for later military toughness, with all the associated problems that were witnessed in Somalia, Bosnia, and elsewhere.

References

1. Convention and Protocol Relating to the Status of Refugees. (Publication HCR/INF/29/Rev.3.) Geneva: U.N. High Commissioner for Refugees; 1968.
2. U.S. Committee for Refugees. World Refugee Survey, 2006. Washington, DC: U.S. Committee for Refugees, 2006.
3. U.S. Committee for Refugees. World Refugee Survey, 1996. Washington, DC: U.S. Committee for Refugees, 1996.
4. Burkholder BT, Toole MJ. Evolution of complex disasters. Lancet 1995;346:1012–1015.
5. Goodhand J, Hulme D. From wars to complex political emergencies: Understanding conflict and peace building in the new world disorder. Third World Q 1999;20: 13–26.
6. Centers for Disease Control and Prevention. Famine-affected, refugee, and displaced populations: Recommendations for public health issues. MMWR Morb Mortal Wkly Rep 1992;41:1–76.
7. Reed HE, Keeley CB (Eds.). Forced Migration and Mortality. Washington, DC: National Academies Press, National Research Council, 2001.
8. Centers for Disease Control and Prevention. Public health consequences of acute displacement of Iraqi citizens: March–May 1991. MMWR Morb Mortal Wkly Rep 1991; 40:443–446.
9. Goma Epidemiology Group. Public health impact of Rwandan refugee crisis: What happened in Goma, Zaire, in July 1994? Lancet 1995;345:339–344.
10. Toole MJ, Waldman RJ. Refugees and displaced persons: War, hunger, and public health. JAMA 1993;270:600–605.
11. Toole MJ, Waldman RJ. Prevention of excess mortality in refugee and displaced populations in developing countries. JAMA 1990;263:3296–3302.
12. Shears P, Berry AM, Murphy R, Nabil MA. Epidemiologic assessment of the health and nutrition of Ethiopian refugees in emergency camps in Sudan. BMJ 1987;295: 314–318.

13. Centers for Disease Control and Prevention. Enterically transmitted, non-A, non-B hepatitis—East Africa. MMWR Morb Mortal Wkly Rep 1987;36:241–244.
14. Boccia D, Klovstad H, Guthmann JP. Outbreak of Hepatitis E in Mornay IDP Camp, Western Darfur, Sudan. Paris, France: Epicentre, 2004.
15. Spiegel P. HIV/AIDS among conflict-affected and displaced populations: Dispelling myths and taking action. Disasters 2004;28:322–325.
16. Toole MJ, Galson S, Brady W. Are war and public health compatible? Lancet 1993; 341:935–938.
17. Centers for Disease Control and Prevention. Status of public health—Bosnia and Herzegovina, August–September 1993. MMWR Morb Mortal Wkly Rep 1993;973: 979–982.
18. World Health Organization Working Group. Use and interpretation of anthropometric indicators of nutritional status. Bull W H O 1986;64:929–941.
19. Yip R, Sharp TW. Acute malnutrition and high childhood mortality related to diarrhea. JAMA 1993;270:587–590.
20. Centers for Disease Control and Prevention. Outbreak of pellagra among Mozambican refugees—Malawi, 1990. MMWR Morb Mortal Wkly Rep 1991;40:209–213.
21. Desenclos JC, Berry AM, Padt R, et al. Epidemiologic patterns of scurvy among Ethiopian refugees. Bull W H O 1989;67:309–316.
22. Centers for Disease Control and Prevention. Nutrition and mortality assessment— southern Sudan, March 1993. MMWR Morb Mortal Wkly Rep 1993;42:304–308.
23. Depoortere E, Checchi F, Broillet F, et al. Violence and mortality in West Darfur, Sudan (2003–2004): Epidemiological evidence from four surveys. Lancet 2004;364: 1315–1320.
24. Coghlan B, Brennan R, Ngoy P, et al. Mortality in the Democratic Republic of Congo: A nationwide survey. Lancet 2006;367:44–51.
25. Collins S. The need for adult therapeutic care in emergency feeding programs: Lessons from Somalia. JAMA 1993;270:637–638.
26. Manoncourt S, Doppler B, Enten F, et al. Public health consequences of civil war in Somalia, April 1992. Lancet 1993;340:176–177.
27. Boss LP, Toole MJ, Yip R. Assessments of mortality, morbidity, and nutritional status in Somalia during the 1991–1992 famine. JAMA 1994;272:371–376.
28. Amnesty International. Bosnia and Herzegovina: Rape and sexual abuse by armed forces. (Amnesty International report EUR 63/01/93.) New York: Amnesty International, 1993.
29. The Sphere Project. Humanitarian Charter and Minimum Standards in Disaster Response. Geneva, Switzerland: The Sphere Project, 2004.

14

Detainees and the New Face of Torture

Leonard S. Rubenstein and Stephen N. Xenakis

Torture violates human rights and assaults human dignity. The mechanisms of torture vary—interrogators pulling out the fingernails of a detainee, applying electricity to a man's genitals, turning thumbscrews, maliciously twisting a burning cigarette into flesh, or describing in excruciating detail to a hooded prisoner the pain that is to be inflicted on his mother, wife, or child—but it always brings pain, degrades people, even deprives them of their humanity. That is why torture has been debated since at least the time of the ancient Greeks and, by the time of the Enlightenment, was banned in most of Europe. Yet it continues today. In 2005, Amnesty International reported that torture was being used in 150 countries, and it was widespread or persistent in 70 of these countries.

Torture is defined in international human rights law to mean the intentional infliction of severe mental or physical pain or suffering for purposes such as obtaining information or a confession, punishing for suspected acts, or intimidating or coercing the individual. The human rights stance against torture has been unequivocal, one of the few absolutes in human rights law: It is never permitted, never excused, never to be balanced against national needs or interests—even in cases of national emergency. Torture is also forbidden under the laws of war. It is considered a war crime under the Geneva Conventions.

Torture has long been associated with political repression and with regimes without any semblance of an independent judiciary or media. The Soviet Union's imprisonment of dissenters and forced use of psychotropic medication on them, the Khmer Rouge's torture of thousands of people in Cambodia, and the Augusto Pinochet regime's brutality against prisoners in Chile all bear witness to the association between totalitarian or authoritarian regimes and their use of torture.

In many countries today, however, torture is not just practiced against political opponents but also against those who are, or are alleged to be, common criminals. And, in the past 50 years, countries with strong democracies that profess deep commitment to human rights have insidiously legitimized the use of torture as a necessary weapon in fighting terrorism. Examples include France occupying Algeria, Great Britain battling the Irish Republican Army, Israel seeking to stop Palestinian attacks on civilians, and now the United States waging its "war on terror."

While eschewing many of the gruesome physical techniques long associated with torture, the governments of these countries have employed abusive interrogation methods, including psychological ones, to compel prisoners to yield information. In Northern Ireland, Great Britain used what it called "interrogation in depth" as part of counterterrorism strategies against the Irish Republican Army, with techniques that included hooding, wall-standing, use of loud noise for long periods of time, and deprivation of food, water, and sleep. In Israel, the security services have used painful stress positions, shaking, hooding, sleep deprivation, and other draconian interrogation methods against Palestinian detainees.

And the Bush administration in the United States, claiming that the "war on terror" required new techniques, has embraced a wide variety of forms of torture against detainees held in Afghanistan, Iraq, and at Guantánamo Bay in Cuba, including stress positions, extremes of temperature, long-term isolation, waterboarding (strapping a person to a board and lowering him into water to simulate the feeling of drowning), sleep deprivation, instilling of fear through use of dogs, threats of death or severe harm, bombardment by loud music, severe humiliation, and physical force (Figure 14-1).[1,1a] With the help of psychologists, it has even adapted techniques used by the Survival, Evasion, Resistance, and Escape (SERE) school for training and inoculating American soldiers against succumbing to torture to design tactics for interrogating prisoners at Guantánamo and elsewhere.[2,2a,2b]

In the past, United Nations agencies, courts, and others responsible for interpreting the law on torture have determined that all of these techniques amount to torture and other forms of cruel, inhuman and, degrading treatment.[1,1a] Moreover, when other countries employed them, they were condemned by the U.S. Department of State.[3] And for good reason. Research on the psychological

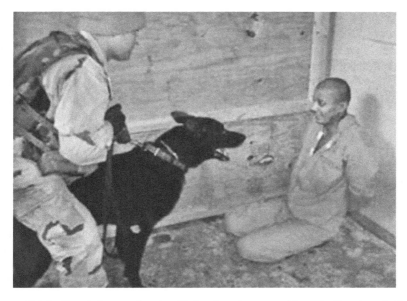

Figure 14-1. Dog being used to instill fear in prisoner at Abu Ghraib prison in Iraq. (Source: Courtesy of Physicians for Human Rights.)

and long-term consequences of torture has been difficult because of methodological problems, including the absence of controlled studies and adequate long-term follow-up.[4] But we know, from clinical experience worldwide in many people subjected to extreme psychological methods, that painful and often disabling symptoms emerge acutely and can persist for years.[1,1a] Sleep manipulation contributes to cognitive impairment and disruption, with psychotic features emerging within 1 week, and can lead to self-harm, including suicide. Sensory deprivation, including hooding and isolation, leads to severe anxiety, depression, and psychotic-like thinking with serious health consequences. Repetitive exposure to frightening and life-threatening circumstances contributes to debilitating posttraumatic stress disorder (see Chapter 4).

Nevertheless, governments experiencing terrorism have convinced themselves that harsher techniques are necessary to protect the nation and its people from a possibly imminent terrorist threat, and this position has gained interest and sympathy.[5] Indeed, it can be argued that the mindset of many of the lawyers, analysts, psychologists and military officials who authorized and developed the Bush administration's interrogation techniques thought they were doing just that: devising techniques that are coercive but do not amount to torture. These officials saw themselves as having a duty to implement interrogation techniques that, in their minds, were consistent with the obligation not to torture but were nonetheless harsh enough to yield information from unwilling detainees.

This attitude was articulated frankly by General Michael V. Hayden, now Director of the Central Intelligence Agency (CIA). In a meeting in 2005 with human rights leaders, at which one of us (L.R.) was present, when he was the Principal Deputy Director of National Intelligence, General Hayden said that the obligation of national security officials is to use all techniques within their arsenal that fall short of violating the law against torture. Invoking the image of a chalk line on a football field, Hayden said that interrogators should come so close to the line that they have chalk on their uniforms. Moreover, recognizing that the use of the techniques could easily get out of control, U.S. national security officials have established limitations, ground rules, safeguards, approvals, and monitoring mechanisms to try to ensure that the techniques used do not cross that line.

It is in this context that new legal justifications were sought for harsh interrogation tactics, especially a reinterpretation of the meaning of "torture." In 2002, the Assistant U.S. Attorney General, J. S. Bybee, was asked by the White House counsel, Alberto Gonzales, to answer a question raised by the CIA: What, exactly, is torture, under U.S. criminal law? His response was that, for conduct to be considered torture, the resultant pain had to be extraordinarily severe. He wrote "[F]or an act to constitute torture as defined in [United States Code] Section 2340, it must inflict pain that is difficult to endure. Physical pain amounting to torture must be equivalent in intensity to the pain accompanying serious physical injury, such as organ failure, impairment of bodily function or even death."[6] In addition, the interrogator had to have a specific intent to cause such pain.

To qualify as mental, or psychological, torture, Bybee wrote in his memorandum, the technique "must result in significant psychological harm of significant duration, e.g., lasting for months or even years"—a requirement contrary to the international Convention Against Torture. Bybee acknowledged that a U.S. criminal statute recognized that mental harm could result from threats of imminent death; threats of infliction of the kind of pain that would amount to physical torture; infliction of such physical pain as a means of psychological torture; and use of drugs or other procedures designed to deeply disrupt the senses or fundamentally alter an individual's personality. But in order to qualify he opined that the suffering must be on the order of a brief psychotic disorder, including delusions and hallucinations; the onset of obsessive-compulsive disorder; or individuals pushed to the brink of suicide. Even when the Bybee memorandum was superseded in late 2004, the U.S. Department of Justice continued to adhere to a very restrictive interpretation of psychological torture and continued to define mental torture as requiring a specific demonstration of prolonged harm—which can be shown only after the fact.[7]

The Bybee memorandum was so ridiculed when it leaked 2 years later that the Bush administration repudiated it. But the drive to identify and justify harsher forms of interrogation in the name of national security remains, even among some who have advocated for civil liberties. Some observers simply deny that the harsh techniques are harmful. For example, a reviewer commented after seeing the film, *The Road to Guantanamo* (about three British citizens detained there for more than 2 years), that the hooding, the dogs, and the forced wakefulness were more equivalent to bad college pranks, not torture.[8] More commonly, to prevent harsh techniques from degenerating into torture, proponents offered elaborate safeguards to ensure that the techniques were limited and were implemented in accordance with law.

For example, Professor Philip Heymann, a Harvard Law School professor and U.S. Department of Justice official in the Clinton administration, and Professor Juliette Kayyem, a former Democratic Congressional staffer now at the Kennedy School of Government at Harvard, developed the concept of acceptable "highly coercive interrogation," using techniques such as hooding, forced standing against a wall for extended periods, and deprivation of food, sleep, and medical treatment.[9]

Let us put aside for a moment whether these techniques constitute torture or other forms of cruel, inhuman, and degrading treatment, or whether they violate the prohibition of the Geneva Conventions on the use of any form of coercion against prisoners of war. The Heymann-Kayyem approach demands that "highly coercive" interrogation methods be regulated by approvals and reviews, limits on duration and repetition, and assessment of the likely impact of combined techniques. Probable cause must be established to ascertain that the individual against whom the highly coercive techniques would be used possesses significant information that could threaten American lives and, more importantly, that there is no reasonable alternative technique for obtaining this information. These findings must be shared with the U.S. Attorney General and relevant members of Congress. Finally, in exceptional, "emergency cases"—a term that is deliberately vague—the President can personally order the use of highly coercive techniques but must notify relevant members of Congress afterward.

In 2003, the journalist Mark Bowden offered another approach to determining whether "coercive interrogation" should be used. He claimed that coercive interrogation could be effective but carries great risks of both overuse and degeneration into torture. He advocated a rhetorical and legal prohibition on coercive techniques, accompanied by implicit approval: "Torture is a crime against humanity, but coercion is an issue that is rightly handled with a wink, or even a touch of hypocrisy; it should be banned but also quietly practiced."[10] In other words, interrogators can be given *explicit* rules to refrain but *implicit* approval to go forward; that message, he stated, would be a means of controlling coercive interrogation while still achieving its ends.

While elegantly argued and increasingly popular as a middle ground, these approaches are extremely dangerous. To start, they rest on some very dubious assumptions, including (1) that useful, accurate information can be obtained, and without an unacceptably high false-positive rate, a proposition for which no evidence exists[11,11a] and (2) that the techniques are actually morally and legally acceptable. They also ignore both the short- and long-term psychological agony that these techniques impose. But, even if all these objections were to be put aside and we accepted, for the sake of argument, that harsh techniques can yield valuable information from "terrorists," the approach would still be profoundly wrong. The very nature of harsh interrogation and the closed and tense circumstances in which it takes place create a logic of expanding the group of people to whom it is applied and the techniques used, and thereby render all the safeguards meaningless. Once the door is opened to harsh interrogation, torture most certainly follows. And not just for some: Policies allowing highly coercive interrogation yield not just *instances* of torture, but *regimes* of torture. Neither regulatory approval nor Bowden's wink-and-nod approach can prevent it.

Historical experience demonstrates the dynamics of the phenomena. In the closed world of detention, with pressures on interrogators to gain information, the exception becomes the rule. The lack of knowledge of what a detainee knows becomes a justification for escalating the force used to gain information. Interrogators become hardened to the harsh techniques, those with sadistic leanings tend to come to the fore, and abuse becomes routinized—and then barely noticed. Values become corrupted. Torture becomes the norm. In the face of these dynamics, a regulatory approach to harsh interrogation is not only ineffective but also corrupting.

Consider the case of Israel. In 1987, the Israeli government created a special commission, headed by former Supreme Court Justice President Moshe Landau, to review interrogation procedures used by the national security service and to make recommendations for future practice.[12] The commission found that physical force was frequently used against detainees to extract confessions and that members of the security service frequently committed perjury to mask the circumstances under which the confessions were obtained. The commission's most notable work, however, was future oriented, as it sought to balance what it saw as the need for information about impending terrorist attacks with the imperative of respecting human dignity. So it authorized the use of psychological techniques and what it referred to as "moderate physical pressure." These techniques, however, could only be used in exceptional cases, such as to prevent imminent murder or to gain information from a suspect thought to possess vital knowledge about a terrorist organization, such as the location of arms or explosives caches or planned acts of terrorism that could not be uncovered by any other means. Moreover, the techniques, which were kept secret, had to be consistent with the core value that the pressure must never reach the level of physical torture or bring about grievous harm to the individual's honor, which would deprive him of human dignity.

The commission also required strict safeguards: (1) the use of harsher measures had to be deemed essential in that the detainee was thought to have vital information and that lesser measures had not worked; (2) the government was instructed to establish permissible techniques in advance and to limit their use through legally binding directives; and (3) supervisory mechanisms were implemented and discipline for violations was established, including criminal prosecution, where necessary.

If the measurement of success was limitation of the use of harsh techniques in accordance with its guidelines, the commission's approach was a complete failure. The techniques became brutal, including hooding, sleep and food deprivation, tying detainees to chairs in positions that caused severe pain, sensory deprivation, use of extremes of heat and cold, and violent shaking. These techniques were often used in combination, and they were not limited to extreme cases. Exceptions became the rule. Torture became routine for political activists, relatives of persons listed as wanted, students suspected of being pro-Islamic, sheiks, and Palestinians in professions with knowledge about preparing explosives.[13] The Israeli human rights group, B'tselem, reported that, based on its interviews, review of testimony, and investigations, about 85 percent of Palestinian detainees in custody after the commission's recommendations were put into effect were subjected to torture—approximately 850 people each year. The elaborate procedural safeguards were disregarded, violators were not disciplined (much less prosecuted), and judicial oversight had failed.[14] More than a decade later, the Israeli Supreme Court held that many of the techniques used were illegal and must end.[15]

The experience of torture of detainees by the United States since the September 11, 2001, attacks on the World Trade Center and the Pentagon is equally illuminating. Even as the Bush administration reinterpreted the law on torture and denied applicability of the Geneva Conventions to alleged Taliban and al-Qaeda detainees, it sent a double message[16]:

- Very harsh interrogation techniques were not only permitted but also welcome.
- At least in the Department of Defense, even as the rules were loosened, legal and policy discussions at the highest levels devoted enormous attention to setting limits to the harsh methods authorized and implementing safeguards against abuse.

According to one key working group appointed by the Secretary of Defense to make recommendations concerning permissible interrogation techniques, even before any of these techniques were used[16]:

- Determinations had to be made that there was a good basis to believe the detainee had critical intelligence
- Interrogators had to be specifically trained for the techniques
- The detainee had to be medically and operationally evaluated as suitable for techniques used, including techniques used in combination
- A specific interrogation plan had to be in place that included reasonable safeguards, limits on duration, intervals between applications, termination criteria, and presence or availability of qualified medical personnel
- Appropriate supervision had to be provided
- Appropriate specific, senior-level approval had to be given for use with any specific detainee after considering the criteria and receiving legal advice.

In addition, specific safeguards were supposed to apply to particular techniques, such as temporal limitation. One of the first memoranda proposing the use of long-term isolation, written for the base commander at Guantánamo Bay in 2002, stipulated that it could not be used for more than 30 days, with extensions requiring approval by the commanding officer.[17] Six months later, the working group of the Secretary of Defense required more elaborate purported safeguards, including specific guidelines regarding the length of isolation, medical and psychological review, and approvals of increases in duration of isolation at the appropriate level in the chain of command. Sleep deprivation was supposed to be limited to four consecutive days.

The high-level approval and legal review that were required for long-term isolation were also intended to apply to forced grooming, sleep deprivation, removal of clothing, use of dogs, waterboarding, and threats of imminent death. In Iraq, Lieutenant General Ricardo Sanchez wrote an instruction that use of dogs, stress positions, sleep management, sensory deprivation, yelling, loud music, and bright light required his case-by-case approval.[1]

Another purported safeguard was medical review. For example, according to a memorandum from the Secretary of Defense to the Commander of the Southern Command, the use of isolation required medical and psychological review.[1] Colonel Thomas Pappas, the head of intelligence at the Abu Ghraib prison in Iraq, testified, in an internal investigation, that a doctor had to approve interrogation plans that included sleep deprivation.[18] Medical involvement was also required at the back end, such as for monitoring of dietary manipulation, sleep management, and sensory deprivation.

Because interrogation records are, with rare exceptions, unavailable to the public, we do not know how many of these purported safeguards were followed. We do know that, even to the extent they were followed, they were totally ineffective in preventing widespread abuse of prisoners, which became routinized. A review published in 2006 by three human rights organizations found at least 330 cases in which more than 600 U.S. military and civilian personnel were credibly alleged to have abused, and in some cases to have killed, more than 460 detainees in detention centers operated by the United States. These cases—more than 1,000 acts of criminal abuse—included assault, severe humiliation, sexual abuse and assault, and the use of stress positions.[19]

These data do not include use of abusive techniques, such as isolation, that became so routine that they were not reported as incidents of abuse. For example, in a review of detention practices at the Abu Ghraib prison in Iraq, Major General George Fay reported the use of isolation as "routine and repetitive."[20] One soldier told investigators for General Fay that when requests were made for isolation, they were rarely turned down, and no one checked to determine whether the recommendation was sound. Isolation, often accompanied by nakedness, became part of the normal course of operations at Abu Ghraib. In 2003, shortly after the authorization for 30-day isolation went into effect, most detainees were isolated in single cells and allowed out of these cells only twice a week for 15 minutes; no physical contact between detainees was permitted.[21] In Iraq, the International Committee of the Red Cross (ICRC) reported that so-called high-value detainees held at the Baghdad Airport in 2003 were held in strict solitary confinement in small concrete cells devoid of daylight.[22] Later in 2003, the ICRC found prisoners kept naked in total darkness in isolation cells at Abu Ghraib and it learned that this practice was simply "part of the process."[22]

General Fay also found, as did the ICRC, that sleep deprivation was a common practice at Abu Ghraib. At Guantánamo, a review of certain abuse allegations by Lieutenant General Randall Schmidt found that some interrogators recommended detainees for a "frequent flyer" program, lasting for more than a year, in which they were moved every few hours from one cell to another in order to disrupt their sleep.[23] The routine use of harsh and abusive practices extended further, including severe humiliation, nudity, and loud and disorienting music.

The logic of harsh interrogation even led to blurring of the boundaries between an instrument of abuse and a purported safeguard, such as medical monitoring.[23a] That medical monitoring of interrogation provides any measure of safety is dubious, because the presence of health professionals may serve to legitimate coercive interrogation rather than restrict it.[24] In one infamous case, a physician provided treatment to a severely dehydrated detainee while loud music was bombarding the detainee to keep him awake.[23] Because of these dangers, physicians are ethically prohibited from monitoring interrogation. But

the monitoring groups established by the U.S. Department of Defense, called
behavioral science consultation teams (BSCTs, or "biscuits") are composed of
medics, psychologists, and physicians and have had dual functions. According
to the Pentagon, the role of these teams is to ensure that interrogation is "safe"
but also "effective." A review of medical operations and detainees ordered
by the Surgeon General of the U.S. Army emphasized that the BSCTs play the
role of "safety officer," whose function is to ensure that interrogations are
conducted in a safe, ethical, and legal manner.[25] At the same time, however,
they are expected to advise interrogators on how to gain intelligence information. In order to perform that function, the BSCTs are supposed to provide
psychological expertise to review information about detainees, such as opinions
on their character and personality and their medical history, with a focus on
depression, delusional behaviors, manifestations of stress, and "buttons" (sensitivities that may elicit an exaggerated response). They consult on the interrogation plan and approach and provide feedback on interrogation technique—
"knowing when to push or not push harder in the pursuit of intelligence
information."[25]

Experiences in Israel and the United States demonstrate that controlling
harsh interrogation techniques by means of various "safeguards" is illusory.
As the BSCTs have demonstrated, the safeguards may lead to further abuse—
which should not be a surprise. Interrogation under the best of circumstances
carries risks of abuse; interrogation is even riskier in closed settings, under
intense pressure to obtain information, with huge power differentials between
the participants. At Abu Ghraib and Guantánamo, the "normalization" of
torture has occurred as a result of inadequate training, overzealous intelligence
gathering, failure of leadership by authorizing the techniques in the first place,
reliance on highly dangerous psychological techniques, and, most profoundly,
the dynamics of harsh interrogation.

Classic psychological studies performed more than 30 years ago by Philip
Zimbardo, who created a simulated prison environment, and Stanley Milgram,
whose subjects were willing to impose severe electric shocks on others, have
helped illuminate these dynamics.[26] These studies demonstrated that Every-
man is a potential torturer and that once restraints are lifted on cruel behavior,
it becomes enormously difficult to control, no matter what "safeguards" are
put in place. In war, the likelihood is even greater. Psychiatrists who looked at
those who perpetrated the abuse suggested that it became "an inexcusable way
of working off their rage, anxiety about their own safety, and their sense of
helplessness."[27]

In another classic psychological study, Herbert Kelman described three
factors as being necessary for torture: authorization, routinization, and dehumanization.[28] Authorization means that someone with power stated that
extreme measures were acceptable. Authorization leads to routinization, a

form of division of labor. In Nazi Germany, for example, one person had responsibility for writing the orders to deport the Jews, and another for shaving their heads. The guards at Abu Ghraib were told they were merely "softening up" the prisoners for interrogation. Dehumanization follows. In Vietnam, the enemy became "slopes"; in Guantánamo and Iraq, they became "towel heads." Covering prisoners' faces with hoods makes it possible for the soldiers to sever any empathic human connection with them. The dehumanization of prisoners in the environments in which they are interrogated further increases the potential for extreme abuse. As human rights scholar Michael Ignatieff, has said, "I don't see any clear way to manage coercive interrogation that does not degenerate into torture."[29]

The impulse to use ever more harsh interrogation in pursuit of intelligence information is strong. And the effort to find a means to reconcile the rights and dignity of human beings with the desire for information often appears compelling. In such an atmosphere, the idea of accompanying harsh interrogation techniques with a range of safeguards is appealing and even seductive. But going down that road will lead to more torture, more devastation to the lives of its victims, and more erosion of human values that should be sacrosanct.

References

1. Physicians for Human Rights. Break Them Down: Systematic Use of Psychological Torture by U.S. Forces. Available at: http://www.physiciansforhumanrights.org/library/report-2005-may.html (accessed June 12, 2007).

1a. Physicians for Human Rights and Human Rights First. Leave No Marks: Enhanced Interrogation Techniques and the Risk of Criminality, 2007. Available at: http://physiciansforhumanrights.org/library/documents/reports/leave-no-marks.pdf (accessed September 10, 2007).

2. Office of the Inspector General of the Department of Defense, Review of DoD-Directed Investigations of Detainee Abuse, dated August 25, 2006. Available at http://www.fas.org/irp/agency/dod/abuse.pdf (accessed July 11, 2007).

2a. Mayer J. The black sites. The New Yorker, August 13, 2007. Available at: http://www.newyorker.com/reporting/2007/08/13/070813fa_fact_mayer (accessed August 31, 2007).

2b. Eban K. Rorschach and awe. Vanity Fair (online) July 17, 2007. Available at: http://www.vanityfair.com/politics/features/2007/07/torture200707 (accessed August 31, 2007).

3. Malinowski T. Banned state department practices. In Roth K, Worden M (eds.). Torture: Does It Make Us Safer? Is It Ever OK? New York: The New Press, 2005.

4. Basoglu M, Jaranson JM, Mollica R, Kastrup M. Torture and mental health. In Gerrity E, Keane TM, Tume F (eds.). The Mental Health Consequences of Torture. New York: Springer, 2001.

5. Luban D. Liberalism, torture, and the ticking bomb. In Greenberg KJ (ed.). The Torture Debate in America. New York: Cambridge University Press, 2006.

6. Memorandum for Alberto Gonzales, re: Standards of Conduct for Interrogation under 18 USC §§2340–2340A, dated August 1, 2002. Available at: http://www .washingtonpost.com/wp-srv/nation/documents/dojinterrogationmemo20020801.pdf (accessed July 11, 2007).

7. U.S. Department of Justice, Office of Legal Counsel. Memorandum for James B. Comey, re: Legal Standards Applicable under 18 USC. 2340–2340A. Available at: http://fl1.findlaw.com/news.findlaw.com/hdocs/docs/terrorism/dojtorture123004mem .pdf (July 11, 2007).

8. Hunter S. This "Road" Leads to Tough Questions. Washington Post, June 23, 2006; p. C1.

9. Heymann P, Kayyem J. Long-Term Legal Strategy Project for Preserving Security and Democratic Freedoms in the War on Terrorism. Available at: http://www.mipt .org/Long-Term-Legal-Strategy.asp (accessed July 11, 2007).

10. Bowden M. The dark art of interrogation. Atlantic Monthly 2003;3:51–76.

11. McCoy AW. A Question of Torture: CIA Interrogation, from the Cold War to the War on Terror. New York: Metropolitan Books, p. 102.

11a. National Defense Intelligence College, Intelligence Science Board. Educing Information. Interrogation: Science and Art, 2006. Available at: http://www.fas.org/irp/ dni/educing.pdf (accessed August 31, 2007).

12. State of Israel. Commission of Inquiry into the Methods of Investigation of the General Security Service Regarding Hostile Terrorist Activity, October 1987. (Excerpts of the official English translations appeared in 23 Isr. L. Rev. (1989) 146. The same volume carries a symposium on the Commission's report.) Cited at: http:// www.ejil.org/journal/Vol8/No4/art4–01.html#P22_2403 (accessed July 19, 2007).

13. B'tselem. Torture: Background on the High Court of Justice's Decision. Available at: http://www.btselem.org/english/torture/background.asp (accessed June 12, 2007).

14. Felner E. Torture and terrorism: Painful lessons from Israel. In Roth K, Worden M (eds.). Torture: Does It Make Us Safer? Is It Ever OK? New York: The New Press, 2005.

15. Public Committee Against Torture v. State of Israel, HCJ 5100/94. Available at: http:// elyon1.court.gov.il/files_eng/94/000/051/a09/94051000.a09.pdf (accessed June 12, 2007).

16. Working Group Report on Detainee Interrogations in the Global War on Terrorism: Assessment of Legal, Historical, Policy and Operational Consideration. Available at: http://www.ccr-ny.org/v2/reports/docs/PentagonReportMarch.pdf (accessed July 13, 2007).

17. Memorandum for Commander, Joint Task Force 170. From Jerald Phifer, LTC, USA, Director J2. Subject: Request for Approval of Counter-Resistance Strategies. October 11, 2002. Available at: http://www.npr.org/documents/2004/dod_prisoners/20040622 doc3.pdf (accessed June 12, 2007).

18. Interview by Major General Taguba, CFLCC Deputy Commanding General, U.S. Army with Colonel Thomas Pappas, Commander, 205th Military Intelligence Brigade. Conducted February 9, 2004, for the Article 15–6 Investigation of the 800th Military Intelligence Brigade. Available at: http://www.publicintegrity.org/docs/AbuGhraib/ Abu14.pdf (accessed July 13, 2007).

19. Detainee Accountability Project. By the Numbers: Findings of the Detainee Abuse and Accountability Project. Available at: http://hrw.org/reports/2006/ct0406 (accessed June 12. 2007).

20. Major General George R. Fay. AR 15–6. Investigation of the Abu Ghraib Detention Facility and 205th Military Intelligence Brigade (Executive Summary). Available at: http://www.defenselink.mil/news/Aug2004/d20040825fay.pdf (accessed June 12, 2007).

21. Van Natta D Jr. Questioning Terror Suspects in a Dark and Secret World. New York Times, March 9, 2003.

22. International Committee of the Red Cross. Report of the International Committee of the Red Cross on the Treatment by the Coalition Forces of Prisoners of War and Other Protected Persons by the Geneva Conventions in Iraq During Arrest, Internment and Interrogation. February 2004. Available at: http://www.globalsecurity .org/military/library/report/2004/icrc_report_iraq_feb2004.htm (accessed June 12, 2007).

23. Lieutenant General Randall Schmidt. Article 15–6 Final Report. Investigation into FBI Allegations of Detainee Abuse at Guantanamo Bay, Cuba Detention Facility. 2005. Available at: www.defenselink.mil/news/Jul2005/d20050714report.pdf (accessed July 11, 2007).

23a. Rubenstein L. First, do no harm: Health professionals and Guantánamo. Seton Hall Law Review 2007;37:733–748.

24. Rubenstein L, Pross C, Davidoff F, Iacopino V. Coercive U.S. interrogation policies: A challenge to medical ethics. JAMA 2005;294;1544–1549.

25. Office of the Army Surgeon General. Final Report: Assessment of Detainee Medical Operations for OEF, GTMO, and OIF. 2005. Available at: www.globalsecurity.org/ military/library/report/2005/detmedopsrpt_13apr2005.pdf (accessed July 11, 2007).

26. Zimbardo P. The Lucifer Effect: Understanding How Good People Turn Evil. New York: Random House, 2007, p. 267–276.

27. Szegedy-Maszak MC. Sources of Sadism. U.S. News & World Report, May 24, 2004.

28. Kelman HC, Hamilton VL. Crimes of Obedience. New Haven, CT: Yale University Press, 1989.

29. Ignatieff M. Moral prohibition at a price. In Roth K, Worden M (eds.). Torture: Does It Make Us Safer? Is It Ever OK? New York: The New Press, 2005.

V

SPECIFIC WARS

15

The Iraq War

Barry S. Levy and Victor W. Sidel

Hundreds of friends, neighbors, and veterans lined the streets here yesterday to mourn the town's first resident to die in combat since the Vietnam War, a car-loving former altar boy named Jared J. Raymond.

Under a fluttering American flag suspended between the ladders of two fire trucks, two chestnut horses pulled a black caisson bearing the remains of Raymond, a 20-year-old U.S. Army specialist who was killed September 19 when an improvised explosive device detonated near the tank he was driving in Iraq.

Dentists in blue scrubs, library workers, elderly people on the senior center porch, firefighters outside a station house, a boys' football team in blue jerseys—all watched as Raymond's flag-draped casket rode past.

People wept, saluted, and waved American flags, as bagpipes played and the caisson proceeded from the church where Raymond was baptized two decades ago to the cemetery where he was buried yesterday.[1]

The Iraq War has had disastrous health consequences. This war needs to be viewed in the context of two previous wars involving Iraq. The first was the Iran–Iraq War from 1980 to 1988, in which the United States sided with Iraq. In that war, between 750,000 and 1 million people were killed, and another 1 to 2 million people were wounded. The Iran–Iraq War uprooted 2.5 million people and destroyed whole cities. It cost more than $200 billion.

The other previous war, the Persian Gulf War, which was fought in 1991, also took a huge toll. Tens of thousands of people died. Many were injured.

And many became chronically ill. But the numbers of deaths and illnesses during this war were far exceeded by those that occurred in the several years after the war. The United Nations Children's Fund (UNICEF) estimated that between 350,000 and 500,000 excessive deaths of children under the age of 5 years occurred in Iraq between 1991 and 1998, largely due to postwar sanctions imposed by the United Nations and enforced by the United States and other countries.[2] (This estimate was based on the assumption that these deaths would not have occurred if the substantial decrease in child mortality during the 1980s in Iraq had continued through the 1990s.) These sanctions restricted food, medicines and medical supplies, and other materials, such as equipment and supplies to ensure clean water, from getting into Iraq for several years, until the Oil-for-Food Program began in 1997. (The Oil-for-Food Program enabled Iraq to export oil worth $10.4 billion a year with which to purchase items to support its civilian population.)

The Iraq War began in March 2003, when U.S. and other Coalition forces invaded Iraq. This was described as a "preemptive" war that was justified by the George W. Bush administration on the grounds that Iraq possessed weapons of mass destruction and had close ties to Al Qaeda (see Box 15-1). Both of these justifications for the war have been proven to be false; in fact, although President Bush has repeatedly considered the Iraq War as the central front in the "war on terror," leading intelligence experts have stated that the Iraq War is increasing terrorism. Military experts, journalists, and others have written extensively on the military and political aspects of the war, including the inadequate basis for the invasion and the incompetent execution of both the war and efforts to rebuild Iraq.[3–5] Others have suggested practical strategies for the United States to end its military presence in Iraq and to rebuild Iraq with a fraction of the resources that are being used to execute the war.[6]

This chapter focuses primarily on the direct and indirect consequences of the war on public health. Two months after the invasion, President Bush declared from the deck of a U.S. aircraft carrier that most hostilities were over. But most health consequences of this war have occurred since then. An outline of the chronology of the war appears in Table 15-1. The status of Iraq, characterized by several parameters, between 2003 and 2006 is shown in Table 15-2.

There are at least seven categories of health consequences of the Iraq War:

- Direct impacts on health
- Adverse effects on health services
- Damage to the infrastructure that supports health
- Refugees and internally displaced persons
- The impact on human rights and the international order
- Diversion of resources
- Impacts on the physical, sociocultural, and economic environments.

Box 15-1 The New American Militarism
Andrew J. Bacevich

We Americans have become infatuated with military power. We have come to have outsized expectations of the efficacy of force. We have come to have a very romantic view of soldiers. We have come to see military power as the preeminent measure of our national greatness. I call this the New American Militarism. It made its appearance during the 1990s and gave rise to the view that we possessed permanent global military supremacy. This was a view shared by neoconservatives as well as liberal Democrats.

But, that was the 1990s. Now it is 2007, and we confront a different reality. Our nation is stuck in an unwinnable war, a war offering no good military or political options. And we are running out of soldiers. How did we so quickly confront the limits of our military power?

1. *These expectations of permanent global military supremacy were based on a very misleading conception of warfare.* In the aftermath of Operation Desert Storm in 1991, national security professionals, both military and nonmilitary, came to see war as the management of target effects, rather than the continuation of politics by other means. War became a matter of putting the right ordnance on the right target—as with "shock and awe" at the beginning of the Iraq War. It became something that "we" did to "them," rather than an interactive process. As a consequence of this flawed view of war, American national security professionals implicitly discounted the entire history of warfare. They persuaded themselves that history had been overturned or rendered irrelevant by the invention of precision weapons and precision targeting. They were therefore unable or unwilling to anticipate the political complications likely to ensue from overturning the existing order in Iraq. Worse still was their failure to grasp the intensely political nature of armed conflict, in which technology plays only a limited role.

2. *In responding to the September 11, 2001, attacks, the Bush administration failed to understand how much our claims of military supremacy rested on the consent of others in the international order.* Our status as the sole superpower after the end of the Cold War depended on the consent of others—on the fact that Western European nations, China, and Russia saw it as in their interests for us to play this role. This paid huge dividends, for example, during Operation Desert Storm, when the United States assembled a broad coalition of nations to eject the Iraqis from Kuwait and to persuade other nations to pay for the war. Our "indispensability" derived not from our omnipotence but from other nations' expectations that we act consistent with their interests—that we would be a responsible, and even conservative, superpower. U.S. actions after 9/11 revealed that we were anything but conservative. Pursuing a revolutionary agenda, the Bush administration launched a pre-

(continued)

ventive war. When other powers saw that we were radical, they sought to punish us, and they did so mainly by refusing to join us in Iraq. We find ourselves in Iraq lacking both adequate numbers of troops and adequate financial support. We are stuck with an enormous bill, which we cannot easily pay.

3. *Our vision of military supremacy discounted the importance of nurturing an intimate and effective relationship between the army and society.* President Bush committed the United States to an open-ended global "war on terror" without making the least effort to mobilize the nation—the first time in our nation's history that we have embarked on a major war without changing the nation's priorities to focus on it. The Bush administration chose not to mobilize the country because it assumed that our existing military forces would suffice. That assumption proved to be wrong. In any nation, military power lies with the people, not with technology.

The implicit contract established at the end of the Vietnam War between Americans and their government remains intact: Military service is a matter of individual choice. Our government no longer possesses authority to require service—even during the global "war on terror." So we still have, as we did on 9/11, approximately 1.4 million soldiers on active duty, even though the nation's population is more than 300 million. This figure of 1.4 million may be near the total number of Americans who are willing to serve in the military. Even if another 100,000 U.S. soldiers in Iraq could guarantee victory in the war, there are not many more volunteer soldiers available, and there is no plausible way of making them available. We indeed are stuck.

Direct Impacts on Health

As of July 11, 2007, 3,610 deaths had occurred among U.S. military personnel in the Iraq War.[7] Of these deaths, 3,470 occurred after President Bush declared, on May 1, 2003, that most hostilities were over, and more than 3,100 of them after the capture of Saddam Hussein. Figure 15-1 shows the number of Coalition and Iraqi police and troop deaths, by month, from the start of the war in March 2003 through June 2007. In addition, as of April 1, 2007, there were at least 917 U.S. government contractors killed in Iraq.[8]

According to the U.S. Department of Defense, 26,558 U.S. military personnel were wounded in Iraq by June 30, 2007—many with serious injuries necessitating amputation of limbs or causing long-term disability (Figure 15-2).[7] At least another 30,000 suffered significant injuries or illnesses.[9] In addition, as of April 1, 2007, more than 12,000 government contractors in Iraq had been wounded in battle or injured on the job.[8] Several physicians and other health professionals who have treated military personnel and others during the war

Table 15-1. Timeline of Selected Events of the War in Iraq

	2003
March	• Coalition air attacks begin.
April	• Baghdad is captured by Coalition forces.
	• Saddam Hussein's statue is pulled down.
	• Gen. Tommy Franks expects a pullout of all but 30,000 of 110,000 Coalition troops by September.
May	• President George W. Bush announces the end of major combat operations in Iraq, while standing before a banner reading "Mission Accomplished."
	• Economic sanctions on Iraq are lifted. Looting sweeps across Iraq; U.S. troops do little to intervene.
	• L. Paul Bremer, head of the U.S.-led occupation government, bans Ba'ath Party members from top positions in politics or education and orders the Iraq army disbanded; these actions fuel widespread resentment, unemployment, and a budding insurgency.
	• Plans to turn control over to Iraqis by the summer are put on hold.
July–August	• Lt. Gen. Ricardo Sanchez takes command of all ground forces in Iraq, but seems unprepared for the random bombings, assassinations, sniping, and growing signs of a guerilla war.
	• First meeting of the Iraqi Governing Council.
	• Saddam Hussein's sons are killed.
	• U.N. headquarters in Baghdad is destroyed by a truck bomb; large car bomb explodes outside Jordanian embassy, killing 17.
	• Increasing scale of insurgents' attacks puts Iraqis on edge.
September	• Madrid Donors Conference pledges about $2 billion per year for reconstruction.
	• Bremer outlines a multiyear plan for rebuilding Iraq, which is rebuffed by the Bush administration and the Pentagon.
November–December	• First U.S. helicopter is downed.
	• Oil-for-Food Program ends.
	• Saddam Hussein is captured.

	2004
January–February	• Organized insurgency, aiming to derail democracy in Iraq, grows, with increased attacks and suicide bombings.
March	• Interim constitution is signed.
April–May	• Four U.S. contractors are killed in Fallujah and their burned bodies are dragged through the streets.
	• U.S. military attacks insurgents in Fallujah, but 3 days into the battle, with outrage over civilian casualties threatening political stability, the attack is called off.
	• Shi'ite uprisings occur in several southern cities.
	• *60 Minutes II* breaks the story of U.S. soldiers' abuse and torture of Iraqis at Abu Ghraib prison; brutal abuse of Iraqi detainees there and elsewhere alienate the Iraqi people.
	• Bremer asks U.S. Secretary of Defense Donald Rumsfeld for 40,000 more troops; Rumsfeld does not reply.

(continued)

	2004
June	• Bremer hands over sovereignty to an appointed Iraqi interim government.
November	• U.S. forces again attack Fallujah, which has again become a safe haven for Sunni insurgents; over 10 days of battle, at least 1,000 insurgents, 54 Americans, and 8 Iraqi soldiers are killed and many more are wounded.
	• A U.S. Marine is videotaped killing an unarmed man inside a mosque.

	2005
January	• Elections are held for the 275-seat Transitional National Assembly; an estimated 58% of Iraq's population votes, but almost all Sunnis boycott the election and are disenfranchised from the political process, dashing hopes of establishing a representative Iraqi government.
February	• Sunni insurgents increase attacks in an effort to undermine the government.
March	• Training Iraqi forces becomes a U.S. priority.
April	• New Iraqi government is approved by parliament.
May	• U.S. troops adopt a new policy of clearing insurgents door-to-door, holding neighborhoods by stationing troops among the people, and rebuilding by distributing construction funds to Iraqis.
June	• President Bush focuses on strategy of training Iraqis to take charge of their country's security.
October	• Despite the opposition of Sunnis, the Iraqi constitution is ratified in a national referendum.
	• Rumsfeld refutes U.S. Secretary of State Condoleezza Rice's position of "clear, hold, and build," asserting Iraqis must be the ones to hold and build.
November	• 24 Iraqi noncombatants in Haditha, including 11 women and children, are reportedly killed by 12 U.S. Marines.

	2006
February	• Bombs destroy the golden dome of the Askariya Mosque in Samarra, one of Shi'a Islam's holiest shrines, igniting a wave of sectarian violence, increasingly perceived as a civil war, in which thousands of Iraqis will die over many months.
March	• Congress announces the creation of the Iraq Study Group, chaired by former U.S. Secretary of State James Baker III and former Indiana Representative Lee Hamilton.
May	• The United States promises to hand over Baghdad security to the Iraqis by the end of the year.
June	• Meeting is held at Camp David to review Iraq war strategy; midway through meeting, President Bush decides to fly to Baghdad to meet the new Iraqi Prime Minister, Nouri al-Maliki.
	• Prime Minister Maliki announces new plan to stem bloodshed in Baghdad with curfews, checkpoints, and Iraqi-led patrols.

(continued)

Table 15-1. (*continued*)

	2006
August	• Random violence plagues Baghdad; violence actually increases in areas handed over to Iraqi forces.
	• Marine Corps intelligence memo concludes that the United States can no longer defeat the insurgency in western Iraq or counter the popularity of Al Qaeda in that area.
November	• Coordinated car bombs kill 144 and wound 200 in the Shi'ite Sadr City section of Baghdad, the bloodiest single day in the capital since the 2003 invasion.
	• U.S. National Security Adviser Stephen Hadley states that much of the sectarian violence links back to the Shi'a-dominated government and Shi'a militia forces.
December	• President Bush states for the first time that the United States is not winning the war in Iraq.
	• Iraq Study Group releases its report calling the situation "grave and deteriorating," and recommending diplomacy with Iraq's neighbors and the handing over of security to Iraqi forces so U.S. troops can withdraw by early 2008.
	• Saddam Hussein is executed.
	2007
January	• President Bush announces a new plan, a surge of 20,000 troops, to secure Baghdad.
April	• Suicide bombings continue, one of which targets the Parliament cafeteria inside the Green Zone, injuring 22 and killing a member of Parliament.
	• Nearly 200 people are killed in a series of bombings in Baghdad on one day, the deadliest in the capital since the start of the U.S. troop surge.
June	• The minarets of the Askariya Mosque in Samarra are taken down by bombs; shortly thereafter, U.S. and Iraqi forces begin a major offensive against Sunni insurgents in and around Baghdad.

Source: Adapted from "Timeline Struggling to Find a Strategy for Success in Iraq." Frontline, WGBH, Public Broadcasting System. Available at: http://www.pbs.org/wgbh/pages/frontline/ngame/cron/ (accessed July 11, 2007).

have written detailed accounts.[10] Although many returning U.S. military personnel who were severely wounded have received highly advanced medical care for their injuries in the United States, others have not received adequate care for their physical or mental disorders, even at the Walter Reed Army Medical Center.[11] Many people believe that the medical care system for returning U.S. military personnel did not adequately anticipate the number and severity of wounds and other injuries among veterans of the Iraq War.

Table 15-2. The State of Iraq: An Update

	August 2003	August 2004	August 2005	August 2006
U.S. troop fatalities	36	65	90	63
U.S. troops wounded	181	891	608	641
Iraqi security force fatalities	65	65	282	233
Iraqi civilian deaths from violence	700	1,500	2,000	3,000
Multifatality bombings	4	13	27	52
Foreigners kidnapped	0	30	24	0
Internally displaced persons (since April 2003)	100,000	200,000	250,000	500,000
Attacks on oil assets	5	21	9	2
U.S./other Coalition troops in Iraq (in thousands)	139/22	140/24	138/23	140/19
Iraqi security forces (in thousands)	35	91	183	298
Iraqi security forces in top two readiness tiers (out of four; in thousands)	0	0	30	100
Oil production (in millions of barrels per day; prewar peak: 2.5)	1.4	2.1	2.2	2.2
Household and transport fuel supplies (as percentage of estimated need)	57	84	96	71
Average electricity production (in megawatts; prewar: 4,000)	3,300	4,700	4,000	4,400
Trained judges (estimated need: 1,500)	0	200	350	750
Registered cars (in millions; prewar: 1.5)	1.5	2.0	3.0	3.5
Children in school (in millions; prewar: 4.6)	4.6	4.8	5.1	5.2
Iraqis optimistic about the future (percent)	60	51	43	41

Source: Kamp N, O'Hanlon M, Unikewicz A. The State of Iraq: An Update. New York Times, October 1, 2006, p. 11.

There has been a high incidence of mental health disorders among U.S. troops. The Surgeon General of the U.S. Army estimated that 30 percent of troops surveyed described stress-related mental health problems during the 3 to 4 months after coming home from the Iraq War (see Chapter 4).[12] A study of U.S. Army and Marine personnel who completed routine postdeployment health assessments between May 2003 and April 2004 found that 19.1 percent

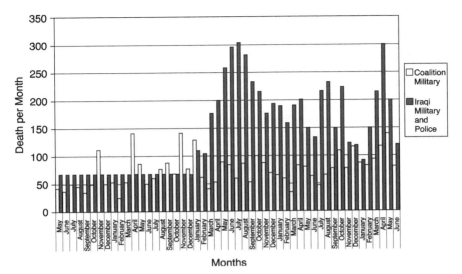

Figure 15-1. Coalition and Iraqi troop deaths, Iraq War, May 2003 to June 2007. (Data on Iraqi troop deaths averaged for May 2003–December 2004 period.) (Source: Richard Garfield.)

of service members returning from Iraq reported mental health problems, and 35 percent of Iraq war veterans used mental health services during the year after they returned home.[13] Another study of U.S. Army and Marine Corps personnel found that approximately 16 percent of those returning from duty in Iraq had responses that met the screening criteria for major depression, generalized anxiety, or posttraumatic stress disorder (PTSD).[14] Related to the clinical aspects of these mental health problems are family and social pathology, including family violence, divorce, behavioral problems in children, and unemployment, and financial burdens on returning veterans.

The health consequences of the Iraq War have been profound—more profound than statistics alone can convey. As we have often said, "Statistics are people with the tears washed off." Boxes 15-2 and 15-3 provide personal accounts of the suffering of U.S. military personnel and their loved ones. Articles in medical journals, newspapers, and elsewhere have also detailed the personal tragedies of military personnel and their families.[15,15a]

The toll on Iraqis has been many times greater than that on U.S. military personnel (Figure 15-3). Figure 15-4 provides a count-based estimate of attacks and Iraqi noncombatant deaths by month from May 2003 to February 2007.

Two studies were performed by researchers at Johns Hopkins University, Columbia University, and the Al Mustan Siraya University College of Medicine in Baghdad, one in September 2004 and the other between May and July

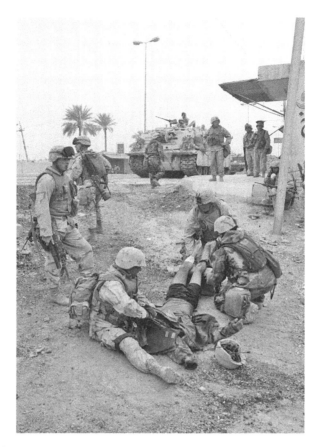

Figure 15-2. U.S. Marines of the 3rd Battalion, 4th Marines, attend to a colleague badly wounded by artillery fire on the Baghdad Highway Bridge in April 2003. (Source: Associated Press Photo: Gary Knight/VII.)

2006.[16,17] The 2004 study was based on a systematic sample survey of almost 1,000 households. Using statistically conservative assumptions, the researchers estimated that about 100,000 excess deaths had occurred among Iraqis since the 2003 invasion. The study also found that most of the excess deaths were among women and children, that the risk of violent death had increased more than 50-fold since the invasion, and that most of these violent deaths were the result of air strikes by Coalition forces.[16]

The 2006 survey estimated that there had been 654,965 (confidence interval: 392,979–942,636) excess Iraqi deaths since the 2003 invasion, approximately 600,000 as a result of violence, most commonly gunfire.[17] The study was based on a national cross-sectional cluster sample survey; 50 clusters were randomly selected, each consisting of 40 households. The study found

Box 15-2 A Soldier's View
Garett Reppenhagen

I was a sniper in Iraq. What I experienced in Iraq directly conflicted with what I was told my mission was supposed to be. This war can be described as "a body parts war," with multiple-fatality bombings, suicide bombings, vehicle bombs, improvised explosive devices, and rocket-propelled grenades that come out of nowhere and sever body parts. I have friends in Walter Reed Army Hospital who are missing arms and legs—all too common injuries. The violence is unimaginable. And there is no front line in this war and no enemy to retaliate against. It is frustrating and stressful. We were isolated on bases that were constantly under mortar attack, and we always had to keep up force protection to ensure base security. No time to rest. No opportunity to get a beer.

Since I've been back, I visit my friends at Walter Reed. One explained to me how he dreams at night. He lost his arm from the elbow down and he lost the use of one of his legs. He dreams every night that his arm is back. When he wakes up in the morning he has to relive the tragedy of losing his arm as he tries to lift himself out of bed. Another friend had his face surgically reconstructed after it was blown apart with shrapnel and severely burned. He looks gruesome. When I spoke to him at Walter Reed, he told me that when he was high school, if he had a pimple, he might stay at home because he was afraid of ridicule and rejection. Now he says, "Look at me. How am I going to go to a job interview? How am I going to go out on a date?" I have seen a lot of these guys start to overcome their disabilities, but eventually what they can't seem to get past are the questions "Why me? Why was I disabled? Why do I look like this? Why do I have mental health problems?" They search for meaning—the basic psychological protection for doing your job in a war. Many of the soldiers who come to Walter Reed severely injured hold onto this ideal to keep themselves sane. If you ask most of the soldiers at Walter Reed if they think they did the right thing in Iraq, they are going to say, "Yeah! Damn right I did!" It is hard to face the soldiers and tell them the truth.

Most of these soldiers don't necessarily have posttraumatic stress disorder. They are considered to have preexisting conditions, so the military is not responsible for their mental health disorders. They are told that they have personality, adjustment, or anxiety disorders that are not considered serviced-related disabilities because they cannot prove there was an incident—a stressor—that caused them psychological damage.

Many of these soldiers feel that they are not victims, but victimizers, criminals, thieves, murderers. But there is no diagnosis for this, and they are shooed away. Because they are not punished by society like criminals, these soldiers often punish themselves—consciously or not—through alcoholism or drug addiction. They abuse members of their families and communities.

(continued)

253

Box 15-2 (*continued*)

Sometimes they kill themselves because they can't find resolution, they can't forgive themselves.

I went to my chaplain the first time I killed an innocent civilian. (The chaplain is not only a religious leader, but also in charge of the battalion's psychological well-being.) I told him that I was frustrated and angry because of what I had done. He told me that I did it because it was the will of God, because it was for democracy. I realized he had premanufactured meaning for me. I have a right to be angry. And this is not only my problem. It is society's problem as well. It is a political problem that cannot be diagnosed psychologically. It is a problem with the reason—the meaning—why I was there. These are some of the costs of war. If we, as a society, can't afford to pay these costs, then we shouldn't have gone to war.

Now, I'm involved in Iraq Veterans Against the War, because it allows me to speak about what I did in Iraq. It allows me to say that I am not that person anymore; I have changed and I will not do it again. And it allows me to empower myself to help others and to help improve the situation in Iraq. Three religious ideals are confession, repentance, and atonement. I am not very religious, but I believe that confession, repentance, and atonement are healing me and can heal our society.

Box 15-3 A Perspective from Military Families
Elizabeth Frederick

I am a member of Military Families Speak Out, an organization of more than 3,000 families nationwide who have loved ones who are serving, have served, or have been killed in Iraq, and who are opposed to the war in Iraq.

The mental effects of this war have hit very close to home. My soldier came home 3 months ago. I had hoped that the stress of his being in a war zone would now be gone. But I quickly learned that it was replaced with a different kind of stress: having him physically home but mentally absent. He was not the same person who left a year before.

I am not an expert in posttraumatic stress disorder. But I've learned about it by reading books and materials provided by the Veterans Administration and talking to other family members who are going through the same thing. But I still feel uninformed and usually not very helpful. The books can tell me that sleeping disorders are common, but they can't tell me if or when they will go away. They also can't tell me what I'm supposed to do when my distressed soldier can't fall asleep at night. They can't tell me how to get over my exhaustion, because when he is not sleeping, I don't sleep either. Both of us end up being restless and exhausted.

(*continued*)

The books can't tell me how to react when he wakes up in the middle of the night to tell me that even though he came back, the man I fell in love with died in Iraq. The V.A. can't tell me how to keep it together when he tells me that he feels dead inside and that he won't blame me if I want to leave and find someone else. Books can't tell me how to keep him from drinking himself to sleep every night. Books can't tell me how to react to his not having been sober for two consecutive days since he has been home. And books can't tell me how to stay calm when I know that on one occasion he seriously considered taking his own life.

Why doesn't he get help from the military? Another soldier's words perhaps hold the answer: "You live a violent year in a hellish place. And when you get back, you feel such animosity for the people who put you there that you don't want to stay there and ask for their help. You want to get away from the people you hate and go home to the people you love."

For us, it's been a matter of learning as we go, trying to figure out what works and what doesn't, and suppressing the rage we feel because this war has thrown the two of us into this situation. This war has taken my healthy, happy soldier and returned him as a broken shell of a human being who may get better with time—or not. I just have to wait and see and hope for the best. Although my soldier experiences nightmares, flashbacks, and other mental health problems, his struggle is mine and our family's as well.

The physical effects of war are just as challenging to deal with. A soldier whom I know conducted missions at an old chemical plant in northern Iraq. The command thought that it would be a perfect hiding place for insurgents. U.S. soldiers spent about 10 hours at a time there, watching roads and looking for insurgents, while sitting on waste and breathing it in. The fumes made them dizzy. And they went back there often. When they were preparing to come home, these soldiers completed questionnaires but were not tested for effects of this exposure. They may not know for another 20 or more years if what they were exposed to in Iraq will have any lasting health effects.

We Americans need to decide if we would be willing to personally bear the costs of war, or if we are content with sending others to bear them on our behalf. If Americans weighed these costs more carefully and fully understood them, perhaps we wouldn't find ourselves engaged in wars of choice.

---

that pre-invasion mortality rates were 5.5 per 1,000 people per year, compared with 13.3 per 1,000 per year during the first 40 months after the invasion. Although U.S. government leaders questioned the methods used in these surveys, highly respected epidemiologists confirmed the reliability of the methods.[17a]

Child mortality has soared. In 1990, Iraq's mortality rate for children under 5 years of age was 50 per 1,000 live births. In 2005, it was 125 per 1,000—a 150 percent increase, the highest increase of any country.[18]

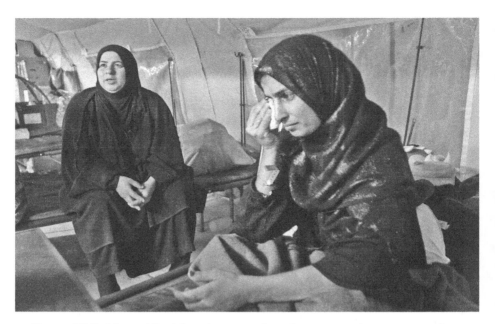

Figure 15-3. Metaq Ali, right, wipes tears from her eyes as she recuperates from injuries to her legs at a U.S. Army combat surgical hospital in April 2003 at an air base near Nasiriyah, while her sister Sahar Ali talks about Metaq's husband, who died when he was caught in a crossfire between Iraqi and U.S. forces during fighting in Nasiriyah. Metaq was wounded in the crossfire that killed her husband. (Source: Associated Press Photo/Julie Jacobson.)

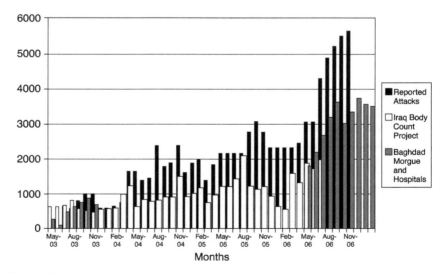

Figure 15-4. Count-based estimate of attacks and Iraqi noncombatant deaths, by source of data, Iraq War, May 2003 to February 2007. (Reported attack information not available for last 3 months.) (Source: Richard Garfield.)

There have been many reports of brutal treatment of civilians by U. S. soldiers. Iraq War veterans have provided vivid accounts of indiscriminate killings of Iraqi civilians.[19] (See Box 1–1 in Chapter 1.)

During the past 15 years, there has been significant childhood malnutrition in Iraq. The prevalence peaked during the mid-1990s, largely due to the sanctions on importing food and medicine. Although malnutrition among children was lower in 2006 than in the mid-1990s, about one-fourth of Iraqi children were, at that time, chronically malnourished, and many more were underweight.[20]

Adverse Effects on Health Services

Health services in Iraq have been profoundly affected by the war. During the initial phase of the war, for example, only two of the hospital emergency departments in Baghdad were functioning. During 2003, approximately 12 percent of hospitals and many other health care facilities were damaged. The two major public health laboratories were damaged and looted. Access to health services has often been restricted, largely due to security issues and inadequate financial resources. Public health programs have also been adversely affected. Initially, there were shortages of essential medications. The cold chain for vaccines as well as vaccine administration were often disrupted. Looting caused extensive damage to equipment and vehicles. And many health workers have left Iraq.[21]

Damage to the Infrastructure That Supports Health

During both the Persian Gulf War and the Iraq War, much damage has been inflicted on water treatment and sewage treatment facilities, which has led to a high incidence of gastrointestinal illness, including many cases of fatal diarrhea in children. In some periods, approximately half a million tons of raw and partially treated sewage have been dumped daily into rivers in Iraq. Food security has been an issue: at least one-fourth of Iraqis have at times been dependent on the distribution of free food. Power generation has been unpredictable. Transportation and communication systems have been damaged or have broken down. And all of this has led to serious health consequences.[21]

Refugees and Internally Displaced Persons

Worldwide, there are about 12 million refugees, many having become so as a result of war. The Persian Gulf War created about 500,000 refugees; in Jordan alone, there may have been as many as 400,000, and some are still there. During the Iraq War, there have been 2 million refugees, but only a small fraction of them have been officially recognized by the United Nations High Commission on Refugees. In addition, approximately 2 million people have been internally displaced within Iraq, and they have often faced greater risk to their health than have refugees who left the country (Figure 15-5).[22] In contrast to the U.S. policy on refugees from Vietnam at the end of the Vietnam War, few refugees from Iraq have been permitted to enter the United States. (See Chapter 13.)

The Impact on Human Rights and the International Order

During the regime of Saddam Hussein, there were numerous serious human rights violations. Many people were killed. Many became political prisoners. Many human rights were violated. We may never know the full extent of

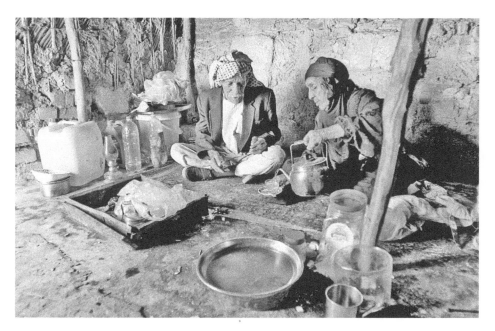

Figure 15-5. Khayriya Shallal pours tea for her husband Hussein Shawkat, both refugees from Fallujah, at their makeshift home at what had been Saddam Hussein's Republican guard barracks in Baghdad, which were destroyed in the U.S bombing at the start of the invasion in 2003. At these barracks, 150 families displaced by sectarian violence and war took refuge. (Source: Associated Press Photo/Samir Mizban.)

these violations.[23] That being said, we want to comment on four sets of human rights violations during the Iraq War:

1. Many experts believe that this war violated the United Nations Charter, weakened the U.N. system, and set a dangerous precedent for the future.
2. At Abu Ghraib and other prisons, detainees have been physically tortured and psychologically abused. This has taken the form of beatings, stress positions, food and sleep deprivation, exposure to extremes of heat and cold, sensory deprivation, isolation, exposure to loud noise, forced nudity, use of dogs to instill fear, cultural and sexual humiliation, waterboarding and other forms of mock execution, and threats of violent death.[24] This torture and abuse has led to many health problems, including memory loss, difficulty in concentration, headaches, back pain, irritability, depression, nightmares, feelings of shame or humiliation, PTSD, and death[24] (see Chapters 4 and 14).
3. Women's rights have been adversely affected. Before the war, women in Iraq had more access to educational and professional opportunities than most other women in the Arab world. Those opportunities are far fewer today (see Chapter 11).
4. Freedom of speech has been curtailed. Laws in Iraq criminalize speech that ridicules the government or its officials, and several Iraqi journalists have been criminally charged under these laws with offending public officials.[25]

Diversion of Resources

More than 50 years ago, President Dwight D. Eisenhower said: "Every gun that is made, every warship launched, every rocket signifies, in the final sense, a theft from those who hunger and are not fed, those who are cold and not clothed."[26] The following are three examples of diversion of resources related to the Iraq War:

1. According to the U.S. Department of Defense, as of April 30, 2007, more than 425,000 members of the National Guard and Reservists had been deployed to Iraq or Afghanistan since 2001, for an average mobilization of 18 months.[27] Many police, firefighters, emergency medical technicians, and other first responders in communities across the United States are members of the National Guard, and their communities have felt the absence of those who have served or are serving

in Iraq or Afghanistan. This became readily apparent in August 2005, when Hurricane Katrina struck. Many National Guard troops who could have been there to help were not available. They and their equipment were in Iraq.

2. Resources used to fight the Iraq War could have been used for health and human services at home, especially during a period when there have been dramatic cuts in these services. The $442 billion spent for the Iraq War by July 11, 2007, could have been used in the United States to provide education, housing, medical care, or other services, such as one of the following[28]:
   - Build almost 4 million additional housing units
   - Enable more than 58 million children to attend 1 year of Head Start
   - Hire more than 7.5 million public school teachers for 1 year
   - Provide more than 21 million students with 4-year scholarships at public universities
   - Provide health insurance for more than 65 million children for 4 years.

3. The $442 billion spent on the Iraq War by July 11, 2007, could have been used internationally for all of the following: to eliminate world hunger and to provide for all developing countries, for 6 years, with enough medicines to treat HIV/AIDS, enough immunizations for all children, and enough clean water and sanitation for hundreds of millions of people in need.[29]

Impacts on the Physical, Sociocultural, and Economic Environments

There have been many adverse impacts on the physical environment. About 10 to 12 million landmines and units of unexploded ordnance have been strewn throughout Iraq. About 8,000 barrels of hazardous substances have been stolen or destroyed. The fragile desert ecology has been disrupted by tanks, military encampments, and battles. And between 1,000 and 2,000 tons of toxic and radioactive depleted uranium (DU), which is used to harden shells and shell casings to permit them to penetrate armor, have been used in Iraq by American and British forces during the war. Radioactive and toxic uranium constitutes a widespread and long-lasting threat to health.[21]

The sociocultural environment has also been adversely affected. In Iraq, there has been damage to religious and cultural institutions, looting of the National Museum, a substantial increase in crime, and disruption of everyday life. Here in the United States, there have also been many adverse sociocultural impacts, such as the tripling of divorces among U.S. Army officers. In addition, the war has served as an example to other nations and to people everywhere that violence is an acceptable way to settle disputes.

Finally, the war has adversely affected the economic environment. For Iraq, there has been high unemployment and lagging oil production. For the United States, $442 billion had been spent on the war by July 2007, and was costing the country more than $2 billion a week. The total cost of the war could surpass $2 trillion,[30] making it the most expensive U.S. military effort since World War II—much more expensive than the Vietnam War.

In sum, the Iraq War has damaged health directly, adversely affected health services, damaged the infrastructure that supports health, made millions of people refugees or internally displaced persons, violated human rights and the international order, diverted resources, and adversely affected the physical, sociocultural, and economic environments.

Comparisons between the Vietnam War and the Iraq War

Although, as of July 2007, the Vietnam War had lasted considerably longer and led to many more civilian and military deaths and nonfatal war injuries than the Iraq War, there are striking similarities between these two wars (see also Chapter 19):

- Both wars were launched for questionable reasons that were later proven to be false, and were continued with overoptimistic assessments.
- Both led to massive numbers of civilian casualties.
- In both wars, many U.S. troops returned with long-term health problems, including widespread psychological problems that necessitated both treatment and measures to integrate these individuals into society.
- In both wars, weapons considered illegal or questionable under international law were used (DU in the Iraq War, and Agent Orange in the Vietnam War).
- In both wars, there were violations of the Geneva Conventions, with confirmed reports of killing of innocent civilians and torture of detainees.
- In both wars, there were calls by many active-duty U.S. military personnel for the withdrawal of U.S. troops and large antiwar protests by the public (larger and more numerous during the Vietnam War).
- In both wars, there were incursions or threats of incursions into neighboring countries (Iran and Cambodia) in which there were alleged routes of weapons.
- And, during both wars, professional organizations such as the American Public Health Association adopted policy statements opposing the war and urging the withdrawal of U.S. troops.[31]

Conclusion

As of July 2007, there were many unanswered questions about the future of the Iraq War. These questions included the ongoing involvement of U.S. and other Coalition forces as well as the potential impact of the war to adversely affect, and possibly destabilize, other countries in the region. But whatever the ultimate outcome of the war, its disastrous impact on the health of military personnel and especially Iraqi noncombatant civilians has been enormous.

Acknowledgment: The authors of this chapter acknowledge Richard Garfield, R.N., Dr.P.H., for his assistance in and contributions to the development of this chapter.

References

1. Levenson M. Swampscott mourns a son. Boston Globe, September 29, 2006, p. 1.
2. United Nations Children's Fund (UNICEF). Information Newsline: Iraq surveys show "humanitarian emergency." Available at http://www.unicef.org/newsline/99pr29.htm (accessed July 12, 2007).
3. Ricks TE. Fiasco: The American Military Adventure in Iraq. New York: The Penguin Press, 2006.
4. Woodward B. State of Denial: Bush at War, Part III. New York: Simon & Schuster, 2006.
5. Fallows J. Blind Into Baghdad: America's Iraq War. New York: Vintage Books, 2006.
6. McGovern GS, Polk WR. The way out of war. Harper's Magazine 2006; 313: 31–39.
7. Iraq Coalition Casualty Count. Available at: http://icasualties.org/oif (accessed July 11, 2007).
8. Broder JM, Risen J. Death toll for contractors reaches new high in Iraq. New York Times, May 19, 2007. Available at: http://www.truthout.org/docs_2006/051907Z .shtml (accessed July 20, 2007).
9. Grady D. Agency says higher casualty total was posted in error. New York Times, January 30, 2007. Available at: http://www.nytimes.com (accessed June 19, 2007).
10. Jadick R with Hayden T. On Call in Hell: A Doctor's Iraq War Story. New York: New American Library, 2007.
11. Priest D, Hull A. Soldiers face neglect, frustration at Army's top medical facility. Washington Post, February 18, 2007. Available at: http://www.washingtonpost.com (accessed June 19, 2007).
12. Survey: 30% of returning Iraq veterans suffer mental ills. USA Today, July 28, 2005. Available at: http://www.usatoday.com/news/health/2005-07–28-Iraq-vets-health_x .htm (accessed July 11, 2007).
13. Hoge CW, Auchterlonie JL, Milliken CS. Mental health problems, use of mental health services, and attrition from military service after returning from deployment to Iraq or Afghanistan. JAMA 2006;295:1023–1032.
14. Hoge CW, Castro CA, Messer SC, et al. Combat duty in Iraq and Afghanistan, mental health problems, and barriers to care. N Engl J Med 2004;351:13–22.

15. Okie S. Reconstructing lives: A tale of two soldiers. N Engl J Med 2006;355:2609–2615.

15a. Carter B. The price of war, front and center: James Gandolfini sits down with scarred survivors of Iraq. New York Times, September 6, 2007, pp. B1, B8.

16. Roberts L, Lafta R, Garfield R, et al. Mortality before and after the 2003 invasion of Iraq: Cluster sample survey. Lancet 2004;364:1857–1864.

17. Burnham G, Lafta R, Doocy S, Roberts L. Mortality after the 2003 invasion of Iraq: A cross-sectional cluster sample survey. Lancet 2006;368:1421–1428.

17a. Reactions to the study. Iraqanalysis.org. Available at: http://www.iraqanalysis.org/mortality/441#faq1628 (accessed September 12, 2007).

18. Buncombe A. Infant mortality in Iraq soars, report says. The Independent, May 8, 2007. Available at: http://www.wunrn.com/news/2007/05_07/05_21_07/052807_iragq.htm (accessed July 19, 2007).

19. Hedges C, Al-Arian L. Confessions from U.S. soldiers in Iraq on the brutal treatment of civilians. The Nation, July 17, 2007. Available at: http://www.alternet.org/module/printversion/56761 (accessed July 17, 2007).

20. World Vision. Iraq: Children Caught Up in War. Available at: http://meero.worldvision.org/sf_iraq.php (accessed July 10, 2007).

21. Medact. Enduring Effects of War: Health in Iraq 2004. London: Medact, 2004.

22. Refugees International. Iraqi refugees in Syria: Silent exodus leaves 500,000 in need of protection and aid. Available at: http://www.reliefweb.int/rw/RWB.NSF/db900SID/KKEE-6J6TEL (accessed June 19, 2007).

23. Amnesty International. Decades of human rights abuse in Iraq. Available at: http://web.amnesty.org/pages/irq-article_3-eng (accessed June 19, 2007).

24. Physicians for Human Rights. Break Them Down: Systematic Use of Psychological Torture by US Forces. Cambridge, MA: Physicians for Human Rights, 2005.

25. von Zielbauer P. Iraqi journalists add laws to list of war dangers. New York Times, September 29, 2006, p. A1, A12.

26. Eisenhower D. Speech before the American Society of Newspapers Editors, April 16, 1953.

27. Tyson AS. Possible Iraq deployments would stretch reserve force. Washington Post, November 5, 2006, p. A01.

28. National Priorities Project. The War in Iraq Costs. Available at: http://www.nationalpriorities.org/costofwar/index-public-education.html (accessed July 11, 2007).

29. Bennis P, Leaver E, Institute for Policy Studies (IPS) Iraq Task Force. The Iraq Quagmire: The Mounting Costs of War and the Case for Bringing Home the Troops. Washington, DC: Institute for Policy Studies and Foreign Policy in Focus, 2005.

30. Regan T. Report: Iraq war costs could top $2 trillion. Christian Science Monitor, January 10, 2006. Available at: http://www.csmonitor.com/2006/0110/dailyUpdate.html (accessed July 11, 2007).

31. Opposition to the Continuation of the Iraq War. APHA policy statement 2006–17. Washington, DC: American Public Health Association, 2006.

16

The War in Chechnya

Khassan Baiev

In August 1994, when Russia massed thousands of troops along the border of its breakaway republic of Chechnya, I was a 31-year-old surgeon in Moscow. I left my surgical career in Moscow then to aid my Chechen countrymen, who I knew would need my expertise.

When the hospital where I worked in Grozny, the capital of Chechnya, was destroyed by Russian shelling, I returned to my nearby hometown of Alkhan Kala and restored an abandoned clinic with help from villagers. Soon I was the only doctor for tens of thousands of residents and refugees in the area. During 6 years of war and intermittent ceasefire, I often worked without gas, electricity, or running water; with only local anesthetics; and dressed wounds with sour cream or egg yolks when supplies ran out. My nurses and I would routinely donate blood for surgical operations. I once performed 67 amputations in 3 days.

The two recent conflicts between the Russian Government and Chechen separatists have killed 20 percent of the Chechen population of 1 million people, made homeless another 350,000 people, and caused the deaths of thousands of Russian soldiers. This chapter is one Chechen physician's account of these conflicts. It was excerpted, with permission, from Baiev K, with Daniloff R and Daniloff N. The Oath: A Surgeon Under Fire. New York: Walker & Company, 2003.

I also worked under a constant threat of execution. Although I mainly treated civilians, I also cared for both Russian soldiers and Chechen rebels, never allowing politics to interfere with my commitment to the Hippocratic oath. For this, both the Russian special forces and Chechen extremists branded me a traitor, and I was kidnapped and nearly killed on several occasions. Each time, with an ever-increasing dedication to the wounded and indifference to my own safety, I returned to my operating room.

The following are some of my experiences during this conflict.

On January 17, 1995, a missile struck the roof of the hospital at 9:30 A.M. I was in the operating room on the first floor along with another doctor, a refugee from Grozny who arrived a week earlier, and two nurses. We were bandaging the leg of a local Chechen fighter. The detonation was terrifying, shattering windows, shaking the walls, and bringing down the roof. We all threw ourselves facedown on the floor. I cradled my head in my hands. I couldn't breathe. Plaster dust clogged my throat, and debris rained down on my back. Another explosion; a woman screamed, followed by the thud of falling beams. I may have passed out—I was not sure. I pressed my body to the floor until the explosions subsided, then staggered to my feet. Stars flashed before my eyes, or maybe it was dust, and I felt dizzy. The door of the operating room lay on the floor. An icy wind whipped through the open windows, flapping the shreds of curtains Zulai had made for us.

I looked around for the nurses and the doctor. I saw one nurse lying unconscious in the corner. I struggled to stand up and hurried over to her, my feet crunching the broken glass. I placed my thumbs in the cavity behind her ears and pressed down. Her eyes flashed open. Then I placed my thumb and forefinger on either side of her brows just above the nose and applied pressure. I had learned about the acupuncture pressure points from a book on Chinese medicine and often used them when a person passed out on the operating table. After she came to, I pulled her to her feet, and together we went out into the corridor, holding on to the wall for balance. The other nurse and doctor had escaped to safety and left for Urus-Martan.

"Anyone there?" I shouted. On the other side of the building, more screams. "Is anyone there?" I repeated. No reply, only the sound of falling plaster and the thud of distant guns. I felt disoriented as if in a nightmare, feeling I would soon wake up. I stumbled to the window overlooking the courtyard and looked out. Below I saw two men unloading someone from a car and carrying the person into the hospital.

"Where's Khassan?" a voice shouted.

I felt my way along the corridor, stepping over the piles of plaster and broken glass. I rounded the corner, and there on the floor not far from the entrance lay wounded men, their blood trickling onto the broken glass and plaster on the floor.

"Doctor, can you help?" a woman called out.

I looked over at the wounded men. There must have been seven or eight of them. I had treated hundreds of emergency cases but always with help and never all at once like this. Fear gripped me. My chest tightened, and I had trouble breathing. I had no idea what to do. It was as though I had forgotten everything I had learned in medical school, as though I had never seen a wounded person before. I was so confused, I didn't know where to start, whom to treat first. At any moment the hospital could take another hit, I thought. I wanted to clap my hands over my ears to muffle the groans of pain and run from the hospital.

"Khassan, you are losing control," I told myself. I took a deep breath. I had to pull myself together. I couldn't leave. The wounded were waiting for me to do something. I stumbled over to the box in the corner and rifled through the bits of broken plaster to pull out the rubber tourniquet straps. *First, identify the seriously wounded, then stop the bleeding.* Gradually, I regained control.

For the next seven hours, I amputated several limbs, removed shrapnel, and sewed up gashes. It turned out I was the only person with medical training left in the hospital. Everyone else had fled. The hospital was out of commission— the work of the townspeople destroyed in seconds. The building had operated for only three weeks, and Zulai's white flag with the red cross lay in tatters under the rubble. So much for the protection of the Geneva Convention. All that the flag had done was to signal to the Russians where to bomb. And about all I could do now was stabilize the wounded so that their relatives or friends could transport them to the hospital in Urus-Martan. The remaining patients I took to my house.

Alkhan Kala was now under constant attack. I managed to persuade my parents to join the rest of the family in Urus-Martan by promising I would look after the livestock. A mass of cars, carts, tractors, buses, and trucks choked the road out of town. Women and children screamed in panic as long-range Russian artillery shelled them; dead and wounded lay at the side of the road. At the entrance to Urus-Martan, the locals met the refugees and took them to their houses. That night, I made another six trips to Urus-Martan, transporting children and the wounded. By the next day, the only people left in Alkhan Kala were old men, a couple of old women, and 100 volunteer fighters who stayed to defend the town.

After the damage to the hospital, I relocated all medical services to my house. I received the wounded in the courtyard and performed operations in the wood-paneled entrance hall on the ground floor. In May 1993 when I began building the house, neighbors made fun of the eighteen truckloads of soil I had removed to build a large root cellar and storeroom. The house was completed in 1994. Two iron doors in the cement floor of the summer kitchen led down into the cellar. I placed triple-decker bunk beds against the basement wall and laid planks in the aisle of the concrete floor for mattresses. With Nana, Malika, and the other women gone, I needed someone to prepare food for my patients, whom I sheltered in the basement. Addi, a 40-year-old cameraman for the local television station, volunteered.

Addi was an enormous help. He prepared meat soups for the wounded men in a large aluminum cauldron outside in the courtyard. He also baked bread in my mother's tandoor-like earthen oven. In addition to Addi, three young boys from the neighboring village changed dressings; passed around the bedpans, cans of water, and soap; and helped turn the patients so they wouldn't develop bedsores. Several patients had to be turned two or three times a day.

The heavy artillery fire continued nonstop. Snipers strafed the town from nearby hills. At night, I put on a white camouflage uniform and went out into the snow with the old men, including our family friend Hasilbek, to bring in the wounded. We also collected the dead and gave them temporary burials until their relatives could give them a proper funeral.

And it wasn't only the Chechens we buried. One day, as I stood in the attic of my house, I observed something which, if I hadn't seen it with my own eyes, I would never have believed. Through the binoculars I saw men scattering in all directions, a helicopter gunship firing on them. At first I thought they were Chechens, but as I looked closer I saw that they wore Russian boots and soldiers' tunics. Russian officers were shooting their own men, probably because these recruits were terrified to enter Grozny, where our fighters waited for them!

A few days later on the outskirts of town, near a bombed-out house, we found dogs devouring several of the corpses. The smell made me gag, and I felt my stomach rise up. If not for the dog tags, we wouldn't have known they were Russian soldiers, because the bodies were so mutilated. We wrapped the remains in sheets and buried them. Hasilbek shook his head in disgust. "What kind of people are the Russians?" he said as we shoveled earth over the remains. "They don't even bother to collect and bury their dead."

Later, we sent word to the Committee of Soldiers' Mothers, a grassroots organization in Moscow, about these dead and urged them to send someone to pick up the remains. Eventually, these courageous mothers journeyed to Chechnya and crossed the front lines with the help of Chechen mothers, to search for their sons or what remained of them.

On January 30, my house was struck by a missile at about 3 P.M. I was standing outside talking to neighbors when I heard the distant sounds of the Russian helicopter. The Russians had apparently found out that I was treating Chechen fighters at home. I had frequently warned people not to enter my house in groups—because the Russians could spot them through binoculars or night-vision scopes—but often they ignored me. At that time, I had 32 wounded men in my cellar and another 8 lying outside, all wrapped up, on cots in the summer terrace of the house.

Something told me that the helicopter was targeting my house. Over the last weeks, I had developed a sixth sense, almost as if I could read the intentions of the pilot. I had noticed that people's survival instinct, like that of animals, becomes acute in extreme conditions. I called it *perestroika* of the organism. It was similar to participating in a judo competition. I could tell instinctively which move my opponent would make.

The engine was faint at first but grew louder. Now the helicopter came into view. A few seconds later, I saw its tail lift upward, signaling the start of an attack dive.

"Into the cellar!" I yelled. The neighbors rushed in. I always kept one of the two iron doors leading to the cellar open, and I literally dove headfirst down the 10 steps. The missile hitting the house was like an enormous thunderclap overhead. The blast threw everyone against the walls. I felt my head hit the concrete. For several minutes I lay unconscious. The reinforced concrete ceiling above us cracked as the house collapsed upon it, showering us with brick dust, which seeped into our hair, nostrils, and between our teeth. The ceiling held, thanks to the reinforced steel rods, but now we were trapped inside. The place was totally dark; we were entombed in a giant coffin. We knew that as long as it was still light outside, no one could dig us out for fear of the helicopter returning. There was no doubt that the direct hit had killed the patients on the summer terrace.

Many hours later—well into the night—some 40 volunteer fighters started to dig us out. At 2 A.M., we surfaced like miners from the pit, our faces covered in red dust. Everyone looked at me to see my reaction to the destruction of the house. My belongings were scattered across the street as if lying in a landfill. I managed to control myself. I said that the important thing was that we were alive and that you could always rebuild a house; but inside I burned with anger. I had only just finished the house. The wrought iron gate with its beautiful scrolling, which I had ordered specially made, now straddled the roof of the little house next door where my parents lived; the medical books I had collected over the years lay in the rubble.

Friends and neighbors, including my sister Raya's 15-year-old son, Ali, helped me go through what was left of the house. I rescued some books and covered them with a plastic sheet. Then, while it was still dark, we packed the wounded into carts with the help of volunteers and drove them to Urus-Martan. Before leaving, I untied Tarzan. With me gone, he would have to fend for himself like all the other stray dogs wandering the streets. As I drove out of Alkhan Kala in pitch darkness, swerving to avoid the bomb craters in the road and the sound of explosions in the background, I wondered how to break the news about the house to the rest of the family. Dada would take it philosophically—he hadn't wanted me to build the house in the first place, saying it would only get destroyed. Nana, on the other hand, would be horrified.

It seemed we Chechens spend our energies building our houses and our lives, only to have them devastated and to start rebuilding them again.

Treating the ill was a Herculean task. The economy had collapsed; 90 percent of men were unemployed. Half the doctors and nurses had left the republic during the war to find work in Russia. Either their nerves had given out, or they couldn't support their families. Unfortunately, war has placed a terrible strain on our traditions, especially relations between men and women. Once the factories had closed, men lost their jobs, forcing many women to become the breadwinners by trading in the bazaar. I knew a number of educated women—doctors, teachers, and others—who abandoned their specialties and went into small-time business to support their families. For a Chechen male, there is no greater humiliation than not being able to support his family. I was fortunate. I still had some savings left, but I knew they wouldn't last forever.

Friends suggested that I would do better to go to Moscow and work there, but my father's voice always reminded me about duty, and I knew I was meant to stay in Chechnya. It was my duty to support my relatives. Most of them had no jobs, and those who did work, like Malika and Razyat, received no salaries. In all, I was responsible for 13 people, not counting all the others who asked for loans they never paid back. I knew I had to make some money, not only to support my family but also to buy much-needed medicines and equipment for the hospitals. My friend Abek Bisultanov, who had made money from a car sales business, which he started after retiring as an athlete, collected more than $12,000. During 1997, I made several trips to Moscow to purchase medical supplies with his donation.

I decided that I would solve my financial problem by taking private patients for cosmetic surgery after-hours at the hospital, as I had done before the war. With the war over, everyone wanted to forget the ugliness. Stress speeds up the aging process, and when women looked in the mirror, they didn't like what they saw. Some of them came to me in secret, ashamed to be worried about their looks when so many people were suffering from the trauma of war. They dug into savings or borrowed money for the operations. I was sympathetic with this postwar desire to look good. Never again would I have a 6-day growth of stubble because there was no water to shave, or wear damp blood-stained trousers, the matted sheepskin coat, or the boots that leaked. Now I took pleasure in shaving each morning and wearing a clean shirt and a tie.

I kept my fees low, which meant I never lacked patients. My price for a nose job, removing crow's feet, or a face-lift were a tenth of what the doctors charged in Moscow at the Institute of Cosmetology. As long as I had strength, I was determined to work. When I returned home, I would find relatives of the injured waiting in the street for me even after midnight, begging for my help. I grew weary; I was one man with limited strength. Once in the house, Dada would tell me of his friends who needed a doctor, mostly people who had been exiled with him in Kazakhstan. I knew his friendships from those times were sacred.

I took no money from my regular patients. Most of them were penniless. To overcome their embarrassment, they felt compelled to tell me their stories. This one had lost two children, that one a wife. This one's brother had been tortured; that one's daughter had been raped. "Please don't tell me," I implored them. "We all lost friends and relatives." I tried to control my irritation, which seemed to be growing with every passing day despite everything I did to curb it.

In addition to caring for civilians, I was called upon occasionally to treat Salman Raduyev, the controversial field commander I had operated on in the mountain hideout. Several months after the original operation, I had removed the scar tissue from the facial reconstruction. Not only was he an exasperating patient, never following instructions, but the association put my life in danger. One time after treating him, I found a note slipped under my door: "If you continue to keep Raduyev alive, the next time you'll be killed."

By the middle of the summer of 1999, it was becoming clear that peace was wishful thinking and that sooner or later Russia would attack again. The signs were there: Russian troops were gathering along the Chechen borders, and Russian planes dropped bombs on what the Russian military spokesmen called "bandit-formation" camps around the republic. President Maskhadov seemed incapable of reining in the radical commanders or arresting gangsters like Arbi Barayev, or persuading Khattab, the radical field commander from Saudi Arabia, to leave Chechnya.

Adding to the unrest, the local police in the neighboring province of Dagestan were launching a campaign against Islamic extremists, forcing them into Chechnya, where anti-Maskhadov groups and criminal gangs welcomed them. The Islamic authorities in Dagestan, threatened by radical Islamists themselves, supported the crackdown. Earlier, many Wahhabi radicals, along with Dagestani opposition groups, had fled into Chechnya and set up operations in the town of Urus-Martan, their idea being eventually to overthrow the pro-Russian government of Dagestan and create an Islamic confederation in the North Caucasus.

Once more, fear gripped the republic. People began hoarding food. Many fled and sent children to relatives. I began dropping by the wholesale food market and picking up 100-pound bags of flour, sugar, and large boxes of macaroni. At the same time, I built up my stocks of basic medical supplies like lidocaine, surgical thread, and Polyglukin. I couldn't find a surgical saw and drill, so I would have to perform amputations and trepanations (holes bored into the skull to relieve pressure from swelling) with ordinary carpenter's tools, which were hard to keep clean and sterile.

Not knowing when Russians would attack put everything on edge. Dada stayed glued to his radio. The only thing that appeared to distract him was little Markha, who toddled through to his room each morning, asking to be lifted on his knee. Nana, Zata, and my sisters became nervous, especially Malika, who lapsed into depression every time she saw the ruins of her beloved Grozny. The bombing panicked Hussein and Rita, who were not used to it. The slightest sound made them whisk Khava and Adam off into the cellar. It would take a while for them to tell where an attack plane was headed by the speed and sound of its engines.

Malika wanted us to go to the neighboring republic of Cherkessiya, buy a house there, and wait out the war. "They don't treat Chechens badly," she said of the Cherkess. We thought about leaving, but it wasn't practical. Nana said she couldn't leave the animals. And I knew many people would be depending on me for medical care when the war started. We decided to stick it out.

By now, kidnapping had reached epidemic proportions. Gangsters like Barayev, in partnership with Russian security services, made millions from ransoms and selling the corpses of the people they had murdered back to their relatives. When the *kontraktniki* signed up to fight in Chechnya, the Russian military promised bonuses. But the army was broke. By all accounts, military commanders gave the mercenaries freedom to loot and kidnap. The outside world heard about the kidnapping of journalists like Andrei Babitsky, a Radio Free Europe correspondent, or a Russian MVD officer like General Gennadi Shpigun, but never about the Chechens who were victimized 80 percent of the time. Back in June, the Chechen public had demanded that Maskhadov name the kidnappers and declare a war against them. He did nothing. The elders were beside themselves, addressing crowds outside the mosque after Friday prayers and going on radio and television, urging people to stop the kidnapping.

Family and friends warned me, "If a guy wears a tie, builds a large house, and is a plastic surgeon, everyone assumes he is rolling in money. How can you drive around by yourself at night? You should carry a gun. You should have bodyguards. You should leave Chechnya!" Early on, I had decided that I couldn't live my life worrying about being shot or kidnapped. I refused to walk around with bodyguards or carry a gun. At the hospital we had only one gun, which we borrowed from the local police. The longer I had avoided death, the more fatalistic I became. As with most things, Allah decides.

Once I thought I had been kidnapped. At 2 A.M., someone hammered on the outside gate. When I opened it, I did not recognize the bearded man dressed in fatigues. A full moon illuminated everything, and on the other side of the street I could see a military jeep with three men inside. "We have a wounded comrade at the Ninth City Hospital," one of them said. "We were told you were a specialist. We need your help."

I told them to wait while I dressed and collected my things. By this time, Nana was up. "Are you sure it is safe to go? You don't know who they are," she said as I went out the door. I shouted not to worry.

The three fighters in the jeep didn't get out to greet me or introduce themselves when I crossed the street. Odd behavior for Chechens, I thought. They usually say hello. The bearded fighter pointed to a front seat. I got in, and he sat in the driver's seat, gunned the engine, and the jeep shot forward, tires screeching. The men in the back seat didn't address me but spoke together in low voices. The needle of the speedometer hovered around 60 miles an hour, with the driver swerving and braking to avoid the potholes in the road. I held on tight and braced myself against being thrown into the windshield. At the approach of the military checkpoint at the edge of Alkhan Kala, the driver accelerated. He's running the checkpoint, I thought. This is it. I'm being kidnapped.

The needle of the speedometer shot up to 72 miles an hour. A guard at the post stepped into the road, then jumped back, never raising his gun. The kidnappers often worked hand in glove with the Russian military. My first thought now was how to behave. Don't let them see any fear, I told myself. Don't anger them. Keep calm. My heart pounded against my ribs, and I took a deep breath.

The words of my judo coach before a match raced through my mind. "Center yourself." Without closing my eyes, I prayed. "Please, Allah, don't let this be a kidnapping."

The idea of another detention scared me. Memories of the pit haunted me. Images flashed before my eyes: my picture on television with the other abducted victims; relatives and friends begging for my release on the air; my patients collecting ransom money. Then I thought of my patients: the old man with the massive gash on his hip, from which I drained gobs of yellowish, foul-smelling pus every day. And what about the three old men with urinary blockages who needed their catheters changed? Or the 12-year-old boy with the wound on the side of his head from an antipersonnel mine? I needed to check for purply red blotches, indicating the onset of infection. If sepsis set in, he could be dead in five days. I was so busy making a mental inventory of my patients that I didn't see that the jeep had turned onto the street toward the Ninth City Hospital. This was not a kidnapping after all. I sank back in the seat and let the tension drain from my muscles.

At the hospital, I reassembled the wounded fighter's shattered jaw while his comrades smoked outside the operating room. Later, driving me home, they broke their silence, telling me how amazed they were that I had agreed to get into the jeep with them. I didn't tell them how terrified I had been.

The calm was too good to last. One afternoon, I sat with my nurse Rumani Idrisova and staff around the table drinking tea and eating soup. On the table was a box of chocolates Nuradi had brought for the nurses. A few days earlier, Rumani's husband had visited the hospital to try and persuade her to return with him to Ingushetia. They went off into an empty room and talked for nearly two hours. When she came out, she was smiling. "I'm staying," she said. "My place is here."

Several streets away, on Mira (Peace) Street, one of the main thoroughfares in the town, people gathered following the funeral of a young boy who had stepped on a mine while collecting wood. A crowd of people on the streets was always an invitation for Russian fire. The mourners should have known better, but the exchange of condolences after a death is one of our important traditions.

Suddenly, there was an enormous explosion. We rushed away from the windows and into the corridor, then squatted on the floor with our backs to the wall. We veterans of the first war were determined to stay calm, to finish our soup. Razyat Almatova, one of our local volunteer nurses, couldn't lift the spoon to her mouth because her hand shook so much. Fear was contagious, so I cracked a few jokes, which I don't think she appreciated.

Within five minutes, the wounded began arriving, some in the arms of relatives, others in carts or on stretchers. There had been no warning—a mortar is silent until it explodes close to the ground, spraying shards everywhere, shredding human flesh. There were at least 70 casualties, some killed and some with limbs hanging off. Relatives elbowed their way into the passageway, stumbling over the bodies strewn every which way on the floor. I was confronted by endless wounded and didn't know where to begin; I felt disoriented; my head began pounding. The first thing to do, I told myself, was to identify the victims who had a chance of survival. Slowly, I pulled myself together.

"Move away; give the doctor room to work!" Nuradi shouted. He never lost his head. Some of the nurses panicked, running aimlessly in all directions, grabbing the stands with hanging drips.

"Forget the stands!" I shouted. "We don't need the drips yet. Grab the rubber tourniquets. Stop the bleeding! First of all, stop the bleeding!"

With Nuradi at my side, I operated along with the other nurses and doctors until 3 A.M. I was only too familiar with this ghastly work: stuffing gauze into wounds, clamping off major blood vessels, cauterizing smaller ones, peeling back skin, and sawing through bone. There was no time to swab the floor, which was slippery with blood. We wrapped up the severed limbs for the relatives.

During this period of intensive bombing, I continued to do my medical rounds, sometimes on foot and sometimes by car. I had learned to read skin and tissue: to interpret discharge from an injury, to know that roughness and a lack of elasticity under my fingers as I probed a wound meant the flesh was damaged. The way a surgeon cuts into the tissue, being careful to save the blood vessels, determines how long the wound takes to mend. Sepsis can progress with lightning speed, so I visited patients like Sultan Ganayev daily to combat his infection. He had a large, open wound at the level of his right hip that had spread to his lower spine. I did battle with his dying flesh. The smell of pus and dead tissue was so strong that visitors gagged and left the room. The constant shelling had undermined Sultan's nervous system, and his body was struggling with the spreading infection.

"Leave me up here. I'm going to die anyway. You get down into the cellar." He would yell at his wife and grown children every time the shelling started. The eldest son never left him, not even through the worst shelling.

One day as I drained the pus into the bowl, Sultan turned to me and said, "Khassan, tell me the truth. Am I going to die?"

"Of course not," I said. "Your wound is getting better."

He grinned. "As soon as I am well, I will take you to my vineyard; then you will have as many grapes as you can use," he said.

"I look forward to it," I replied.

I never told my patients they were dying, because I felt that it destroyed all hope, and healing needs hope. I believe that telling the truth often encourages death. Especially the onset of cancer. There is no word for cancer in the Chechen language. The Russians call cancer *rak,* the same word as crab. In Chechen we call cancer "the unmentionable" and hide it from the patient.

I never gave up on Sultan, though I didn't hold out much hope for those grapes. I continued to struggle for his life, believing in miracles. Under different conditions, I might have saved him, though he would have spent the rest of his life in a wheelchair.

As the weeks passed and the casualties streamed in, our medical supplies started to dwindle. I turned to Dada's age-old remedies. I cleaned wounds with sour milk and applied honey to help close them. On burns, I used egg yolk and sour cream. I advised people to urinate in a container, let the urine stand for a week, and apply the sediment, which settled at the bottom, to their wounds. I also used herbal solutions made with oak bark, coltsfoot, or sage as dressings. When our surgical thread was gone, I appealed to the townspeople for ordinary thread, which we disinfected by boiling. When the disinfectants gave out, we mixed weak, medium, and strong salt solutions. To dress wounds, I used ordinary household supplies.

During this period, our team experienced tragedies of its own. One night when Nuradi walked me home, he told me that he hadn't heard from his older son, Akhmed, in weeks. Nuradi always insisted on accompanying me, even though I would tell him it wasn't necessary.

"I tried to get messages to him," he said. "I want to go to Grozny and look for him."

"It's too dangerous," I said. "Too many Chechens have been shot going to Grozny to look for their relatives."

In the end, Nuradi agreed not to go. Then one day he asked me to go home with him. When he stopped in front of his house, eyes downcast, I guessed what was coming.

"Some local fighters came from Grozny," he said. "They reported that several young men from Alkhan Kala were buried in the central stadium." The Dinamo Stadium in Grozny had become a temporary burial ground for Chechens until it was safe enough for the relatives to remove the bodies for a proper burial. The news of Akhmed's death was closely held. Nuradi's elderly mother was not informed for fear it would give her a heart attack. One day when she sat outside in the street, friends approached with condolences. She died a month later from the shock.

Alavdi's 18-year-old sister died when a shell hit their courtyard. She was sweeping the yard, and he was inside the house. The shock wave knocked over the young woman, shredding her body before his eyes. He rushed to the hospital with her mutilated corpse, in a state of shock, thinking I could help, but it was far too late. Nuradi tried to calm him down. Alavdi didn't know how he was going to inform his parents, who lived in another town.

Sometimes I felt that the whole population was verging on nervous collapse. Children walked around in shock, either retreating into silence or crying nonstop. The milk of nursing mothers dried up. One day, I saw a 9-year-old boy with half a head of white hair. His mother said it had happened overnight. Another, a 7-year-old boy, had been so frightened by bombardments that the left side of his face twisted over to the right, leaving him with a disfigured, wry mouth. I had no tranquilizers or medication to calm people down, nothing to curb the outbreaks of violence brought on by stress, as in the case of Salavdi Kadirov, a weight lifter, whose brothers asked me for help. My only advice was to tie him to the bed, which, with such a bull of a man, required the help of several men. On the street, the first Russian sniper would have picked him off. Some people treated their nerves with alcohol, for which I couldn't blame them.

November 25, 1999, brought a harrowing bombardment. I thanked God that most of my family was safe in Ingushetia. "From the sound of the explosion, the shelling is following a full-coverage pattern," I told Nuradi. "The Russians have mapped the town into squares and are systematically directing their barrage from quadrant to quadrant. They'll probably hit the hospital, and in another few minutes my house will fall in the target square."

"I'll hold the fort here," Rumani volunteered. "Go home quick and warn anyone who is there."

I ran home as fast as I could. There I found Nana, friends, and neighbors gathered around my television, which I had managed to hook up to an old Japanese generator. The electricity had been out for months. My friends were waiting for the 9 P.M. Moscow news, anxious to learn how the Russians were reporting the war.

"Get into the basement," I yelled. "The shelling is moving this way."

"Can't it wait until after the news?" one of my neighbors asked.

"No!" I ripped the plug from the generator. "Get down there immediately!"

About 9:50 P.M., a missile smashed into the house with a deafening explosion. Two minutes later, a second rocket hit, smashing through the top of the basement. A blinding flame flashed through the cellar as the rocket rammed through the ceiling. That was followed by an explosion that tore off the corner of my house, causing the basement ceiling to crack. The women screamed; we all crowded into the far corner, praying out loud.

A third hit, and it would be over. People clung to one another in silence, eyes closed, waiting for the end. But we were lucky. Allah heard our prayers. There was no third missile. I struggled to push open the steel door, which had crashed shut, but it was blocked by rubble that had fallen on it. Above, I could hear voices, and when our neighbors finally freed us, I stumbled out, tripping over fallen bricks and what used to be the table of the summer kitchen, choking on the dust and acrid smoke. What greeted me was a terrible sight: My house was partially destroyed; the upper floors and roof were gone, and only the ground floor, constructed of reinforced concrete, was left standing. My parents' house was leveled. So much time and energy rebuilding the house! One minute, and it was rubble. Nana had taken such pride in the wooden roof I had built out over the courtyard at the back of the house.

Where do we live now? I thought as I looked at a broken dinner plate lying under a fallen roof beam. We build; the Russians destroy. Then we build again; the Russians destroy again. Some people can't take it; they have heart attacks and die. Others are defiant: "We will rebuild our house, and this time it will be an even better house than the one the Russians destroyed," they say. The process becomes a way of life. We have been doing it for centuries. But right now, rebuilding wasn't on my mind. The wounded would be pouring in.

Fallen bricks, plaster, and collapsed beams blocked the front of the house. I scrambled over the mess into the back and climbed over the fence. The road and path behind the house had disappeared under fallen debris. Houses burned on either side of me as I ran. Men with buckets of water were trying to extinguish the fire at Hussein's house. At the time Hussein and Rita were in Ingushetia, along with their children. He and Malika returned to Alkhan Kala a little later.

In those awful days, we all expected tragedy, even death. When death arrived, it wasn't the kind of shock someone experiences with a plane or car crash. For people surrounded by tragedy, death is a natural event, something happening to everyone. You are not alone. In the house across the street, someone was killed yesterday. In the house next door, three people last week; and in one house, a whole family. Every Chechen family had its deaths. In these extreme circumstances, you realize the fragility of life. You recognize what is important, what is superficial. What is true, and what are lies.

I eventually managed to make my way through the debris and arrived at the hospital, which was only partly damaged. It was now past 10 P.M., and I went back immediately to the operating table. I worked throughout the night and into the next morning. . . . Fourteen hours later, I left the operating room, exhausted. My last operation before taking a break was to extract pieces of shrapnel from a young boy's back, a tricky job since four of the shards were close to the spinal column. I didn't want to risk paralysis, so I decided to leave them in.

I worked all that day, and throughout that night, to the groans of the wounded and the dying as the mullah and the elders intoned the words of the Koran. During those hateful hours, many of the famous field commanders passed through my hospital. Abdul Malik was brought in wounded; others like Hunkar-Pasha Isparilov and Lecha Dudayev were brought in dead; Ruslan Gelayev survived and hung around the corridors. Ali, Razyat, and my other volunteers moved among the living, adjusting the tourniquets and cleaning wounds.

I received word that several nurses and doctors, including Oumar Khanbiev, the Chechen minister of health, were on their way from Grozny to help. That was cheering news, because my strength was fading, and my arms ached from sawing. In addition to the amputations, I performed brain surgeries using a carpenter's hand drill.

Before long, I had cut through so much bone that the teeth at the center of the hacksaw blade became dull. I didn't have a second blade, so I started bearing down hard on both ends of the saw, easing up on the middle. I got so used to this three-part stroke that the sawing motion became automatic. For 24 hours, I didn't leave my operating room; not did I drink or eat. I couldn't face the scene in the corridor. Finally, someone placed a cup of strong tea laced with sugar in my hand, and I squatted in the corner for a few minutes. Every second, every minute was a man's life. I lost all sense of time. My hands felt increasingly heavy, dead weights, reluctant to obey. My fingers fumbled with the thread. I prayed that I wouldn't pass out in the middle of an operation.

About 27 hours after the crisis hit, I heard a roar overhead. "Please, Allah, let me finish this patient," I said under my breath. I felt dizzy. I quickly stitched the flesh together and tied off the thread. Then I sensed myself falling. The next thing I knew, I was outside and Rumani and Razyat were rubbing my face with snow. The cold revived me, and I stumbled back to the operating room.

We had run out of surgical thread, and I was now using ordinary thread soaked in alcohol. Working with the wet thread proved difficult and annoying. By this time, I had sewed so many wounds without gloves that cuts developed between my fingers. The blisters on my hands were bursting and turning into small wounds. And still no sign of the doctors and nurses from Grozny. I feared they had been unable to reach Alkhan Kala.

On the second day, February 1, I operated without a break until about midnight, when I fainted a second time. Again, the nurses rubbed my face with snow, and I went back to work. By the third day, I had performed 67 amputations and 7 brain surgeries. The severed limbs piled up for Nuradi to bury in the corner of the hospital grounds with a quick prayer near the fence.

After two days with hardly a break, my strength gave out. I could no longer control my hands, and my arms developed spasms. There was still no sign of the doctors and nurses from Grozny, and Rumani insisted I get some sleep. She said I was of no use in my current state. Stumbling home at 4 A.M. February 2, I breathed in cold air and ash. A fresh snow had fallen, and the sky was clear. Flames and rebounding flashes of artillery fire mingled with the stars. I was indifferent to the gunfire and explosions around me. All I could think about were the dead and the mangled in the corridor with their dangling extremities.

When the Russian army ordered my immediate arrest in early 2000, I finally fled Chechnya and sought political asylum in the United States, where I now live with my wife and children.

17

War in the Democratic Republic of Congo

Les Roberts and Charles Lubula Muganda

In 1994, a spasm of ethnically motivated violence resulted in the deaths of more than 600,000 Rwandans, killed by a military and government comprised primarily of the Hutu majority ethnic group, who were determined to eliminate the ethnic Tutsi minority from their population. Rwandan Tutsis who had left Rwanda during earlier periods of ethnic tension had been staging a low-intensity conflict in the northern part of the country. When the genocide efforts began, this Tutsi rebel group, called the Rwandan Patriotic Front (RPF), invaded Rwanda in earnest and drove the military and government from power, probably driving most of the perpetrators of the genocide into Tanzania and Zaire.

Coerced by fleeing soldiers and militia and fearing reprisals from the RPF, hundreds of thousands of Rwandan Hutus accompanied the perpetrators into exile. The largest concentration of these fleeing Hutus arrived in Goma, Zaire, over a 3-day period in July. Little was done to round up and bring to justice those who had taken part in the genocide. For example, in spite of the presence of French, United States, and Zairian troops in Goma, approximately 200 uniformed Hutu soldiers with guns were allowed to jog through Mugunga camp on July 20, 1994, while chanting about the inevitability of their victorious return to Rwanda.[1]

Eventually, these Hutu extremists controlled resources and political influence in the three Goma camps with a refugee population of almost 1 million. Aside from creating a security threat to the Tutsi-led postwar government in Rwanda, armed men who may have resided in the camps began violent sorties into Rwanda, and stealing cattle and attacking ethnic Tutsis inside Zaire. In late October 1996, Rwanda, with support from Uganda, Burundi, and rebel Zairians opposed to the Kinshasa-based government, invaded eastern Zaire. The Zairian military hardly posed resistance, and within months the invading forces had overrun all of Zaire, placing Laurent Kabila as the new head of state.

In the newly renamed Democratic Republic of Congo (DRC), the euphoria of a new government quickly gave way to pessimism about the continued economic disarray and open hostility by the Congolese toward the Rwandan and Ugandan troops. President Kabila recognized the popular disdain for the foreign troops and attempted to consolidate a power base with Congolese troops.[2] In August 1998, Rwandan and Ugandan forces withdrew from the country, with some of the departing troops literally reinvading the next day to overthrow the government they had recently put in place. President Kabila found military support in neighboring Angola, Zimbabwe, and Chad.

Eventually, seven foreign armies and a host of Congolese rebel groups were fighting in Congo, resulting in what has reportedly been the most deadly war anywhere since World War II.[3,4] Adding to the complexity of the conflict was the rise of indigenous rebel groups, which aligned and opposed the various invading armies, sometimes changing allegiance over the course of the conflict. DRC is particularly rich in diamonds, gold, and the mineral columbium tantalite (coltan), which is used in microchips. Once groups gained control of mineral-rich areas, they often were more focused on maintaining control of these areas than on pressing ahead with the military campaign. Thus, within a couple of months after the August 1998 reinvasion, the country was divided, with the line of conflict changing little over the next 3 years.

Many striking issues were displayed in this conflict, including the lack of press coverage given the magnitude of the crisis, the importance of mineral resources in fueling the conflict, and the profound importance of infectious diseases in manifesting the human misery of this war. A peace accord signed in 2002 laid out a framework for the invading armies to be withdrawn and for a government of reconciliation to be formed. Although the armies did formally withdraw in 2002, reunification and the process of establishing a functional, centrally based government has been problematic in many parts of the Eastern section of the country. Elections in 2006, as set out in the 2002, U.N.-brokered accord, have further solidified the peace process and the reconciliation of the East and the West. Some exploitation of diamonds, gold, timber, and coltan is still ongoing at the hands of Congo's neighbors, but this is no longer openly associated with state-backed military forces. Thus, the war has ended in DRC, although, in many of the Eastern areas, peace and prosperity have yet to come.

This chapter focuses on the period from August 1998 through December 2002, the period of the "internationalized" war in DRC. Although foreign influence and the social disruptions caused by the war continue to contribute to elevated mortality in many areas, the period after 2002 has been characterized by a lower level of violence and conflict based on local forces and by dynamics that have tended to vary among the provinces.

A series of mortality surveys, which were performed by the International Rescue Committee (IRC), provide unique, population-based mortality data from rural areas obtained while the conflict was occurring. The purpose of this chapter is not to describe specific events in the DRC, but rather to explore these data to better understand the nature of the relationship between infectious diseases and armed conflict.

Geographic Analysis of Armed Conflict and Infectious Disease Mortality

Between 1999 and 2002, 23 surveys were conducted in the eastern DRC to determine the crude mortality rate (CMR) among health zones with populations that ranged from 62,000 to 345,000. (The methods employed in these surveys are described elsewhere.[5,6]) In all of these surveys, respondents in each household were asked several questions about the household composition and recent births and deaths in the household. If a death had occurred, the cause of death, month of death, and age and gender of the decedent were recorded. The family's ability to diagnose some causes of death may be limited in specificity, but these data enabled the separation of violent from nonviolent deaths. For this analysis, all violent deaths involved armed combatants (all male, by chance) inducing the events that directly led to a civilian death. Among the nonviolent deaths, major categories, such as febrile illness and diarrhea, were listed individually, with less common causes of death, such as measles, meningitis, tuberculosis, and typhoid, lumped together as "other infectious" deaths. Ten of these surveys in 2002 provided a sample of the accessible health zones in eastern DRC. The other surveys from earlier years were conducted in areas that were considered safe when little of eastern DRC was accessible.

Over the 3 years in which these surveys took place, the average CMR observed was 2.5 to 3.7 times the assumed baseline rate of 1.5 deaths per 1,000 population per month. Table 17-1 shows the causes of 2,223 reported deaths from these 23 surveys. Although certain distinctions in causes of death,

Table 17-1. Causes of 2,223 Deaths Reported by Interviewed Families, Democratic Republic of Congo, 1999–2002

Febrile illness	27%
Diarrheal disease	12%
Acute respiratory infection	4%
Other infectious diseases	19%
Malnutrition	10%
Violence	8%
Other noninfectious diseases	14%
Other or unknown	6%

such as febrile illness as opposed to acute respiratory infection, may be questionable, it was clear that violence accounted for only a small fraction of deaths and that infectious agents accounted for most of them. The two most common noninfectious causes of death, as reported by the families, were anemia and malnutrition. In many cases, these conditions may have also been caused by infectious diseases. Among the category of "other infectious" causes, measles, tuberculosis, and meningitis were the most commonly reported causes.

Figure 17-1 shows rates of nonviolent deaths and violence-specific deaths for the 23 surveys. This scatter plot demonstrates that areas with the greatest rates of violence also tended to experience the most deaths from nonviolent causes. There was a statistically significant correlation between violence and death from other causes. The data projected onto the scatter plot imply that excess deaths in this war were occurring from two mechanisms: (1) a general elevation of the death rate even where violence was not occurring, and (2) an additional increase in the death rate with an increasing rate of violence. The

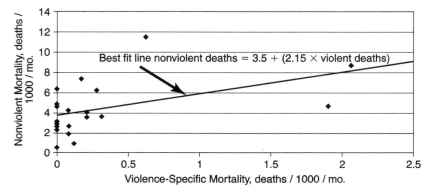

Figure 17-1. Nonviolent and violence-specific mortality rates for 23 surveys, Democratic Republic of Congo, 1999–2002. (Source: Les Roberts)

best-fit regression line indicates that, in wartime eastern DRC among the surveyed populations, the baseline CMR was 3.5 per 1,000 population per month, even in the absence of violence—2.3 times the baseline rate of 1.5 per 1,000 per month assumed to exist before the war. The slope of the line indicates that there were an additional 2.15 nonviolent deaths for every violent death within the areas surveyed. Overall, within the study areas (which were disproportionately the safest and least violent areas within eastern DRC), there were approximately four excess deaths (above the baseline) for every violent death that occurred. A summary analysis by the IRC of the first 11 surveys, which were conducted between 1999 and 2001 (when the war was at its peak), indicated that there were six excess nonviolent deaths for every violent death.[6]

Temporal Analysis of Armed Conflict and Infectious Disease Mortality

In November 1999, Rwandan and allied Congolese Rally for Democracy (RCD) troops withdrew from Kalonge, an area of South Kivu Province with a population of 62,000. Their withdrawal led to an immediate takeover by counterinsurgents, both Congolese Mayi-Mayi rebels (local militias), and former Rwandan soldiers who had fled to Congo after the 1994 genocide. Killings of civilians were widespread, and interviewees reported that virtually the entire surviving population fled the area.

Figure 17-2 shows the violence-specific mortality rate, the rate of death attributed by the interviewed families to fever (febrile illness), and the CMR— all expressed as deaths per 1,000 population per month. What is striking about this figure is not that the political turnover was associated with a simultaneous

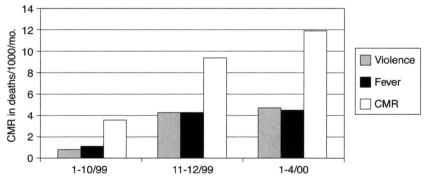

Figure 17-2. Violence-specific mortality rate, fever-specific mortality rate, and crude mortality rate, Kalonge, DRC, January 1999–April 2000. (Source: Les Roberts)

six-fold increase in the rate of violence, but that it corresponded to a four-fold increase in the rate of death related to fever and a more than three-fold increase in the CMR. Interviewees reported that their families fled into the jungle with inadequate clothing and often with no blankets or buckets. Thus, the main health consequence for these people was not specifically the violence but rather the disruption that the violence induced.

The converse of this phenomenon was also observed. In early 2002, a ceasefire agreement was signed between the Kinshasa-based government and the Government of Rwanda. Over large areas of southern and east central DRC, Rwandan troops withdrew during 2002, with the Rwandan government claiming that all of its troops were withdrawn by September. Two of these areas of withdrawal were surveyed in 2001 and, by chance, picked at random to be resurveyed in 2002, using a similar questionnaire and methods. The results of these surveys are summarized in Figures 17-3 and 17-4.

In both Kalemie and Kalima, the violence-specific mortality rate and the CMR were exceptionally high in 2001, while the area was occupied by Rwandan forces, and were significantly lower in 2002, when those troops were initially withdrawing and eventually withdrawn. Although this temporal association does not prove causality, it is consistent with anecdotal reports that the withdrawal of foreign forces was associated with improved security and with an overall analysis which showed a marked reduction in the overall CMR in eastern DRC with the advent of the ongoing peace process.[4]

The relationship between violence and infectious diseases is probably different in every war. Indeed, it was probably different within DRC during the 1999–2001 period than while the war was waning during 2002. As seen in Figure 17-1, the mechanisms by which violence makes a society susceptible to deaths from infectious diseases are multiple and complex. The war in DRC showed that prolonged conflict makes a population extremely susceptible to

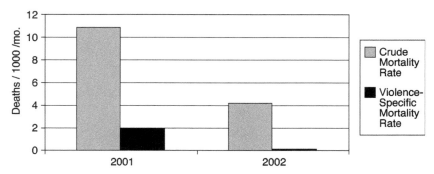

Figure 17-3. Crude mortality rate and violence-specific mortality rate, Kalemie, DRC, 2001 and 2002. (Source: Les Roberts)

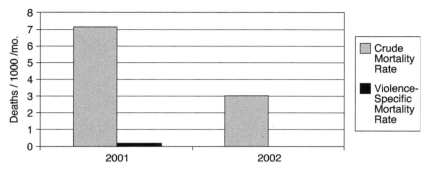

Figure 17-4. Crude mortality rate and violence-specific mortality, Kalima, DRC, 2001 and 2002. (Source: Les Roberts)

death from those pathogens that were endemic among the population before the violence began. In this war, the link between violent death and death from infectious disease was strong—both when comparing places and when observing the same population over time as the rates of violence changed. Within the populations surveyed, there were approximately four excess deaths, primarily from infectious diseases, for every violent death. During the 1999–2001 period, this ratio was probably closer to six for the 20 million people in eastern DRC. A larger follow-up survey by IRC in 2004 documented a CMR of 2.3 per 1,000 population per month—almost 2 years after the formal end of hostilities. The war in DRC showed that documenting the effects of wars by counting only violent casualties underestimates the consequences of war in settings of high disease transmission—enabling people worldwide to continue ignoring those wars occurring among the most impoverished populations.

Perhaps the most interesting observation over this series of IRC mortality surveys in the East was not among the many areas with overwhelming association between violence and bad health but was an example in which refusal to accept violence was associated with good health. The health zone of Butembo had less than half the CMR of any other area visited during the war: 0.4 deaths per 1,000 per month, lower than that of the United States or Europe. The area of North Kivu near the Ugandan boarder had been occupied early on by Rwandan forces. Local residents closed their shops, bars, and restaurants and did not openly fight the Rwandans, but refused to cooperate with them. Local officials were respectful but elusive. Because the area had no mineral resources and no goods or food could be obtained there, the occupying forces moved on after several weeks. Later, the same process occurred with Ugandan forces. With no military occupiers there, local merchants began importing goods through Uganda for distribution throughout eastern DRC. Local merchants did so well that in 2002 a new children's hospital was opened, paid for entirely with local contributions. Perhaps because of the luck of having no minerals, but perhaps more because of the collective will of the public, Butembo thrived at a time when the areas around them suffered.

Preventing Future Similar Conflicts

At least three lessons can be learned from the disastrous course of events in DRC. First, this war arose as the direct result of the international community's unwillingness to arrest and control the perpetrators of the genocide in Rwanda once they had fled to neighboring countries. Second, once Rwanda and Uganda had invaded Congo in 1996, it was a mistake that their second invasion was met with little protest from the community of nations; they were overthrowing a government that they themselves had established and should not have been permitted to do so. Third, for public health and human rights workers, this conflict shows the importance of documenting and publicizing the public health consequences that usually accompany armed conflict.

Before the first IRC survey (2000), an article in the *New York Times* estimated the death toll from this conflict to be under 100,000[10]; in contrast, the IRC survey 3 months later put the estimate at 1.7 million. IRC struggled with the most effective way to release the 2000 report: through the news media or through a peer-reviewed journal. In the end, a deal was struck with the *New York Times,* whereby it would be given an exclusive on the report in exchange for front-page coverage. This approach was not favored by many scientists who believed that scientific information requires peer-review endorsement to be credible. However, in retrospect, the media-based release appeared to be the right approach.

The published report triggered a United Nations resolution calling for all foreign armies to withdraw from DRC and a dramatic rise in humanitarian funding to address the crisis. The media stopped referring to the war as a political quagmire and started referring to it as a humanitarian crisis. Coverage of the war in the Western media increased dramatically. Reporters could informally visit war-torn areas and easily confirm that about 10 percent of the population had died. The second report estimated that, by mid-2001, 2.5 million people had died; it triggered even more media and political attention. In the months that followed the second report, a successful effort to get the presidents of Rwanda and DRC to meet, followed by a U.N.-brokered accord, led to the withdrawal of foreign troops and an end to the seven-nation war. It is not possible to quantify the role of the IRC reports in the political processes that led to the peace accord, but they helped to create a political environment in which allowing the war to continue was unacceptable. Therefore, in this case, the most important public health service to the people of the DRC might have been simply documentation of the health consequences of the war.

Over the past 40 years, population-based estimates of civilian death tolls from most major armed conflicts have not been provided until after wars were over. The responsibility for this falls squarely on the shoulders of the public health community. The IRC surveys in DRC, and more recent similar studies in Iraq and Darfur, demonstrate that such estimates can always be developed if the public health community is truly determined to serve the victims of armed conflict.

References

1. Personal observation by the author (LR), July 20, 1994.
2. Edgerton RB. The Troubled Heart of Africa: A History of the Congo. New York: St. Martin's Press, 2002.
3. Africa's Seven Nation War. ICG Democratic Republic of Congo report no. 4, May 21, 1999. Available at: http://crisisgroup.org/home/index/cfm?id=1643&l=1 (accessed June 19, 2007).
4. Roberts L, Ngoy P, Mone C, et al. Mortality in the Democratic Republic of the Congo: Results from a nation-wide survey. New York: International Rescue Committee, March 2003. Available at: http://www.theirc.org/resources/documents.html?page=2 (accessed July 2, 2007).
5. Elevated Mortality Associated with Armed Conflict—Democratic Republic of Congo, 2002. MMWR Morb Mortal Wkly Rep 2003;52:469–471.
6. Roberts L, Hale C, Belyakdoumi F, et al. Mortality in Eastern Democratic Republic of Congo: Results from Eleven Mortality Surveys. New York: International Rescue Committee, 2001. Available at: http://www.theirc.org/resources/documents.html?page=2 (accessed July 2, 2007).
7. Roberts L. Mortality in Eastern DRC: Results from Five Mortality Surveys. New York: International Rescue Committee, 2000. Available at: http://www.theirc.org/resources/documents.html?page=2 (accessed July 2, 2007).
8. Depoortere E, Checchi F, Broillet F, et al. Violence and mortality in West Darfur, Sudan (2003–2004): Epidemiological evidence from four surveys. Lancet 2004;364: 1315.
9. Roberts L, Lafta R, Garfield R, et al. Mortality before and after the 2003 invasion of Iraq: Cluster sample survey. Lancet 2004;364:1857–1864.
10. Fisher I, Onishi N, Swarns R. et al. Chaos in Congo: A Primer: Many Armies Ravage a Rich Land in the "First World War" of Africa. New York Times, Feb. 6, 2000, page 1.

18

Wars in Latin America

Charlie Clements and Tim K. Takaro

After several decades of civil wars that affected a number of countries in Latin America, during the 1995–2005 period there have been only two armed conflicts in the region: the continuation of the protracted war in Colombia and a 12-day armed confrontation in Chiapas, Mexico, that continues to smolder in the zone of conflict.

The effects of decades of civil war in Guatemala, El Salvador, and Nicaragua continue with devastating impact. In contrast, peace and the lack of military expenditures have had positive impacts on public health in Costa Rica.

Countries in Latin America and the Caribbean have long been plagued by internal armed conflicts as well as economic exploitation, which has been both a cause and a consequence of armed conflict. There has been a pattern of interference and intervention—military and economic—by the United States in the region.

Since 1995, conditions in many countries of Latin America have changed dramatically. Whereas major armed violence continued in Colombia and threatened in Chiapas, several countries, including Venezuela, Bolivia, Peru, and Brazil, have changed leadership through electoral processes that were notable for dramatic increases in electoral participation by lower economic classes and/or indigenous populations. However, the region still suffers enormous debt burdens and structural adjustment policies (SAPs) of major credit organizations, the instability in Haiti, and the U.S. economic blockade of Cuba, any one of which could be a tripwire for conflict.

The fruits of peace, economic recovery, and improved health have not been uniformly achieved in the region. Disadvantaged and often indigenous populations lag well behind the dominant cultures in health and economic status. A review published in 1997 by the Pan American Health Organization (PAHO) provided confirmation that major inequalities in health remain a significant barrier to the advancement of the sizable indigenous populations in Latin America.[1] Although these populations were virtually wiped out in much of Latin America by the European invasion of the 15th and 16th centuries, they have re-emerged as a significant demographic and political force in some countries. The population of indigenous people in Latin America was estimated to be 48.5 million in 2003.[2]

The Venezuelan- and Mexican-led *contadora* peace process and the collapse of the Soviet Union coincided to help bring an end to several decades of armed conflicts in Central America. These armed conflicts in Guatemala, El Salvador, and Nicaragua were often referred to by political analysts as "low-intensity conflicts"—total war at the grassroots level, including political, economic, and psychological warfare.[3] Unlike in Vietnam (see Chapter 19), the United States could engage in proxy wars in these countries, providing arms, intelligence, and advisors without committing its own armed forces. For the civilian victims, who far outnumber the military casualties in these kinds of wars, there is nothing "low-intensity" about landmines, napalm, rocket-propelled grenades, or electronic "gattling guns" capable of putting a bullet in every square foot of a football field every minute. Both of us worked for brief periods as health care providers in rural communities in conflicted areas of Central America during that era; we will not demean the civilians whose wounds we treated by using the term "low-intensity conflict."

There were lasting public health consequences for the countries involved, both those in which the wars were fought and bordering countries that were used as staging areas or as places of uncertain refuge for fleeing victims. There are continuing public health consequences to the millions of internally displaced persons and refugees.

Two wars in South America often paralleled these three Central American wars in tactics: the 1973 military coup of the democratically elected Socialist regime of Salvador Allende in Chile, which was followed by a decade of officially declared "states of siege" or "states of emergency"; and the so-called "Dirty War" in Argentina between 1976 and 1983. What the five wars have in common is that the United States was a protagonist in each. Beginning with the so-called Andean Strategy of President George H. W. Bush in 1989 and later with Plan Colombia championed by both Presidents Bill Clinton and George W. Bush, the United States provided billions of dollars in military assistance, law enforcement, economic aid, and intelligence support to Colombia, Bolivia, and Peru in an effort to eradicate the primary source of imported cocaine. These "drug wars" have resulted in severe economic disruption, widespread human rights violations, and unknown public health effects due to spraying of herbicides by aircraft.

A conflict that had been simmering for decades and came to the attention of the world in the mid-1990s was the confrontation between the Zapatistas and the government of Mexico in Chiapas. While it remained mainly just a threat of war to the outside world, to the indigenous communities who were involved in the 12-day "hot" war and who remain affected by the presence of the Mexican military and covert economic and political policies of the government, it continues to feel like an endless smoldering war, one that is intermittently intensified by economical, political, and other winds. Several studies have documented the consequences to the health of these indigenous communities.

El Salvador

Although the civil war in El Salvador began in 1980, it was preceded by a decade of attempts at nonviolent social change, which were met with a brutal response at the hands of death squads, security forces, and the military. Every attempt at loosening the economic monopoly of the oligarchy and the political monopoly of the rightist political parties was considered a "communist threat." Before the war, 1,000 Salvadoran civilians were "disappeared" or killed each month—union leaders, student activists, peasant organizers, health care workers, Catholic priests, nuns, and lay church leaders inspired by liberation theology to respond to the plight of the poor. The United States at that time had a population almost 50 times that of El Salvador's 5 million people. To place these losses in perspective, this small, impoverished country was losing the U.S. equivalent of 50,000 lives per month.[4]

By the late 1980s, despite several billion dollars of military and economic assistance, military advisors and training, advanced weapons systems, and sophisticated intelligence support from the United States, the armed forces of El Salvador were fought to a virtual stalemate by the guerrilla forces, known as the Farabundo Marti Front for National Liberation (FMLN). The end of the Cold War and the concerted efforts of Venezuela, Mexico, and Costa Rica to create a framework for regional peace accords finally led to an end of the civil war in 1992. The cost was horrendous.

During the war, almost 1 million Salvadorans were internally displaced or internationally displaced as legal and illegal refugees. A U.N.-appointed truth commission attributed 95 percent of the almost 80,000 Salvadoran deaths to the death squads and military and security forces, and about 5 percent to the FMLN, which included extrajudicial killings of informants, mayors, and judges.[5] During the civil war, 80 percent of government forces and 20 percent of opposition forces were estimated to be children (younger than 18 years of age).[6]

Public health measures, such as immunizations and vector control for malaria, as well as primary care services and well-baby care previously available in rural clinics, were no longer provided by the Ministry of Health in contested areas of the country. Other health care services were militarized in attempt to "win hearts and minds" of populations sympathetic to the guerrillas. Ministry of Health budgets shrank during most of the civil war.

Malnutrition was already a serious problem in El Salvador, because so much land previously used for subsistence farming had been slowly converted to cotton or coffee production or used to graze cattle. Domestic food production was reduced by almost 30 percent during the war, creating more dependence on imports and leading to further malnutrition.

Early in the war (1980), the army invaded, ransacked, and closed the nation's only medical school. Throughout the war, there were murders of physicians in hospitals or clinics, disappearances of nurses and other health care personnel, intentional targeting of medical facilities or transports, and summary executions of people discovered with medicines and medical equipment.[7]

The Peace Accords signed in Mexico City in 1992 were sophisticated and far reaching; they included a truth commission, land reform, restructuring of the judiciary, a new national civilian police force, disbanding of the notorious Treasury Police and National Guard, reduction in the size of the military and its return to barracks, and internationally supervised elections with political parties formed by the former guerrillas.

Although the Peace Accords were successful in shifting the armed struggle into a parliamentary/political struggle, the continued control of vast economic resources by a small and powerful business elite, stalled land reform, trade agreements that resulted in large "free-trade zones" with few labor protections, and corruption left the country impoverished.

Although statistics are unavailable for Haiti, El Salvador has the second largest percentage of population (31.1 percent) below the international poverty line in the hemisphere. Its ratio of the incomes of the highest 20 percent to the lowest 20 percent of the population is among the highest in the hemisphere.[8]

The worst legacy of the civil war may be the kidnapping, robbery, murder, and gang-related violence that remain prevalent because of the failure after the war to disarm the combatants on both sides. El Salvador's estimated homicide rate of 43.4 per 100,000 population is exceeded in the hemisphere only by that of Colombia.[8]

Nicaragua

Shortly after achieving independence from Spain in 1821 and from Mexico 2 years later, Nicaragua joined the other new Central American nations as targets of "manifest destiny" and opportunities for U.S. business interests. Mercenary armies swept through the country during the 1850s, with the leader of one, William Walker, declaring himself president in 1855. He was deposed a year later by the U.S. Navy supported by Cornelius Vanderbilt. U.S. Marines landed again in 1912 to support a conservative party revolt and occupied the country until 1933. Augusto Cesar Sandino led the resistance to this occupation. Before departing, the U.S. Marines helped establish the National Guard and the government of Anastasio Somoza Garcia, which assassinated Sandino.

The Somoza family was loyal to the United States, and its power was consolidated over the following decades. By the 1970s, it controlled Nicaragua economically and politically. The family rule was ended by the triumph of a popular insurrection led by the Sandinista Front for National Liberation in 1979. The new government of Nicaragua was quickly recognized by the world community, including initially the United States. With its capital, Managua, virtually still in ruins from the 1972 earthquake, the country was further devastated by the insurrection. An estimated 50,000 people (2 percent of the total population) died in the 5 years leading up to Somoza's overthrow.[9] The World Bank reported that "per capita income levels of 1977 will not be attained, in the best of circumstances, until the late 1980s."[10] Three months after the new government was established, it suffered its first losses in the next war for its independence when 20 militia members were killed in a cross-border ambush by former members of Somoza's National Guard. By mid-1980, the nature of the war to come was already clear.[9] Despite the initial support of the Sandinista government by the United States, it was soon labeled "a communist threat" by the U.S. right wing, and the election of President Ronald Reagan in 1980 further fanned the flames of the Cold War. For the next 8 years, while attempting to bring literacy, land reform, and basic public health care to the lowest income groups in the country, the Nicaraguan government fought a cross-border counterinsurgency force, which would come to be known as the *contras*, that was funded, trained, and supported by the United States.

When considered against this postwar/prewar backdrop, the improvement in health indicators for Nicaragua's rural poor was particularly remarkable during the first half of the 1980s. By 1983, the number of primary care facilities had tripled, endemic polio had been eliminated, and the incidence of other vaccine-preventable illnesses had been dramatically reduced, in part through the widespread use of volunteer lay-trained "health brigadistas."[11] In 1982, Nicaragua received recognition from the World Health Organization (WHO) for the most improved health system. Oral rehydration campaigns as well as latrine and water system improvement helped to halve between 1975 and 1986 the rate of diarrheal disease, the leading cause of death for children younger than five years of age.[11]

The Reagan administration's support to the networks of Nicaragua's deposed elite in Miami, who ostensibly led the contras, included mining Nicaragua's harbors, hiring mercenary pilots as "soldiers of fortune" to provide logistical support, using vastly increased military aid to enlist the support of the Honduran military to turn a blind eye to contra bases in their country, and undermining the sovereignty of Costa Rica by establishing contra bases there. In an ironic twist, to avoid Congressional restrictions on funding the contras, the Reagan administration traded arms and spare parts to the government of Iran in return for its support to the contras in what became known as the Iran–Contra Affair. The irregular force, led by former Somoza-era National Guard officers and other anti-Sandinista operatives, established bases along the northern border inside Honduras and covert bases in Costa Rica. The covert flow of money was officially sanctioned when the U.S. Congress approved the first $24 million in 1984. Soon, additional recruits were readily found among Nicaraguan farmers and indigenous peoples who were disillusioned with Sandinista policy and the slow pace of reform in rural areas.

With this financing, training materials provided by the U.S. Central Intelligence Agency (CIA), and U.S. military advisors based in Honduras, the contras launched a relentless campaign against the social fabric of Nicaragua's mountainous rural communities. Farm cooperatives, schools, clinics, and the civilian transportation system were frequent targets. Health care workers and teachers were systematically killed or kidnapped, and their unprotected rural posts were burned to the ground. Many of the kidnapped health workers were teenagers who were force-marched to the Honduran camps. Intimidated by threats to their families, they were pressured along the journey into joining the contra forces.[12]

By the mid-1980s, the relentless state-sponsored terrorism and economic pressures from Washington began to wear down the economy. Medical, nursing, and dental visits peaked in 1983 at 2.3 per capita before beginning a steady decline to 1.7 by 1990. Prescriptions filled followed a similar pattern, with a peak at 4.8 per capita in 1985 and a fall to 2.0 by 1990. The famed vaccination campaigns faltered, leading to a measles epidemic in 1990 that was worse than any recorded in the previous two decades.[11] After hovering near zero for the first half of the 1980s, inflation reached 3,500 percent just before the 3,000 percent devaluation of the currency in 1988. The devastating Hurricane Joan struck the Atlantic Coast in October 1988, destroying another three hospitals and 29 clinics, killing more than 400 people, and leaving 230,000 homeless. The health system was estimated to have lost more than 180 health workers and more than 20 percent of its 600 health facilities to the war. By 1988, an estimated 6,760 Nicaraguans had been killed in the conflict, more than half of whom were civilians.[11]

Nicaragua had few options remaining when the five Central American leaders in the region, led by Costa Rican President Oscar Arias, were finally able to complete a negotiated agreement in 1989, which included the disarming of the contra forces and an end to the war. As part of the agreement, the Sandinistas agreed to early elections. One year later, President Daniel Ortega was defeated by the U.S.-supported candidate, Violetta Chamorro. There was widespread fear that, if the Sandinistas were re-elected, the war might continue.

President Chamorro inherited a devastated economy and a divided country. Notably, the health system inherited from the Sandinistas received high marks from the U.S. Army–sponsored Federal Research Division of the Library of Congress Country Studies/Area Handbook Series[13]:

> Despite the problems of the late 1980s, however, the Sandinista decade left behind an improved health care system. According to a 1991 assessment of Nicaraguan development needs by the U.S. Agency for International Development (USAID), the Chamorro government inherited a health care system that emphasized preventive and primary care; targeted the principal causes of infant, child, and maternal mortality; provided broad coverage; and elicited high levels of community participation. The USAID report noted the effectiveness of the oral rehydration centers, the wide coverage of vaccination campaigns, and the key role of the health *brigadistas,* three programs maintained by the new government. The report concluded that the major problem of the health sector was lack of budgetary resources.

Unfortunately this last caveat, in conjunction with the SAPs mandated by the International Monetary Fund (IMF), continued the war-induced erosion in health. Efforts to decentralize health services and increase the role of the private sector in the health system began in earnest. Between 1992 and 1996, the Chamorro government reduced spending on health by 12 percent and introduced user fees, effectively reducing access to care. The volunteer health campaigns that were popular during the Sandinista period could not be effectively maintained in the new climate. Malaria control was particularly affected, and malaria rates had tripled by the 1995–1997 period.[11] By 2000, market reform efforts had transformed the Nicaraguan health care system from a WHO model for primary care delivery to a multitiered system similar to that of the Somoza era, based on ability to pay or employment status, with some new twists including managed care organizations. Decentralization of health care services to local health authorities with no political accountability continued to insulate the central government from responsibility for meaningful reforms in health.[11]

After decades of global activism advocating debt relief for impoverished nations, Nicaragua enjoyed a dramatic restructuring of its external debt in late 2005. The IMF's Multilateral Debt Relief and Heavily Indebted Poor Countries Initiatives forgave all of Nicaragua's external debt of $204 million to the United States. The relief was specifically to reward "satisfactory recent macroeconomic performance, progress in poverty reduction, and improvements in public expenditure management." On the surface, this relief appears favorable to Nicaraguans, as it reduces service payments on the debt, but the relief was won by legislating reductions in social services. The poorest and most indigenous rural areas of Nicaragua continue to suffer from poor health, with the mortality rate for children younger than 5 years of age being higher than 57 per 1,000 in the 1996–2000 period, twice the rate of the country's four most populated and Ladino provinces.

In late 2006, Daniel Ortega was again elected president. It remains to be seen whether his leadership will affect the future direction of the country.

Guatemala

Negotiations that began in 1991 and concluded in 1996 ended almost four decades of armed conflict between the government of Guatemala and the largely Mayan resistance movements, which toward the end of the conflict had jointed together as the Guatemalan National Revolutionary Unity (URNG). The Peace Accords of 1996 were actually eight distinct agreements, the first of which (the Framework Accord) set up the rules and parties for the subsequent accords. While the United Nations verification commission (MINUGUA) remained in the country, there was fitful implementation by the government of its obligations. When MINUGUA's mission ended in 2004, implementation all but halted. In contrast to the postwar transition in neighboring El Salvador, the Guatemalan resistance has been unable to create a political party to represent its collective interests and thus hold the government accountable to its commitments under the Peace Accords.

The establishment of the Commission for the Historical Clarification of Human Rights Violations and Acts of Violence, a United Nations–assisted truth commission, was one of the few accords fully implemented.[14] The separate REMHI Commission was a parallel effort by the Catholic church to establish an historical record of what happened during the conflict and who was responsible.[15] (In Spanish, REMHI stands for Interdiocesan Project for the Recovery of Historical Memory.) The truth commission attributed 93 percent of the estimated war-related deaths to the military and death squads, and 3 percent to the guerrillas. Neither commission considered other war-related deaths, such as excess child mortality caused by lack of medical attention, food, and shelter among the more than 1 million internally displaced persons and an estimated 250,000 refugees who fled into neighboring Mexico.

Within 2 days after publication of the report, Bishop Juan Gerardi, who led the REMHI Commission, was bludgeoned to death. Although it was known who ordered and who committed the murder, the case would come to represent the impunity of the Guatemala military, which granted itself official amnesty. This period of brutality, officially characterized by the truth commission as genocide, had its roots in the Cold War. The U.N. Truth Commission stated that, "in the context of the counterinsurgency operations undertaken between 1981 and 1983, the agents of the Guatemalan state carried out acts of genocide against groups of Mayan people."[14] The Commission rejected the excuse that the violations were the result of "excesses" or "errors" committed by subordinates and recognized the fact that no high- or middle-ranking official was tried or condemned for human rights violations over such a long period of time as evidence that the violations represented an institutional policy that guaranteed impunity at the highest level of government.

Exploitation and marginalization of the indigenous people of Guatemala began more than 500 years ago with the arrival of the Spanish conquistadors. An aberration on that historical timeline was the 1945–1954 period, so hopeful that it is sometimes referred to as the "Mayan renaissance." Led by a teacher turned president, the government introduced massive literacy campaigns, legalized unions, abolished vagrancy laws that allowed landowners to virtually enslave indigenous peasants, and introduced universal suffrage. His successor was elected with a strong mandate to continue reforms. In an effort to thwart repeated coup attempts, he incited militancy in students and unions and mobilized peasants with massive land reform. The government seized land of the great monopolies that was either idle or in arrears in taxes, turning it over to more than 100,000 landless families.[16]

Since the turn of the 19th century, the United States had been granted concessions, which left the ports, transportation services, power companies, and huge amounts of land controlled by U.S. corporations. The United Fruit Company, which had planted only 15 percent of its vast holdings, quickly lost almost half its land. The legalization of the Communist Party, which won four seats in the Parliamentary elections of 1952, was the beginning of the end of the government of Jacobo Arbenz Guzmán. At the time, Allan Dulles, the Director of the CIA, sat on the board of United Fruit, and his brother, John Foster Dulles, was Secretary of State. In 1953, President Dwight Eisenhower approved a CIA plan to overthrow the government of Guatemala. The coup itself was almost bloodless, but not so the four decades of violence and human rights violations that followed, abetted by U.S. counterinsurgency support in arms, training, and intelligence sharing.[16]

Of the estimated 200,000 wartime deaths, about half occurred in 1982, after the seizure of power by General Rios Montt. He quickly implemented a "scorched-earth" campaign that destroyed more than 600 villages. Survivors were relocated into strategic hamlets, guarded and informed upon by indigenous militias known as civil patrollers. Any male who refused to serve in the civil patrols could be accused of being a "communist" and subjected to summary execution. The anti-communist banner was also used by urban death squads as a pretext to murder hundreds of union leaders and "disappear" thousands of political dissidents and students.

A paragraph from the U.S. State Department Country Reports on Human Rights, released in 2005, provides a snapshot of the consequences of the war[17]:

> There were credible reports of individual police officers' involvement in kidnappings for ransom. Security forces tortured, abused, and mistreated suspects and detainees. Prison conditions remained harsh. In most cases, the prosecutorial and judicial systems did not ensure full and timely investigations, fair trials, or due process. Arbitrary arrest and lengthy pretrial detentions were problems. Judges and other law enforcement officials were subjected to intimidation and corruption. Impunity was pervasive....Members of the media were targets of attacks and intimidation.... Violence increased, and discrimination against women persisted, as did societal abuse of children and discrimination against persons with disabilities and indigenous people. Trafficking in persons was a problem. There were reports of retaliation by employers against workers who sought to form unions and participate in union activities, and the Government did not enforce consistently laws to protect workers who exercised their rights. There was widespread employment of minors in the informal sector.

Given the power of the oligarchs and the business sector, it is not surprising that the Central American Free Trade Agreement (CAFTA) passed in Guatemala despite very strong popular opposition. Ten years' experience with the impact of the North American Free Trade Agreement (NAFTA) in Mexico left little doubt that heavily subsidized U.S. agricultural imports, especially corn, would ruin the country's subsistence farmers.

The tilt toward large business interests did not begin with the CAFTA debate. Médecins Sans Frontières (MSF) complained in 2003 that the Guatemalan government, by granting five years of exclusivity to originators of pharmaceutical products, would prevent generic equivalents from being registered even if there were no patents on those drugs. Guatemala is the only country in the hemisphere with such a law, which will directly affect poor people's access to inexpensive medicines.[18]

Guatemala has the lowest tax base in the hemisphere—too low, according to the United Nations, for the provision of basic services, such as health services, education, and public security. Guatemala has the lowest health expenditure (as a percentage of gross domestic product [GDP]) and the fewest hospital beds per capita in both the region and the hemisphere. In the hemisphere, it ranks behind only Haiti and Nicaragua in illiteracy. Along with Colombia and El Salvador, it leads the hemisphere in homicides.[8] Although the war has ended, Guatemala today is one of the most violent countries with the greatest disparity of wealth in the hemisphere and a country where the majority indigenous population remains politically and economically marginalized.

Colombia

A discussion of the protracted civil war in Colombia begins with the period called "La Violencia"—a decade of sustained warfare from 1948 to 1958 between the Liberal and Conservative parties, the same parties whose elites had alternately competed and cooperated with each other throughout the 19th and 20th centuries. Claiming more than 200,000 lives, La Violencia was ended by a bipartisan agreement called the National Front, which called for alternating power between the two parties every four years. The two leftist guerrilla movements that are still prominent in today's conflict—the Army of National Liberation (ELN) and the Revolutionary Armed Forces of Columbia (FARC)—emerged during early years of the National Front. They resulted from a number of factors, including a reaction to endemic political corruption; the aggrandizement of power by elite interests of the two parties (which all but ignored the needs of the poorest sectors); ineffective, U.S.-assisted pacification programs; and revolutionary fervor that swept through much of Latin America after the triumph of Fidel Castro in Cuba.[19]

This period marked the beginning of the Colombian government's loss of control over much of its territory, an underlying cause of today's intractable conflict. The FARC was the most active militant group, operating in rural areas in a number of departments as a de facto state—establishing its own schools, judicial system, health care, and agrarian economy. During the 1970s, a third, largely-urban guerrilla movement, M-19, was formed partly in response to national electoral fraud. During this period, the illicit narcotics industry emerged as a parallel financial market, placing much of the national economy beyond the control of legitimate authority. The drug lords and guerrillas often worked together during these years, with the guerillas controlling coca-growing regions and the cartels controlling cocaine production and trafficking.

At the end of the 1970s, the government declared a state of siege directed at combating the growing narcotic trafficking and the guerrilla movements. The military began creating paramilitary units to assist the administration of President Belisario Betancur. He had been elected in the early 1980s and faced an economic abyss caused by inflation, foreign debt, domestic deficits, economic recession, unemployment, and increasingly powerful narocotics cartels allied with the guerrilla movements. He sought peace with the guerrillas, offering unconditional amnesty and legitimate participation in the political process. Disarmed guerrillas, former communists, and liberals formed the Patriotic Union, a party that was soon targeted by both death squads associated with narcotraffickers (MAS) and emerging rightist paramilitary forces (AUC). In the following decade, the deaths of more than 3,000 party members, mayors, and political candidates, including two presidential candidates, led the FARC to once again take up arms as the means to political reform. In the meantime, having seized control of coca and poppy fields throughout the country, they began to "tax" the farmers and small producers. As the Cali and Medellin cartels invested their drug profits in cattle ranches, they became the largest land owners in Colombia, which equated them with the guerrillas' traditional enemies.[19,20]

The paramilitaries allied with the armed forces began to target not only guerrillas but also anyone suspected of "leftist tendencies," which included unionists, peasant organizers, human rights workers, and clergy. Judges who attempted to investigate rightist death squads or cooperate with the U.S. "war on drugs" to extradite narcotraffickers were themselves targeted as the paramilitaries turned against the government itself. The next victims were reporters who attempted to expose the cartels, human rights violations of the death squads, or their links to the military. Kidnapping of cartel members or their relatives and profiting from coca production became primary means of financing, and thus rearming, the FARC.[21]

President George H. W. Bush's Andean Plan in the early 1990s committed $2.2 billion of U.S. military and economic aid to Colombia, Peru, and Bolivia but conditioned the economic portion of assistance on acceptance of military aid. Only the Colombian government agreed, and therefore the United States, in the name of the "war on drugs," strengthened its ties to the region's most brutal military, which had for a decade worked hand in hand with the Cali and Medellin cartels, and began its involvement with the counterinsurgency. By 1997, a year when more than 24,000 people were killed, Colombia was labeled one of the worst human rights violators in the world. With more than

3 million people displaced from the countryside to cities since 1998, Colombia has the second highest number of internally displaced persons in the world. About half of these internally displaced persons, according to United Nations High Commissioner on Refugees (UNHCR), have no access to health care; many of them do not have access to housing, education, and work.[22]

The health sector in Colombia is divided into two worlds: urban and rural. Most government and private investments in the health sector have been in urban areas, where causes of morbidity are increasingly similar to those of developed countries, such as cardiovascular disease and cancer. The huge disparities in maternal and infant mortality between urban and rural Colombia reflect the lack of services in rural areas and account for Colombia's overall high rate of maternal and infant mortality.[24]

The Inter-American Commission on Human Rights calculated that 1.7 million people were displaced due to violence in the 1985–1999 period. Among young men aged 15 to 19 years, violence accounted for 69 percent of the deaths; there were 13 male deaths for each female death in this age group.[25] Colombia's homicide rate is almost twice that of any other country in the hemisphere.[8]

The question of how spending on public services and allocation of resources would have been different without a half-century of violence looms in any discussion of Colombia. For example, according to the Ministry of Health, 60 percent of the inhabitants in the municipal seats run a medium to high risk of developing infectious diseases because of the poor quality of the water. In 2000, 76 percent of municipalities did not have potable water. Barely 5 percent of 1,076 municipalities treat their wastewater before they dispose of it, according to the Ministry of Development. This situation has essentially turned the Cauca and Magdalena river basins, which receive more than 80 percent of the nation's wastewater, into open sewers.[26]

The pollution of groundwater by domestic and industrial effluents and solid waste of all kinds is threatening not only the supply of water available for human consumption and production but also the nation's flora and fauna. One of the worst pollutants is oil, which has leaked into the soil and water sources as a result of attacks on the country's petroleum infrastructure. In 1998, the Ministry of Health and other sources estimated that leakage of 2 million barrels of oil had affected 70 municipalities, including 2,600 km of rivers and streams, 6,000 hectares of land with agricultural potential, 1,600 km^2 of marshes and wetlands, and transnational catchment areas such as the Catatumbo and Arauca river basins.[26]

With increasing fears in the United States that much of its supply of Venezuelan oil may be imperilled, considerable military resources supplied under Plan Colombia have now been diverted to guarding oil pipelines. In the fall of 2006, publications ranging from the *New York Times* to *Newsweek* finally began to describe Plan Colombia as a failure: "But despite all the bullish spin coming out of Bogota and Washington, Plan Colombia has failed in most categories of the war on drugs. The crackdown on coca farming in Putumayo had the effect of dispersing growers: the number of departments where the plant is cultivated has risen from a dozen five years ago to 20 today. The total amount of acreage planted with coca may be down nationwide, but the supply of cocaine clearly hasn't been disrupted."[27,28]

Little is likely to change until the U.S. government realizes that the debate must shift from Colombia to the United States. For example, a study from the RAND Corporation in 1994 estimated that treating heavy cocaine users in the United States was three times more effective than implementing mandatory minimum sentencing, and 23 times more cost-effective than eradicating drug crops such as coca.[29]

Chiapas, Mexico

On January 1, 1994, thousands of indigenous people of southern Mexico's state of Chiapas supported an armed uprising led by the Zapatista Army for the National Liberation (EZLN). A 12-day armed confrontation with the Mexican Army ensued, leading to a standoff and an ongoing conflict that continues today. Chiapas, with almost 4 million inhabitants, has one of the largest indigenous populations in Mexico (approximately 25 percent of the population in the state as a whole, and 80 percent in the zone of conflict). In 2000, it also had the lowest per-capita spending on health in Mexico—just one indicator of the marginalization of the population.[30] This marginalization is particularly acute in the indigenous zone of conflict in the north. Jungle and highland regions make up about half of the land area of this state (73,724 km², or 28,465 square miles, slightly smaller than the U.S. state of South Carolina). Here the Mexican Army and the paramilitary forces connected with it continue to spar with EZLN for control and loyalty of the thousands of small farming settlements in the zone.

Unfortunately, health "came to be held hostage" in the conflict zone as Zapatista communities rejected government overtures of assistance in an expression of autonomy and strength. The army tried to impose health and social services through the establishment of army health posts.[31] Dispersion to smaller communities, extrajudicial killings, the introduction of alcohol by the army, paramilitary activities, travel restrictions, and other kinds of intimidation contributed further to social erosion in the conflict zone. Reportedly, individual health practitioners refused to provide health services to people because of their political affiliation or ethnicity, further contributing to the lack of access.[32]

In 2000, the army health posts were removed after a complaint by the United Nations Committee on Economic, Social and Cultural Rights. An office of the UNHCR was established in part to ensure that the Mexican government would honor its obligations to guarantee the right to health for people in the zone of conflict.

In its 2006 study of health care utilization, Physicians for Human Rights demonstrated that these populations continue to live under deplorable conditions without access to basic services and with health indicators well below those of Mexico as a whole.[32] In this study of almost 3,000 households, clear disparities were demonstrated between settlements in the zone of conflict and those in other parts of Chiapas. The infant mortality rate in the zone of conflict was 39.4 per 1,000 live births, more than three times that of Chiapas as a whole in 2000.[33] The study's findings underscored the fact that the "unfortunate synergy" of civil resistance in isolated rural settlements and highly politicized provision of health services to government-controlled settlements interspersed in the same zone is both a result of, and contributes to, the ongoing conflict in Chiapas.

Costa Rica

The story of Costa Rica's progressive government began in 1940 with the election of Dr. Rafael Angel Calderon. His United Social Christian Party enacted legislation that established a minimum wage, land reform, and progressive taxation. His party refused to leave office in 1948, claiming that voting fraud had led to its defeat at the polls.

Jose "Pepe" Figueres, a remarkable and charismatic politician, had been in exile in Mexico since being arrested after an antigovernment radio broadcast in 1942. In Mexico, he formed a party in exile and accused the Calderon government of corruption. By 1947, he had begun training a volunteer army on one of his farms, and the refusal of the incumbent government to step down provided him the pretext he needed. Supported by the governments of Cuba and Guatemala, his forces launched a "civil war" that lasted only 40 days.

The military junta that Figueres led promised to step aside after 18 months. During that time, it established reforms that would change the course of the nation. It disbanded the army that brought Figueres to power as well as the national army he defeated. The junta extended voting rights to women and Costa Ricans of African origin and granted them full civil liberties. It continued the land reforms of the previous government, nationalized the banking and insurance sectors, established the Supreme Electoral Council to prevent electoral fraud, and set presidential term limits. The socialist-leaning junta paradoxically banned the Communist Party.[34]

The Costa Rican people later showed their appreciation of Figueres by granting him two separate terms as president, 1953 to 1957 and 1970 to 1974. His lasting legacy to Costa Rica was the sense of fairness and democratic values that his leadership and governments represented. However, during the 1950s, the U.S. CIA was actively trying to foment his overthrow. Figueres, like Arbenz in Guatemala, was an avowed socialist, but he was considered a threat because of his hostility to neighboring dictator Somoza and because he was providing exile to hundreds of leftists fleeing right-wing military dictatorships throughout Latin America. Figueres gave them not only shelter but also encouragement in returning to overthrow their repressive governments.[35] Oscar Arias, who served as president of Costa Rica from 1986 to 1990, searched for a negotiated settlement to the wars that engulfed Nicaragua, El Salvador, and Guatemala in the 1980s. His tireless efforts led to his receiving the Nobel Peace Prize in 1987. But the prize for Costa Rica over the decades since the triumph of Figueres' rebel army has been stability and good government.

By any measure, Costa Rica's achievements in health, education, and economic security are remarkable, and they are all the more so in comparison with other countries in the region or hemisphere. The life expectancy at birth of Costa Ricans is exceeded only by that of Canadians. With only 2 percent of its population below the internationally established poverty level, it leads the hemisphere. Costa Rica's maternal and infant mortality rates are surpassed only by those of Canada, the United States, and Cuba. Its expenditure of 4.9 percent of its GDP for health ranks it in the top five nations of the hemisphere, but with better longevity than countries whose governments spend greater percentages of their budget for health.[8]

Modern Costa Rica, although born of violence, has eschewed it as a political instrument of the state. Several factors may have contributed to Costa Rica's success as a nation, but one of them has to be the legacy of stability and peace bequeathed by Figueres.

Chile

On September 11, 1973, the democratically elected government of Chile was overthrown by a military junta led by General Augusto Pinochet. Chile's president, Dr. Salvador Allende, a public health physician, was murdered during the coup, which was supported by the U.S. government. The coup led to the arrest of thousands of Chileans, many of whom were killed or "disappeared" and thousands of whom were tortured. General Pinochet ruled Chile until 1990. After his resignation, a democratically elected government was installed, but a law adopted during the reign of the junta gave amnesty to members of the junta for crimes committed.

In September 1987, the government of Chile signed the Convention against Torture and Other Cruel, Inhuman or Degrading Treatment or Punishment. Less than two months later, its president, Augusto Pinochet, sent the military junta, composed of four generals in charge of the army, navy, air force, and police (who represented the legislative power), a communication requesting the ratification of this Convention. In that communication, he specifically stated that the Convention was "an important step in the process of humanization of international law [and] destined to become an adequate mechanism to promote a more effective enforcement of the rights that are guaranteed in several multilateral international instruments." The Convention against Torture was ratified by the government of Chile in 1988 and received the necessary approval of the junta.[39]

A decade later, when Pinochet traveled to Great Britain for medical care, both he and the government of Chile were stunned when Scotland Yard served him an arrest warrant and an extradition order. Baltazar Garzon, a judge in Spain, noting that the Pinochet government had continued to torture, murder, and "disappear" political enemies after signing the Convention against Torture, invoked its definition of state-organized torture as a crime against humanity, thus establishing his court's claim of universal jurisdiction. The indictment had been sealed until a headline in the British newspaper, *The Guardian,* warned, "A Torturer in Our Midst!"[39]

The charter of the court at Nuremberg, after World War II, had first established that crimes against humanity would have universal jurisdiction and no statute of limitations.* The promises of that court were largely forgotten for a half-century until collective guilt about what the world had allowed to unfold in the former Yugoslavia, and soon after in Rwanda, led the U.N. Security Council to establish two special tribunals for crimes against humanity, genocide, and war crimes. European courts in the 1990s had begun to remember the promise of Nuremberg as well, and several national courts began testing jurisdiction for crimes committed outside their borders.

---

*After the Allies occupied Germany in 1945, several trials were held in the city of Nuremberg. The first trial, of the wartime leaders of Nazi Germany, was called the Trial of the Major War Criminals and was conducted by an International Military Tribunal composed of representatives of all four occupying powers—the United States, Soviet Union, the United Kingdom, and France. The Charter of the International Military Tribunal defined "crimes against humanity," "crimes against peace," and "war crimes." The Charter and the trials that followed led to the formulation by an international law commission of a set of Nuremberg Principles, which held that these crimes would be universally recognized and would have no statute of limitations. The second trial, which was called the Doctors Trial, was conducted by a U.S. military tribunal and tried those responsible for medical experiments on prisoners during the war. The trial verdict adopted 10 points that defined legitimate medical research; these points are known as the Nuremberg Code.

Pinochet was held under house arrest while the case worked its way to the highest judicial authority in Great Britain, the Court of the House of Lords. There, after a ruling against him and a subsequent appeal, a panel of British law lords ruled six to one that Pinochet did not enjoy immunity from prosecution as a former head of state and could be extradited to Spain. However, Pinochet's personal physicians claimed that he had suffered a series of strokes during that year which left him with moderate dementia and unable to stand trial. Three court-appointed physicians examined him; two of the three concurred. He was allowed to return to Chile on humanitarian grounds.[39]

Pinochet's indictment and arrest and the judgment of the Court of the House of Lords were collectively a shift of tectonic plates in the world of human rights, the aftershocks of which are still being felt today. The Supreme Court of Chile eventually stripped Pinochet of the immunity he and others of the military junta granted themselves with an amnesty decree in 1978, as well as the further parliamentary protection that he received when he assumed a nonelected lifetime seat in the Chilean senate after stepping down as commander-in-chief of the Chilean armed forces in 1997.[40]

In 2005, the Supreme Court of Argentina overturned a pair of amnesty laws that blocked the prosecutions of crimes committed under the country's last military dictatorship during the "Dirty War." These laws were enacted under duress by President Raúl Alfonsín in 1986 and 1987 to quell military rebellions against human rights trials. Trials for a few of the horrific abuses committed by military and police officials—murders, kidnappings, torture, rapes, and the abduction and sale of infants—unpunished for nearly 30 years, have now begun.[41]

Many legal analysts believe that the Pinochet indictment and extradition by the Spanish judge and subsequent events in several countries around the world are perhaps the most important development in international law since the Nuremberg trials. In 1999, the *New York Times* coined a new verb when it suggested that dictators and thugs around the world might hesitate to travel so freely, lest they be "pinocheted."

The fear of being "pinocheted," of eventually being held accountable for grave abuses of human rights, genocide, and crimes against humanity, is also the hope of the International Criminal Tribunal (ICT), which was finally established in 2003. The slowly emerging reality of remedies for grievous violations of human rights could play an increasingly important role in prevention of war.

In 2006, Dr. Michelle Bachelet, a public health pediatrician, was elected president of Chile. Dr. Bachelet's father, a general in the Chilean army, had been tortured and killed after the coup, and she and her mother had been imprisoned by the junta. After the death of General Pinochet in late 2006, Dr. Bachelet asked the Chilean legislature to repeal the amnesty law.

Preventing Wars

What can contribute to the prevention of wars? To answer this question, we examine developments affecting interstate and internal conflicts in Latin America.

Interstate Conflicts

Other than border disputes, there have been only two wars between Latin American countries in the last half century—the "Soccer War" in the late 1960s between Honduras and El Salvador, and the 1995 Condor Cordillera War between Ecuador and Peru. (We do not consider the war between Great Britain and Argentina over the Malvinas, or Falkland Islands, in the early 1980s to be a Latin American war.) The Honduran–Salvadoran war, sometimes called the "100 Hours War" was quickly concluded with the assistance of an urgent meeting of the Organization of American States (OAS), which was called within 24 hours after the outbreak of hostilities. OAS brokered a ceasefire, dispatched monitors, and threatened economic sanctions if El Salvador refused to withdraw its forces.

The Condor Cordillera War, also known as the Alto Cenepa War, between Peru and Ecuador in 1995, resulted in approximately 1,000 deaths. It paved the way for a definitive diplomatic solution to a problem that had plagued Peru and Ecuador since almost the time of their independence. Mediation by the United States, Brazil, Argentina, and Chile resulted in the Rio Protocol, which ended one of the longest territorial disputes in the Western Hemisphere.[37]

By international standards, Latin America was relatively free from interstate war in the 20th century. Why was this so? What lessons can be drawn from the region that might be applicable to prevention of interstate wars in other countries?

Jorge Dominguez, Professor of International Relations at Harvard and one of the founders of Inter-American Dialogue, observed the following about Latin America[38]:

- Territorial, boundary, and other disputes endure. Interstate conflict over boundaries is relatively frequent.
- Disputes sometimes escalate to military conflict because states recurrently employ low levels of force to shape aspects of bilateral relations.
- Such escalation rarely reaches full-scale war.
- Interstate war is infrequent.

One of his conclusions, evident in the short duration of both wars mentioned earlier, is that regional institutions and procedures that began to develop in the 19th century and matured in the 20th century have played an important role in providing effective international mediation when wars did occur.[38] As evidenced by the Contadora process and the awarding of the 1987 Nobel Peace Prize to Oscar Arias of Costa Rica, these same traditions also played critical roles in the regional negotiations that eventually led to the end of the civil wars in Nicaragua, El Salvador, and Guatemala.

Another of the conclusions by Dominguez may have been even more important in fostering interstate peace and, conversely, may be a factor in the frequency of civil wars. He stated that more than a century of shared identity has meant that Latin Americans do not perceive their neighbors as their enemies. This has contributed to a use of relatively small force when there were border disputes and prompt acceptance of mediation to resolve them. In the historical context of Latin America, the recent example of the United States in its global "war on terror"—discarding international law, disregarding long-standing treaty obligations, and openly disdaining international institutions in favor of unilateral interests—would be behavior that could aggravate rather than help prevent interstate conflict.

Internal Conflicts

Dag Hammarskjöld, former Secretary-General of the United Nations, cautioned that words are important and that their use implies moral categories. There was nothing "civil" about the internal conflicts in Guatemala, Chile, Argentina, Peru, Nicaragua, El Salvador, and Colombia, although they are often referred to as "civil wars." Today, Mayans in Guatemala refuse to use the term "civil war" and instead speak of the "armed conflict," even though most of the arms belonged to one side. The kind of collective brutality evidenced in these conflicts certainly has its roots in a lack of shared identity that allowed one side, or both, to dehumanize the other as subversives, communists, or, more recently, terrorists.

Another element common to all of these countries is economic and political marginalization of much of the population, sometimes by race, almost always by poverty. This situation was typically accomplished through a political system, which may have been democratic only in name. It consistently concentrated authority in the hands of powerful elites, who were usually backed by the police and military. The powerlessness of marginalized populations, the oppression that they experienced in attempting to bring about change, and their recognition of their own rights were common to all these internal conflicts. These "awakenings" had different origins, such as liberation theology, political ideologies of Marxism and socialism, and literacy campaigns based on sources such as Freire's *Pedagogy of the Oppressed,* but they each inspired attempts at altering the status quo.

The failure of democracy in each instance was probably the most significant factor that led to internal armed conflict. In most cases, the United States sided with the privileged elites or military forces in these countries as part of its Cold War strategy, especially when the political opposition espoused Marxist or socialist leanings. Human rights abuses, often on a large scale, were overlooked in the name of anticommunism, and the conflicts were fueled by massive amounts of U.S. foreign and military assistance. Smaller amounts of assistance from Cuba, the Soviet Union, and other socialist-bloc countries played a role in some of the conflicts.

The most promising development of the past 50 years that could contribute to prevention of the kinds of human rights abuses that were precursors to these internal conflicts has been the slow emergence of remedies for egregious violations of human rights. For much of the last half of the 20th century, the hopes embodied in the 1948 Universal Declaration of Human Rights (UDHR) were a half-empty glass. For human rights to have any lasting impact, there must be remedies for their violation. The role of remedies is especially important in prevention of war.

The UDHR, which has given rise to more than 20 treaties or conventions based on its 30 simple articles, had no standing in law at the time of its adoption by the fledging United Nations in 1948. When nations sign a treaty, they indicate their willingness to bring it back to their legislatures for review and ratification. Usually, ratification means modifying a nation's domestic laws to be consistent with the treaty or registering exceptions. When 60 nations have ratified such a human rights convention, it enters into force as international law. A decade later, if the community of civilized nations is adhering to the convention, it can be accepted as customary international law, binding signers and nonsigners alike.

"War Is Merely a Continuation of Politics"

The statement by Carl von Clausewitz, that "war is merely a continuation of politics," remains relevant in Latin America today, because SAPs and free trade agreements are accomplishing much of what the United States previously accomplished by force.

The Free Trade Agreement of the Americas (FTAA, not yet enacted), CAFTA, and NAFTA SAPs are part of the economic stabilization efforts deployed by the IMF, the United States Agency for International Development (USAID), and other international funding agencies. Their primary goals are to reduce government spending and control inflation by privatizing so-cial services and other state functions, deregulating the business environment, and reducing tariffs to promote foreign investment.[42] The degree of control exercised by the external monetary agencies is remarkable. For example, in Nicaragua in 1992, the Nicaraguan government was ordered to "reduce public sector employees by 15,000," which they proceeded to do.[43] The money squeezed from public services such as health care was then available to service the national debt. By the year 2000 in Nicaragua, these annual payments were more than six times the entire budget for health services. Debt relief for Nicaragua (Honduras was the only other Central American nation to qualify) came in late 2005, but only after the country had capitulated on demands for social service reductions and privatization of electrical and some water resources, by passing legislation to that effect. Under these conditions, it remains an open question whether Nicaragua or other nations under similar pressures can come close to achieving the U.N. Millennium Development Goals by 2015.

The NAFTA, CAFTA, and FTAA are all part of a U.S.-dominated effort to reduce barriers to trade. Too often this is at the expense of workers, small businesses and farmers, and the environment. By 2004, when NAFTA cele-brated its first 10 years, it had a very mixed record. Both the relative and the absolute levels of poverty had risen in Mexico during this period. Even the World Bank noted that NAFTA had not done enough to produce the sustained economic growth it promised. Economics Nobel laureate Joseph Stiglitz re-ferred to "broken promises" for the broad social development on which NAFTA was sold to the people of the three participating nations.[44] Multi-national corporations have benefitted and have remained key supporters of these agreements. The NAFTA side agreements, negotiated due to concerns for the absence of protections for labor rights and the environment, have completely failed to protect either. As of 2004, none of the 31 filed complaints had succeeded in getting past the second of seven steps in the process, no workplace hazards had been corrected, no illegally fired worker had been reinstated, and not a single independent union had been established and bargained collectively.[45] There are no labor or environmental-protection side agreements or similar restrictions within the World Trade Organization.

These failures did not go unnoticed as the U.S. Congress debated CAFTA, its most recent trade agreement, and passage was possible in July 2005 only after significant behind-the-scenes arm-twisting, which resulted in a razor-thin margin of two votes. Since then, shifting politics in Latin America and dissatisfaction with existing trade agreements have delayed consideration of FTAA. It remains to be seen whether these changes are representative of a backlash in the region against U.S. domination and what impact such changes will have for public health.

References

1. Pan American Health Organization. Health of Indigenous Peoples. Washington, DC: PAHO, 1997.
2. Montenegro RA, Stephens C. Indigenous health in Latin America and the Caribbean. Lancet 2006;367:1859–1869.
3. Waghelstein JW. Post-Vietnam insurgency doctrine. Military Rev 1985;1:42.
4. Clements C. Witness to War. New York: Bantam Books, 1984.
5. Betancur B. From Madness to Hope: The 12-year War in El Salvador. New York: U.N. Security Council, 1993.
6. Coalition to Stop the Use of Child Soldiers. Child Soldiers Global Report 2001. New York: Human Rights Watch, 2001.
7. Gellhorn A. Medical mission report to El Salvador. N Engl J Med 1983;308:1043–1044.
8. Periago M. Basic Indicators 2005: Health Situation in the Americas. Washington, DC: Pan American Health Organization, 2005.
9. Sklar H. Washington's War on Nicaragua. Boston: South End Press, 1988.
10. World Bank. Nicaragua: The Challenge of Reconstruction, Washington, DC, October 9, 1981, p. 11. (Cited in Conroy ME. Economic Legacy and Policies, in Thomas Walker, (ed). Nicaragua: The First Five Years. New York: Praeger, 1985. pp. 232–233).
11. Garfield R, Williams G. Health Care in Nicaragua. New York: Oxford University Press, 1992.
12. Honorable Les Aucoin. Extension of Remarks, April 11, 1989. Congressional Record 135(42):E1146.
13. Federal Research Division, U.S. Library of Congress. Country Studies/Area Handbook Series: Nicaragua. Washington, DC: U.S. Library of Congress (data as of December 1993). Available at: http://lcweb2.loc.gov/cgi-bin/query/r?frd/cstdy:@field(DOCID+ni0037) (accessed on July 20, 2007).
14. Tomuschatof C. Guatemala: Memory of Silence. New York: U.N. Historical Commission of Clarification, 1999.
15. Archdiocese of Guatemala Human Rights Office. Guatemala: Never Again! Maryknoll, NY: Orbis Books, 2000.
16. Schlesinger S, Kinzer S. Bitter Fruit. Cambridge, MA: Harvard University, 2005.
17. U.S. State Department. Human Rights Country Reports. Washington, DC: U.S. State Department, 2005.
18. Cohen R. Open Letter Concerning Intellectual Property and Access to Medicines in the US-Central American Free Trade Agreement (CAFTA), October 15, 2003. Available at: http://www.essentialdrugs.org/edrug/archive/200310/msg00046.php (accessed June 19, 2007).
19. Leech G. Fifty Years of Violence. May 1999. Available at: http://www.colombia journal.org/fiftyyearsofviolence.htm (accessed June 19, 2007).
20. Livingstone G. Inside Colombia: Drugs, Democracy, and War. London: Latin American Bureau, 2003.
21. Crandall R. Driven by Drugs: U.S. Policy Toward Colombia. Boulder, CO: Lynn Rienner Publishers, 2002.
22. Redmond R. Global Report 2005. Geneva: United Nations High Commissioner for Refugees, 2006.

23. Yamada S. Militarism and the social production of disease. In Fort M, Mercer MA, Gish O (eds.). Sickness and Wealth: The Corporate Assault on Global Health. Boston: South End Press, 2004.

24. Federal Research Division, U.S. Library of Congress. Health and welfare. In Country Studies/Area Handbook Series: Colombia. Washington, DC: U.S. Library of Congress, 1988. Available at: http://lcweb2.loc.gov/cgi-bin/query/r?frd/cstdy:@field(DOCID+ co0061) (accessed July 20, 2007).

25. Inter-American Commission on Human Rights. Third Report on the Human Rights Situation in Colombia. (OEA/Ser.L./V/II.102). Washington, DC: Organization of American States, 1999.

26. Federal Research Division, U.S. Library of Congress. The politics of health: Priorities, institutions, and public policy. In Country Studies/Area Handbook Series: Colombia. Washington, DC: U.S. Library of Congress, 1988. Available at: http://lcweb2.loc .gov/cgi-bin/query/r?frd/cstdy:@field(DOCID+co0063) (accessed July 20, 2007).

27. Forero J. Colombia's coca survives U.S. plan to uproot it. New York Times, August 19, 2006.

28. Contreras J. Failed plan. Newsweek, November 24, 2006.

29. Harman D. Rethinking Plan Colombia: Some ways to fix it. Christian Science Monitor, September 27, 2006.

30. Inequality in Income or Consumption. Human Development Reports 2005. United Nations Development Programme. Available at: http://hdr.undp.org/reports/global/ 2005/pdf/HDR05_chapter_2.pdf (accessed June 19, 2007).

31. Physicians for Human Rights. El Colegio de la Frontera Sur, Centro de Capacitación en Ecología y Salud para Campesinos: Defensoría del Derecho a la Salud. (Excluded People, Eroded Communities: Realizing the Right to Health in Chiapas, Mexico.) Boston: Physicians for Human Rights, 2006.

32. Yamin AE, Penchaszadeh V, Crane T. Health Care Held Hostage: Violations of Medical Neutrality and Human Rights in Chiapas, Mexico. Boston: Physicians for Human Rights, 1998, pp. 25–29.

33. Estadísticas demográficas: Cuaderno de población, no. 13. Aguascalientes, Mexico: Instituto Nacional de Estadistica Geografia e Informática (INEGI), 2001.

34. Ameringer C. Don Pepe: A Political Biography of Jose Figueres of Costa Rica. Albuquerque: University of New Mexico Press, 1978.

35. Wise D, Ross T. The Invisible Government. New York: Vintage Books, 1974.

36. Kapuscinski R. The Soccer War. New York: Vintage, 1992.

37. Parodi C. The Politics of South American Boundaries. Westport, CT: Praeger Publishers, 2002.

38. Dominguez J, Mares D, Orozco M, et al. Boundary Disputes in Latin America. Washington, DC: U.S. Institute of Peace, 2003.

39. O'Shaughnessy H. Pinochet: The Politics of Torture. New York: New York University Press, 2000.

40. Vivanco J. Chile: Pinochet held on torture charges. Washington, DC: Human Rights Watch News, October 31, 2006.

41. Rohter L. After 30 years, hope for justice in Argentina. New York Times, August 20, 2006.

42. Collier P, Guillaumont P, Guillaumont S, Gunning JW. Redesigning conditionality. World Development 1997; 25:1399–1407.

43. Evans T. La Transformacion del Sector Publico. CRIES, Managua, Nicaragua, 1991.

44. Stiglitz JE, Charlton A. Fair Trade for All: How Trade Can Promote Development. New York: Oxford University Press, 2006.
45. Brown G. NAFTA's 10 Year Failure to Protect Mexican Workers' Health and Safety. Maquiladora Network, 2004. Available at: http://mhssn.igc.org/NAFTA_2004.pdf (accessed June 19, 2007).

19

The Vietnam War

Myron Allukian, Jr., and Paul L. Atwood

In the United States, mention of Vietnam still invokes painful memories of the 10-year military conflict that began more than four decades ago in Southeast Asia over 9,000 miles away, in an impoverished nation the size of New Mexico. The impact of the Vietnam War, also known as the Second Indochina War or the American War (as it is called by the Vietnamese), exemplifies the consequences of armed conflict. Consider the following: About 5.3 million Vietnamese were killed, of whom 4 million were civilians.[1] Millions more were wounded or maimed. Large numbers of people were dislocated. Vietnam sustained the most massive bombing campaign in the history of warfare and defoliation of an area the size of Massachusetts (8,284 square miles, or 21,455 square kilometers)[2,3] More than 58,000 U.S. military personnel died, 313,616 were wounded, and about 10,000 lost at least one limb—more loss-of-limb injuries to U.S. military personnel than in World War II and the Korean War combined[4] (Table 19-1).

It is sometimes difficult to distinguish between the consequences in Vietnam of the war with the United States and the effects of the First Indochina War, with France, and of Vietnam's conflicts with China and Cambodia shortly after U.S. withdrawal. Further compounding this analysis are the effects of the U.S. trade embargo, the inexperience of Vietnam's government in economic management, the devastation of Vietnam's infrastructure, the effects

Table 19-1. Estimated Immediate Effects of the Vietnam War
on Vietnam, 1965–1975

5,300,000	killed (4,000,000 civilians and 1,300,000 military of both North and South Vietnam)
4,400,000	wounded (Vietnam)
1,000,000	widows (South Vietnam)
360,000–500,000	war invalids
800,000	orphans (South Vietnam)
300,000	military personnel missing in action (MIAs)
83,000	amputees (South Vietnam)
15,000	Amerasian children
10,000,000	refugees and evacuees (South Vietnam)
1,900,000	cattle killed
20,000,000	bomb craters
150,000–600,000	tons of unexploded munitions

of a century of colonial exploitation, the reliability of the data, and natural disasters that occurred (such as typhoons and floods that caused increased damage because of erosion related to deforestation caused by Agent Orange).

Background

History

Vietnam, which means "Land of the South," had conflicts with China, directly to its north, for 2,000 years, and with France for a century preceding U.S. involvement.[5] After the French defeat at Dienbienphu in May 1954, Vietnam, which then had a population of about 24 million, was divided temporarily at the 17th Parallel, by the Geneva Accords of July 1954, into two republics: the Democratic (Communist) Republic of Vietnam (DRV) in the north (62,066 square miles), and the Republic of Vietnam in the south (67,108 square miles).[5–7] About 928,000 Vietnamese, primarily Catholics, soon moved from northern to southern Vietnam.[8] Essentially refugees, these people strained already inadequate services in the South. The Geneva Accords also provided for reunifying elections to be held throughout both territories in 1956. With the approval of the United States, South Vietnam later refused to participate in these reunifying elections, seeking to separate permanently. In 1954, the United States, along with Australia, France, Great Britain, New Zealand, Pakistan, the Philippines, and Thailand, established the Southeast Asia Treaty Organization (SEATO), by which it promised to defend any nation in the region from attack by "foreign" communist governments.[9]

Many Vietnamese on both sides of the 17th Parallel did not approve of the permanent division, and in the South a guerrilla insurgency, led by southern communists, began. This armed movement, officially known as the National Liberation Front but called "the Viet Cong" by U.S. forces, was successful because, in contrast to the South Vietnam government, it had an extensive network of committed support among peasants in the countryside. The government of South Vietnam was in danger of collapsing. The United States first responded by committing American advisers to the Army of the Republic of South Vietnam (ARVN), about 12,000 by 1962. In response to two alleged attacks on U.S. naval ships by North Vietnamese in international waters (still unproven), the U.S. Congress adopted the Gulf of Tonkin Resolution in August 1964. This resolution gave President Lyndon Johnson authority to use armed force in Vietnam. The U.S. military initiated large-scale bombing of the North in 1964 and escalated the bombing throughout 1965. U.S. Marines landed in Danang in March 1965, the first American combat troops in Vietnam.[5] The People's Army of Vietnam (PAVN), of the North, then became committed to the goal of forcible reunification of Vietnam. By 1968, more than 540,000 U.S. troops were in South Vietnam, waging a ground war they did not bring to North Vietnam for fear of antagonizing China.[10] Unable to win without virtually annihilating the country they were sent to "save" and facing a very determined fighting force, U.S. troops were withdrawn in March 1973. In April 1975, the troops of the Viet Cong and PAVN captured Saigon. After the communist victory, the members of the ARVN and their families, who were seen as agents of foreign occupation, were severely persecuted. Many were imprisoned, and more than 1 million sought exile.

Demographics and Geography

In 1965, the population of Vietnam was estimated to be 34.8 million; in 1975, it was 43.4 million.[11] The populations of North and South Vietnam were about 26 million people each in 1979, when the first modern nationwide census was performed, making Vietnam the 13th largest country in the world with a total population of 52.7 million.[11,12] Average life expectancy at birth was 66 years. (In 2005, the population of Vietnam was 83 million people, and the life expectancy at birth in 2004 was 68 years for males and 73 years for females.) The literacy rate was about 85 percent. Vietnam had 55 to 60 minority groups that comprised 15 percent of the population. Most were of Chinese descent or were aborigines. Located on the Gulf of Tonkin and the South China Sea, with China to the north and Laos and Cambodia to the west, Vietnam is a tropical country with a 1,400-mile coastline. Most people live in the Red River delta in the north or the Mekong River delta in the south, both quite fertile. These two deltas comprise about 24 percent of Vietnam's land area and 62 percent of its population. Another 19 percent of Vietnamese live in urban areas. The rest of the country consists of mountains, high plateaus, and jungle.[11]

The Immediate Effects of the War

More than 12 million tons of high explosives were discharged by the United States in Vietnam—5 million tons of bombs and 7.4 million tons of artillery shells. More than 1,000 pounds of explosives per person were discharged in South Vietnam, the territory of the U.S. ally, where the most intensive bombing of the war took place[3,13] (Figure 19-1). More bombs were dropped by the United States in Vietnam than by all combatants during World War II. The result was massive destruction and approximately 10 million war victims, representing about 25 percent of the population at that time in North and South Vietnam combined.[8] In addition to the estimated 5.3 million people killed, victims included refugees and evacuees, those suffering from physical and mental disabilities, orphans, and elderly people whose children were killed (see Table 19–1).

There are no reliable data on the immediate effects of the war because of bias, poor recordkeeping, destruction of records, and massive forced migrations. Quantitative estimates of these effects vary according to the source. The estimated 5.3 million war deaths among civilians and military personnel of both North and South Vietnam represented about 14 percent of the population. If the United States had the same proportion of deaths, war invalids, and refugees for its population of 205 million in 1970 as did Vietnam, there would have been about 28.9 million American deaths, 2.3 million war invalids, and 45 million refugees.

All five of North Vietnam's industrial centers were demolished. All 29 of its provincial capitals were bombed, as were 2,700 of its 4,000 villages.[13] Virtually every railway and highway was destroyed. There was extensive destruction of irrigation dikes and water conservancy projects.

In South Vietnam, 9,000 of 15,000 rural villages were destroyed or damaged, displacing millions of people into urban areas.[14] Consequently, Saigon's population swelled from 1.4 to 4.2 million. In 1975, South Vietnam had 800,000 war orphans (with another 500,000 in the North), 400,000 people disabled by the war, 600,000 commercial sex workers, 500,000 addictive-drug abusers, and 3,000,000 unemployed people.[13] A 1987 report estimated that 300,000 Vietnamese were still disabled (incapable of working) and totally dependent on the government for their livelihood.[15] Approximately 60,000 of these people with disabilities were amputees in need of rehabilitation and prostheses, although only 15 percent could be provided with them.

At the end of the war, 150,000 to 600,000 tons of unexploded bombs and landmines remained spread across Vietnam[16,17] (see Chapter 7). In an initia-

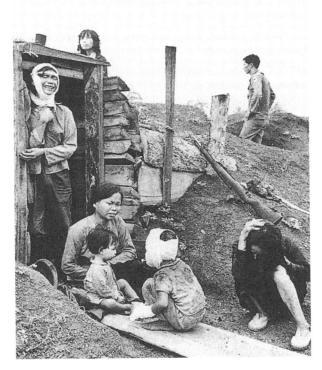

Figure 19-1. Wounded and shocked civilian survivors of the battle at Dong Xoai outside of fort-bunker where they had survived the ground fighting and air bombardments of the previous two days (1965). (Source: Associated Press/Wide World Photos.)

tive to remove them between 1975 and 1977, the Vietnamese suffered an additional 12,000 deaths and 20,000 nonfatal injuries.[18] Between 1975 and 1984, the Vietnamese government cleared about 59,000 land mines from the central province of Quang Tri alone. From 1985 to 1995, in Quang Tri Province, there were 25 deaths and 449 serious nonfatal injuries due to landmines. These figures underestimate the actual numbers of deaths and injuries.[19]

Health Services During the War

South Vietnam

Health services for the South Vietnamese in the early part of the war were abysmal, both qualitatively and quantitatively. In 1965, there were about 800 physicians: 500 were in the military, and 150 treated only private paying patients, leaving 150 physicians to treat more than 15 million people, a physician-to-population ratio of about 1 to 100,000.[20] Of the 28 provincial hospitals with surgical suites, only 11 were being used, due to inadequate numbers of medical personnel.

Medical care for civilians was severely compromised, and limited public health programs were brought to a halt.[20] Not one of 43 provincial hospitals in South Vietnam met minimal standards for a developing country. Almost all hospitals lacked electricity, drinking water, and sanitation facilities. The medical-supply logistics system had broken down; even soap was unavailable in many hospitals. There was a serious shortage of surgeons. In hospitals, hundreds of wounded South Vietnamese were living in sheds and corridors, on floors, and sometimes in open courtyards, awaiting surgery that might be delayed for 1 to 2 years. Conditions of extreme overcrowding existed in some hospitals, with two or three patients to a bed. Often, hospitals were virtually closed at night and on weekends because medical personnel were unavailable or unwilling to work then. With 36,000 amputees awaiting prosthetic devices and only a few hundred devices being produced each month, most people needing such devices faced very long delays.

There was no system to bring war-injured people to hospitals; those who did reach a hospital often had to wait 24 to 36 hours to be admitted. Between 20,000 to 50,000 of those wounded each year died immediately or before reaching a hospital. Civilian medical programs in South Vietnam were inadequate to meet even the peacetime needs of the country. Destruction of villages, uncontrolled movements of refugees, and squalid conditions in refugee camps promoted the spread of disease, causing a rising incidence of tuberculosis, intestinal parasite infestations, leprosy, and malaria as major causes of morbidity, along with marked increases in the incidence of cholera, plague, and human rabies.[20–22]

Although much health assistance was provided to South Vietnam by the United States and other countries beginning in 1964, it was not until 1969 that a major government initiative was implemented, so that each province would have at least one adequate general hospital for both military personnel and civilians.[22,23] Preventive and clinical services for children younger than 15 years of age were also inadequate until 1975, as indicated by the percentage of those *not* vaccinated for diphtheria, pertussis, and tetanus (83 percent); polio (82 percent); tuberculosis (70 percent); and smallpox (50 percent).[7]

In the early 1970s, the infant mortality rate was 100 per 1,000 live births. Life expectancy at birth was 54 years for males and 60 years for females. South Vietnamese women had an average of 5.8 children, compared with 3.9 for Korea, 2.0 for Japan, and 1.9 for the United States.[7] The South Vietnamese government in 1973 spent 53 percent of its total budget on national defense but less than 1 percent on public health. U.S. aid to South Vietnam that year amounted to $2.5 billion, of which 76 percent went to support the South Vietnamese military and only 0.5 percent was used for public health.[16]

Dental care was also inadequate in South Vietnam, which had a dentist-to-population ratio of less than 1 to 100,000. There were about 150 dentists in the country: 70 were in the military, and most of the rest practiced in Saigon. Another 5,000 "sidewalk dentists," who had little or no education or training, also practiced "dentistry," but their work was generally considered more detrimental than helpful.[24]

North Vietnam

In contrast, health services in North Vietnam during the war appeared to be better organized and more effective than those in the South, although documentation is limited. This was primarily due to the fact that North Vietnam, beginning in 1954, made access to health services and preventive medicine a national priority and establishing a socialized health service that implemented mass vaccination campaigns for cholera, typhoid, smallpox, plague, tuberculosis, and polio.[25,26] The effectiveness of these programs is not known. By 1965, about 66 percent of rural villages were served by their own assistant doctor—a nurse with 3 years of practical experience and 2 years of additional training.[27] In contrast, health services in South Vietnam had deteriorated in rural areas by 1965, so that it was "almost impossible to effectively manage, control, direct, or support any kind of medical supply."[22]

Despite great constraints during the war, North Vietnam continued to make health services a high priority. By 1974, there were 5,566 community health centers or infirmaries, a 28-fold increase from the 200 present in 1955.[28] The number of polyclinics and specialized clinics also increased, from 51 in 1955 to 441 in 1974. In addition, 58,000 hospital and 46,000 infirmary beds were added, although these did not satisfy minimum standards. Primary care and prevention were emphasized throughout the health care system. Each family was assigned a "health activist," or health promoter, who made home visits to ensure family sanitation, immunization, proper medications, and health education. By 1973, there were 7,000 physicians, for a physician-to-population ratio of 1:3,500, in addition to 20,000 assistant physicians.[29] About 71 percent of the doctors were primary care physicians. Most deliveries in the villages were performed by midwives, sometimes with the aid of assistant physicians. In 1972, there was, on average, 1 dentist for every 6,000 people, an inadequate number to serve the population's needs but better than the situation in South Vietnam. All health care was free, as were training and education for health care personnel.

Despite wartime conditions, North Vietnam seems to have developed an impressive health care system, with a major focus on prevention and public health at the family and community level. In 1973, malnutrition was rare in North Vietnam. Cholera, plague, smallpox, malaria, and sexually transmitted diseases were controlled, and the incidence of trachoma was greatly reduced.[29]

The bombing of North Vietnam resulted in the destruction of many health facilities: 533 (10 percent) of the community health centers, 94 (28 percent) of the district hospitals, 28 (60 percent) of the provincial hospitals, and 24 research and specialized hospitals.[28] Bach Mai Hospital in Hanoi, the largest diagnostic and therapeutic institution in North Vietnam with more than 1,000 beds, was bombed three times in 1972, resulting in the deaths of 31 people, including a physician and other health care workers.[29] Due to a comprehensive evacuation plan and air raid shelters in North Vietnam, deaths of patients and other civilians were minimized. From 1965 to 1968, about 34 million individual shelters, thousands of group shelters, and approximately 30,000 miles of trenches were built to keep civilians below ground in order to avoid shrapnel and to minimize targets for U.S. aircraft.[8]

Immediate and Long-Term Effects of Herbicides

Between 1961 and 1971, the U.S. military sprayed almost 19 million gallons of herbicides and defoliants over approximately 5 million acres of farmland and forest in South Vietnam, more than one third of the total land mass.[30–32] These chemicals were used to deprive the Viet Cong and the North Vietnamese Army (NVA) of food crops and jungle cover and to denude the perimeters of U.S. base camps to prevent enemy infiltration. The chemical most sprayed was the herbicide Agent Orange, the use of which came under heavy criticism from the American Academy for the Advancement of Science (AAAS) because its active ingredient, 2,4,5-trichlorophenoxyacetic acid (2,4,5-T), had been shown to cause birth defects in laboratory animals.

In 1970, 20 to 50 percent of South Vietnam's mangrove forests, vital to marine life, had been totally destroyed, and half of the commercial hardwood trees and many rubber trees on Vietnam's famed plantations had been killed.[33] Shortly thereafter, it was discovered that 2,4,5-T was contaminated with 2,3,7,8-tetrachlorodibenzo-p-dioxin (2,3,7,8-TCDD), or dioxin, a potent toxicant and carcinogen.[34–36] Because 2,4,5-T had been shown to be a teratogen, the use of Agent Orange in Vietnam was stopped by the U.S. Department of Defense in 1970.[37]

An AAAS team traveled to Vietnam and demonstrated easily measurable amounts of dioxin in fish and in human milk. Simultaneously, a large increase in the rate of primary liver carcinoma was found, and later there were increases in the rates of hydatidiform mole and choriocarcinoma. Offspring of spouses of North Vietnamese soldiers who served in the South were more likely to suffer abnormalities, such as anencephaly, oral clefts, and stillbirths, than the offspring of wives of soldiers who served north of the 17th Parallel, where herbicides were never used.[38]

Studies have since demonstrated increased risk for soft tissue sarcomas and malignant lymphomas with exposure to dioxin, either through military service in Vietnam or from agricultural herbicides contaminated with dioxin. In 1991, the U.S. Congress passed a bill that provided permanent disability benefits to Vietnam veterans suffering from soft tissue sarcomas, non-Hodgkin's lymphoma, and other malignancies. Vietnam veterans' children with birth defects are also eligible for compensation, because a strong risk relationship has also been shown between parental Vietnam exposure to Agent Orange and birth defects, including spina bifida, cleft lip, congenital neoplasms, and coloboma (an eye anomaly).[39–41]

The Institute of Medicine (IOM) completed in 1994 an exhaustive review of studies of Agent Orange and its potential effects on the health of Vietnam veterans in the United States, which found sufficient evidence of association with soft tissue sarcoma, non-Hodgkin's lymphoma, and Hodgkin's disease, as well as limited suggestive evidence of association with some respiratory cancers, prostate cancer, and multiple myeloma.[42] A 1995 study showed that dioxin blood levels among southern and central Vietnamese living in sprayed areas was six times greater than for northerners in unsprayed areas. In addition, the mean dioxin level in adipose tissue in these areas was three times greater than in the United States. Dioxin may be persistent in the environment and in the food chain, putting some Vietnamese at increased risk for cancer.[43,44] In 1996, the IOM added spina bifida and acute and subacute peripheral neuropathy to the category of limited or suggestive evidence of an association.[45]

In 1984, in a landmark class action lawsuit in a federal court in New York, Vietnam veterans were awarded $180 million in compensation for illnesses attributed to dioxin exposure from the seven major chemical companies that had produced Agent Orange on contract to the U.S. government.[46]

When the United States initiated normal relations with Vietnam in 1995, it stipulated that Vietnam drop all claims of war reparations or compensation.[47] The United States then agreed to conduct joint research on lingering questions about the effects of dioxin on the population of Vietnam. In March 2002, the first United States–Vietnam conference in Vietnam on Agent Orange was convened.[46]

The Vietnamese government still allowed private Vietnamese veterans organizations to continue efforts to get redress from the United States. In 2004, the Vietnam Association of Victims of Agent Orange (VAVA) filed a lawsuit, based on the Alien Tort Claims Act, against the herbicide manufacturers in the same New York federal court and with the same judge who had presided over the 1984 case. VAVA claims that 3 million Vietnamese were exposed to Agent Orange and that at least 800,000 suffer serious health problems, including 150,000 children with severe or extreme birth defects. Two weeks before the suit was scheduled to be heard, the United States unilaterally cancelled its contract to conduct an epidemiological study of Agent Orange–related health effects in Vietnam.[48]

In 2005, the Court dismissed the lawsuit, claiming that: (1) although it is toxic, Agent Orange did not fit the definition of "chemical warfare" and did not violate international laws such as the Geneva Conventions, and (2) the "proof of causal connection depends primarily upon substantial epidemiological and other scientific data."[49] It is unclear what is meant by "substantial." The body of scientific evidence causally associating Agent Orange exposure with adverse health effects is large and has been growing. In 2001, the National Institute of Environmental Health Sciences attempted to list dioxin as a carcinogen but was thwarted by chemical industry opposition.[47] In 2001, the leading U.S. researcher on dioxin and researchers in Vietnam conducted a study in Bien Hoa, a city that was a major site of U.S. storage tanks of Agent Orange during the Vietnam War. They found that 95 percent of people tested had elevated blood dioxin levels that were, on average, 135 times higher than controls. They also sampled soil in 2003 in Bien Hoa and found the soil level of dioxin to be about 1,000 times greater than the safe level set by the U.S. Environmental Protection Agency.[50]

A 2003 study demonstrated that (1) many spraying missions in the U.S. military during the war had been overlooked, (2) new estimates of the amount of dioxin sprayed were almost twice previous estimates, and (3) millions of Vietnamese were likely to have been sprayed."[51] A 2002 Canadian study found "a consistent pattern of food chain contamination" by dioxin in Agent Orange, including soil, fish, ducks, and humans.[52] And a 2006 meta-analysis concluded that parental exposure to Agent Orange appeared to be associated with an increased risk of birth defects.[53] This meta-analysis found that the summary relative risk of birth defects associated with exposure to Agent Orange was 1.95, a statistically significant increase.

The continuing effects of Agent Orange in Vietnam, more than 30 years after the Vietnam War, appears to be one of the most serious public health consequences of the war. One author contends, "Some of the victims may not even have been born yet."[54]

Herbicides also completely destroyed about 14 percent of southern Vietnam's merchantable timber, the primary source of housing materials and an important source of foreign exchange. About 10 more years will be required to make up this loss. Before the war, rubber production accounted for 60 percent of exports and employed more than 100,000 people. By 1973, 40 percent of plantation trees had been destroyed, and overall production had been reduced by 70 percent. By 1983, rubber export had reached only half of prewar levels, and full reattainment of production appeared many years away.[13] The reduction of such valuable export commodities limited Vietnam's capacity to earn foreign currencies, which, in turn, had deleterious effects on investment in public health.

Herbicides were also directed extensively at the coastal mangrove forests, the primary breeding grounds for shrimp and many fish, staples in the Vietnamese diet, causing the annual marine catch to keep declining. Such declines contributed to malnutrition problems after the war.

Postwar and Long-Term Effects of the War

Once the war ended and Vietnam was reunified in 1975, it had to cope with the results of the war: millions of dead, wounded, disabled, unemployed, and orphaned individuals and traumatized families, together with massive destruction of homes, villages, the environment, and the nation's infrastructure. With an agenda for rebuilding under socialist principles, the ravaged nation initially had few friends or allies. Unhappy with the forcible reunification of Vietnam by communist troops in 1975, the United States extended an existing embargo with North Vietnam to the entire country. Hanoi also quickly lost the support of China, its former ally, over territorial issues and Vietnam's opposition to the Khmer Rouge regime in neighboring Cambodia. Because most of the other nations of Southeast Asia were aligned with or economically dependent on the United States, most of them participated to some extent in the embargo. Vietnam, therefore, had to attempt its reconstruction primarily with limited assistance from the Soviet Union. Nations that had long opposed U.S. intervention in Vietnam, such as Sweden and Finland, provided some aid, but this too was limited because of U.S. opposition to such assistance.[55]

In South Vietnam after the war, malaria, tuberculosis, leprosy, viral hemorrhagic fever, trachoma, cholera, plague, sexually transmitted diseases, and parasitic infections were reported to be serious public health problems.[28] Malaria was reported to be the most serious public health problem in 1976, with 75 percent of the population living in malarial areas. Tuberculosis was also a major problem; one survey reported a prevalence of 9 cases per 1,000 people older than 10 years of age, a rate twice that of neighboring countries.[28] A prevalence of between 80,000 and 160,000 cases of leprosy were estimated, and in some areas there were 55 cases per 1,000 people. The prevalence of trachoma in 1971 was 75 percent in the northeastern provinces and 57 percent in the Mekong River delta.

Already one of the poorest countries in the world, Vietnam had to develop governmental structures and public health institutions over half of its territory, struggle to overcome its huge losses during the war, and, as a result of the U.S.-imposed embargo, endure isolation from the global economy and humanitarian aid. Simultaneously, it started a war with the Khmer Rouge in neighboring Cambodia in order to stop Khmer incursions into Vietnam and persecution of ethnic Vietnamese in Cambodia. In the process, Vietnam overthrew the regime in Cambodia, one of the bloodiest in modern history, which was responsible for the "killing fields." Nevertheless, the U.S. government accused Vietnam of attempting "military conquest" in Cambodia and further tightened the embargo. In 1979, Vietnam also became involved in a war with China over disputed territories, which resulted in the exodus of most of Vietnam's commercially vital ethnic Chinese population, almost 500,000 people.

After reunification in 1976, the government of Vietnam began a massive relocation of at least 5 million people to try to break up the existing social order and to raise class consciousness by downgrading the middle and upper classes through communication and education programs.[14] In addition, at least 700,000 people a year were placed in reeducation camps to educate and/or coerce those in certain social classes to accept or conform to the new social norms. In 1982, there were still about 120,000 Vietnamese in these camps; the camps are now closed.

Because of the change in government, massive relocation, and social ostracism, many middle-class Vietnamese fled their country. Between 1975 and 1990, an estimated 1.5 million people left Vietnam,[56] of whom about 910,000 reached a destination and about 142,000 refugee "boat people" were lost at sea. Now, about 1.2 million ethnic Vietnamese live in the United States.

Although the revolutionaries were successful in the war against the United States, their abilities at running the government and the economy of Vietnam were sorely tested, especially given its isolation from the "community of nations." Subsequently, the rigidly Stalinist model of economic growth proved unsuccessful, and, throughout the 1980s, famine occurred in some provinces due to the destruction that had occurred during the war, poor government practices, and natural disasters. Once the "rice bowl of Asia," Vietnam could no longer feed itself.

The United States rebuilt ravaged Germany and Japan after World War II, spending more to restore these nations than the war cost the United States. By comparison, the U.S. government did little to restore Vietnam after the war. For example, the Pentagon did not provide maps of mine fields in South Vietnam to enable the Vietnamese to disarm landmines that, together with enormous quantities of unexploded ordnance, continue to kill people more than 20 years after the war. It is estimated today that 3 million landmines and between 350,000 and 800,000 tons of unexploded ordnance are still present in approximately 20 percent of the area of Vietnam (see Chapter 7).

Vietnam desired normalization of relations, but the U.S. government continued to use the issue of prisoners of war (POWs) and those missing in action (MIAs) to exact political concessions. Meanwhile, in 1993, there were about 300,000 Vietnamese MIAs, compared to 2,261 U.S.-soldier MIAs (fewer than 4 percent of U.S. soldiers who had been killed during the war).[57] As of mid-2006, because of recovery efforts, there were 1,805 U.S. MIAs in Vietnam and areas of Laos, Cambodia, and China where Vietnamese forces operated during the war; for 651 (36 percent) of them, there is evidence that they perished and their remains cannot be recovered. For Vietnam alone, there are 1,376 MIAs.[58] By contrast, there are still more than 78,000 American MIAs from World War II (equivalent to 19 percent of the more than 405,000 soldiers killed during the war) and more than 8,000 MIAs from the Korean War (equivalent to 15 percent of U.S. soldiers killed in that war).

The U.S. Trade Embargo: The Long-Term Effects of War by Other Means

During the peace negotiations held between the United States and North Vietnam in 1972 and 1973, President Richard Nixon promised U.S. participation in the reconstruction of Vietnam. In a secret memorandum sent to Premier Pham Van Dong on February 1, 1973, $3.25 billion of aid was promised, and a Joint Economic Commission began planning for the reconstruction of ports, water facilities, agriculture, and transportation.[59] However, no amount for such reconstruction was included in the formal Paris Agreements signed in July 1973. President Nixon's promise was not kept. Indeed, from 1975, when Vietnam was forcibly reunited under communist rule, until 1994, the United States imposed a trade embargo against Vietnam. (The trade embargo was made more stringent by the Reagan Administration. The United States also froze Vietnam's bank accounts in the United States.) In 1994, President Bill Clinton lifted the embargo, and, in 1995, the United States normalized diplomatic relations with Vietnam. The embargo had played a significant role in the difficulties Vietnam faced in recovering from decades of war. Probably the most significant effect of the embargo was to keep Vietnam poor and isolated, because many U.S. allies also participated in economic sanctions against Vietnam. Although poor internal planning and the government's bureaucratic rigidities also hampered Vietnam's recovery, Vietnam raised social indices against overwhelming odds, an accomplishment that even won the praise of the World Bank.[6]

Population

Despite its relatively small geographic area, Vietnam in 1994 was the 13th most populous nation, with about 73 million people.[60] Today, the population is about 84.4 million.[61] Because more than half of the people were born since 1975, most Vietnamese citizens have no memory of the destruction and chaos of the war.

Despite losses to war, famine, and migration, Vietnam's population has increased rapidly, with a high fertility rate and a moderate to low overall mortality rate. The infant mortality rate fell from 156 per 1,000 live births in 1960, to 83 in 1979, to 42 in 1989, and to 25 in 2006—due to a solid commitment to health care by the government.[6,61] In 1979, 70 percent of Vietnam's population was younger than 30 years of age.[12] There were about 1.5 million more females than males[12] as a result of huge numbers of male deaths during almost 30 years of war with the United States and France. Consequently, there have been more women in the labor force and more single mothers having children out of wedlock, as well as a decline in the fertility rate. The Democratic Republic of Vietnam introduced Western family planning measures, although supplies and training were limited. Nevertheless, the population growth rate fell from 3.1 percent during the 1960–1976 period to 2.2 percent in 1993.[6] Economic devastation caused by the war and emigration have also played major roles in the falling population growth rate. Despite these factors, the population grew to more than 84 million by 2006 and will likely approach 100 million by 2015.

Nutrition

Vietnam, with a subsistence agricultural economy, was an important rice exporter until the beginning of the war in 1965. After the war, food shortages were estimated to be 1 to 2 million tons a year, resulting in rationing of basic foods, which, in turn, caused long-standing nutritional deficits.[62] Although food production has since increased, differentials in productivity have varied widely among regions, so that populations in some provinces have suffered more chronic malnutrition and even famine. The proportion of malnourished children in the early 1990s was 45 percent for weight-for-age and 57 percent for height-for-age—rates comparable to those in Bangladesh[6]—with 80 percent of these children in the age group of 1 to 3 years.[63] Although short-term acute food deficits appeared throughout Vietnam, the chronic problem was undernutrition. One fifth of all infants born in 1990 weighed less than 2,500 grams at birth.[6] Food deficits began at birth and continued for most Vietnamese throughout life due to low caloric intake and to cultural beliefs in the inferiority of colostrum as a food, with resultant early weaning. Infants were introduced to solid foods at 2 to 3 months of age, greatly increasing the rate of infection due to malnutrition. Traditional dependence on rice as a staple of diet has long contributed to caloric, lipid, and micronutrient deficiencies—especially of vitamin A, iron, and iodine—which were increasing throughout Vietnam. Adult malnutrition was shaped in part by the unavailability of productive arable land and flooding resulting from defoliation by herbicides, natural disasters, and poor economic performance.

Health Care under the Socialist System

Vietnam was able to provide better health care services than some of its equally poor Southeast Asian neighbors that had not suffered the ravages of war. For example, the average per-capita income in Vietnam in 1996 was $220, compared with $2,085 in Thailand, which had been the recipient of steady U.S. investment since the 1950s. Vietnam did not have adequate medical and dental equipment because of the embargo and the state of the economy. By 1994, Vietnam had 1 doctor for every 2,857 people; Thailand had 1 for every 4,361 people. Vietnam's average life expectancy of 65 years was almost one decade longer than that for Bangladesh in 1989, although the two nations were almost equally poor[64] and both had devoted the same percentage of their gross national product (GNP), 0.7 percent, to health care. Vietnam's achievements in health indicators were far better than those of most countries at its income level. Vietnam's infant mortality rate in the 1990s was better than that of neighboring countries with four times its gross national product.[6] Nevertheless, there were economic impediments compromising health care, and these good survival rates were not evenly distributed throughout Vietnam, particularly with respect to the nutritional status of children. Owing to income differentials throughout Vietnam, infant mortality rates were three times higher in the poorest provinces than in the richest. Whereas adult literacy averaged 88 percent nationwide, it was only 66 percent in the poorest province.

North Vietnam had developed a free, but highly centralized, five-tier health system, which was financed entirely by state funds. However, this system was weakened by the staggering demand put on it during the decade after the war's end, by the outflow of doctors and other medical personnel from South Vietnam to the West, and by the underfinancing of the health sector due to intrinsic economic weakness. After 1975, there was also a severe shortage of medical and dental equipment, supplies, and pharmaceuticals in Vietnam due to the U.S. trade embargo and the overburdened economy.[65] With the adoption of market mechanisms and an open policy for foreign investment, by 1993 drug imports were at $132 million per year, or $1.80 per capita, compared to

$0.50 in 1989, and local drug production increased dramatically, resulting in an uncontrolled market with nonessential drugs, irrational drug use, extensive overprescription, and profiteering.

Impact of Economic Reform on Health Services

Economic reform in Vietnam was hailed by Western nations in the 1990s and by the World Bank as a first step in Vietnam's reintegration into the "community of nations." Market mechanisms replaced central planning, and, in line with World Bank guidelines, Vietnam arrested inflation, stabilized its currency, and reduced foreign trade imbalances. Agriculture and farming was privatized. Although this system has raised food production substantially and growth in personal income has averaged more than 5 percent annually, these advances hid growing imbalances across the nation in 1995.[6,66]

More than half of the population was below the official poverty level in 1995, with incomes declining among the poorest.[66] As a result of reforms essentially dictated by Western financial institutions, 500,000 soldiers had been released from service and 800,000 public-sector workers had been laid off.[6] Meanwhile, in line with economic retrenchment, prices had risen while wages were cut. Rapidly changing economic and social conditions produced an "extremely dynamic epidemiological and health transition."[67] Physicians and pharmacists had been allowed to establish private practices, producing higher prices for health care both in private practice and in state-run clinics. Health care professionals left state institutions to work in private practice. Although health care had improved for those with disposable income, for most Vietnamese, who lived in poverty, health conditions had worsened and access to quality care had diminished. The wealthiest quintile of households had 4.4 times the income of the lowest and spent 4.6 times as much on health expenditures. Public expenditures on health had decreased from 6.1 percent to 4.4 percent of Vietnam's budget, although the total size of the budget had grown.[67] Underinvestment in state-supported medical schools and other training facilities continued, with the consequence that these institutions lacked qualified instructors and teaching aids. Although the government had decided to raise the salaries of health care workers, this increase was made possible only by laying off many employees. Of the 9,788 doctors who graduated between 1977 and 1988, 2,715 remained unemployed in 1994.[65] The collapse of the public-sector health network, in tandem with growing poverty in the bottom half of Vietnamese society, also produced an upsurge in the incidence of disease. Childhood immunization rates remained high (70 to 75 percent), but malnutrition contributed strongly to increased incidences of diarrheal disease and respiratory tract infection. Malaria and tuberculosis remained widespread. Cardiovascular diseases and cancer were said to be increasing.

The World Bank recommended strengthening the public health sector, but this would be possible only by heavily taxing the private sector. Vietnam had avoided taxing the private sector or implementing fair labor standards, child labor laws, and environmental standards that are commonplace in the West. The absence of such standards was the primary reason that Western capital wished to invest in Southeast Asia.[68] By 2004, Vietnamese exports to the United States were between $5 and $6 billion a year. In 2006, the United States and Vietnam reached agreements to pave the way for Vietnam to join the World Trade Organization and trade with the United States reached almost $10 billion a year.

Assistance for Vietnam

There were important exceptions to the isolation of Vietnam after 1975. Many nongovernmental organizations (NGOs), including religious groups and some nations that provided humanitarian aid to either North or South Vietnam during the war, continued in these efforts. Many, including some U.S. Vietnam veterans groups, took the lead to help restore and rebuild Vietnam. They helped build clinics, houses, and schools; assisted in population planning, nutrition, and education; and provided prosthetics for disabled Vietnamese.

In 1987, Vietnam and the United States agreed to improve cooperation to address the humanitarian concerns of both governments.[69] This became known as the Vessey Initiative, named after General John W. Vessey, Jr., former Chairman of the Joint Chiefs of Staff, who was the Special Presidential Emissary to Hanoi for POW/MIA Affairs and who was key to these discussions. The U.S. government chose not to provide assistance directly to Vietnam or through specific NGOs, due to legal and policy constraints, until 1989, when President George H. W. Bush hailed a "new openness" with the Vietnamese. Over some opposition, the U.S. government decided to send Vietnam more than $250,000 in surplus medical equipment, taken from excess and obsolete stock, as a goodwill gesture for help in accounting for the 1,705 American MIAs.[70] In 1989 in New York, a conference on Vietnam with about 100 NGOs from the United States was held,[69] which helped improve NGO activity in Vietnam. The Vietnamese government soon began granting 6-month, multiple-entry visas to American NGOs.

Some groups, including American veterans groups, had also been in the forefront to help restore diplomatic relations between the United States and Vietnam, as the most rational and effective means to heal the wounds of both sides. In 1990, as president of the American Public Health Association

(APHA), one of us (M.A.), a Vietnam veteran, went to Vietnam to visit health departments, clinics, schools, and hospitals in Ho Chi Minh City (Saigon), Hue, Danang, and Hanoi. On his return, he wrote an open letter to President George H. W. Bush urging normalization of relations and the promotion and encouragement of humanitarian aid. In 1990, APHA formed a Vietnam Caucus, and in 1991 the APHA Governing Council adopted a policy statement calling for normalization of relations with Vietnam, the promotion of humanitarian aid, and additional resources for U.S. Vietnam veterans. The International Council of the International Physicians for the Prevention of Nuclear War (IPPNW) adopted a similar resolution. In 1994, after a U.S. Senate nonbinding vote of support, President Clinton lifted the U.S. trade embargo. In 1995, the United States and Vietnam formally restored full diplomatic relations, ending four decades of hostility. In 2004, former President Bill Clinton visited Vietnam. In 2005, Vietnam's Prime Minister visited the United States for the first time since the end of the war. And in 2006, President George W. Bush became the first sitting U.S. President to visit Vietnam, and the U.S. Congress voted to allow Vietnam to join the World Trade Organization.[71] In 2007, Nguyen Minh Triet, president of Vietnam, became the first Vietnam president to visit the United States since the end of the war. At that time, he signed a Trade and Investment Framework Agreement, which is sometimes considered a roadmap to free-trade negotiations. During that visit, President Bush pressed him on the importance of having a strong commitment to human rights and democracy.[72]

The Effects of the War in the United States

The dead. The injured. POW-MIAs. Agent Orange. Posttraumatic stress disorder (PTSD). Shameful treatment of veterans. Homelessness. The Vietnam Memorial. Civil disobedience. The Pentagon Papers. Student unrest and the killing of student demonstrators at Kent State. Draft resistance and draft-card burnings. Flight to Canada. Families torn apart. The rioting at the 1968 Democratic National Convention. The downfall of a U.S. president. Vietnamese "boat people." The My Lai Massacre. Amerasian children abandoned in Vietnam. Distrust of government, and cynicism toward power and authority. Many of these effects and public reactions still affect our people, policies, and national psyche today.

The Vietnam War cost the United States at least $130 billion in direct costs and at least that amount in indirect costs, which continue to this day,[4] or about $584 billion in 2005 dollars, according to the Congressional Research Office. The United States also lost President Johnson's War on Poverty, both economically and politically. As federal funds were redirected toward the war in Vietnam, public health programs originally designed for the poor in the United

States suffered cutbacks. Furthermore, the war in Indochina spurred serious inflation, which adversely affected low-income Americans.

The burden of the Vietnam War was borne mainly by soldiers from low-income families. Twenty-six million young men reached draft age during the war in Vietnam, but only 10.9 million served in the military, because draft deferrals were available to those who could afford college or graduate school.[73] Of these, about 2.6 to 3.8 million served in Vietnam. Dropping the usual entry criteria, the army enlisted more than 300,000 young men, under a special program called Project 100,000, between 1966 and 1972. Eighty percent of these recruits were African Americans who read below sixth-grade level, and they often were suffering from learning disabilities. They were promised benefits after the war. More than one third served in combat. They had double the death rate of other soldiers, and many were so disabled physically or psychologically that they were never able to use government funds available for housing or college under the GI Bill. About 80,000 men recruited under this program were discharged with less than honorable discharges, receiving no benefits.[74] Many of these veterans became homeless, of whom 40 percent had serious mental illness[75] and 10 percent suffered from PTSD.[76] The needs of homeless veterans far exceeded the Veterans Administration's capacity to serve these needs.

The official U.S. estimate of the number of U.S. deaths in Vietnam is 58,253, but this does not include many who were killed in Laos and Cambodia (who were there "illegally"), nor does it count servicemen who were killed in accidents outside the official combat zone or trainees killed by "friendly fire" at home bases.[77] It does not count those who have died since the war, often as a result of wounds incurred in Vietnam or by self-destructive behavior resulting from PTSD. More than 20,000 Vietnam veterans have taken their own lives.[78] No accurate accounting of U.S. civilians killed in Vietnam has ever been made. The probability of getting killed in Vietnam for U.S. troops who served there was 85 per 1,000, compared with 31 per 1,000 for those who served in World War I, World War II, and the Korean War.[79]

More than 300,000 Americans were wounded, with 153,300 classified as seriously wounded. Because of rapid helicopter evacuation techniques and advanced medical facilities, only 2.6 percent of the wounded reaching hospitals died, but some 10,000 servicemen lost at least one limb, more than in World War II and Korea combined. More than 700,000 U.S. veterans of the Vietnam War have suffered severe PTSD, and many of them have been hospitalized for long periods and lost much work time. Acute drug and alcohol abuse, violent or antisocial behavior, high divorce rates, broken families, and homelessness have been closely associated with this disorder.[80-83] More than 1.5 million veterans were estimated to eventually need psychiatric care.[83] During the first 5 years after discharge from the military, Vietnam veterans had a 45 percent excess of deaths, due primarily to external causes such as motor vehicle injuries, homicides, and suicides.[84] In addition, about 15 percent reported having symptoms of combat PTSD. There was a high prevalence of alcohol abuse or dependence, anxiety, and depression. The ramifications of the war in Vietnam have been widespread in our society, although concentrated among the poor and working-class populations. Finally, the Vietnam War also affected the credibility of U.S. presidents and the U.S. government in general, creating deep distrust and resentment, which, in turn, has seriously affected our society's ability to solve numerous pressing problems. As former Secretary of State under President Nixon, Henry Kissinger, admitted[5]:

> Vietnam is still with us. It has created doubts about American judgment, about American credibility, about American power—not only at home but throughout the world. It has poisoned our domestic debate. We paid an exorbitant price.

In his memoir, *In Retrospect: The Tragedy and Lessons of Vietnam,* which was released in April 1995, former U.S. Defense Secretary Robert S. McNamara asserted 30 years after his stewardship of the Vietnam War, "We were wrong, terribly wrong. We owe it to future generations to explain why."[85]

The Vietnam Memorial, popularly known as "The Wall," has been the most visited monument in Washington, D.C., since it was unveiled in 1982. Inscribed on it are 58,253 names of U.S. military personnel killed during the war.[77] The Wall has reminded Americans of the sacrifices made during the war and has helped to heal the nation. However, the immense losses to Vietnam, Laos, and Cambodia remain almost invisible in the United States.

Opponents of the Vietnam War used the slogan, "War is hazardous to the health of children." The Vietnam War has been hazardous and destructive to generations of Americans and Vietnamese.

Acknowledgment: The authors acknowledge the assistance of Ms. Natalie Grigorian in the updating and revision of this chapter from the first edition of this book.

References

1. Wikipedia. Vietnam War Casualties. http://en.wikipedia.org/wiki/Vietnam War Casualties. Accessed June 3, 2007
2. National Academy of Sciences, National Research Council, Committee on the Effects of Herbicide in Vietnam. The Effects of Herbicide in Vietnam: Part A. Summary and Conclusions. Washington, DC: U.S. Government Printing Office, 1974.
3. Stockholm International Peace Research Institute. Ecological Consequences of the Second Indochina War. Stockholm: SIPRI, 1976.

4. Brennan JS (ed.). The Vietnam War: An Almanac. New York: World Almanac Publications, 1985.
5. Karnow S. Vietnam: A History. New York: Penguin Books, 1983.
6. World Bank. Viet Nam: Population, Health and Nutrition Sector Review (Updated). Washington, DC: World Bank, Population and Human Resources Operation Division, July 30, 1993,
7. Dan PQ. The Republic of Vietnam's Environment and People. Saigon: Republic of Vietnam, 1975.
8. Wiesner LA. Victims and Survivors: Displaced Persons and Other War Victims in Viet-Nam, 1954–1975. Westport, CT: Greenwood Press, 1988.
9. U.S. Department of State. The SEATO Treaty: American Foreign Policy, 1950–1955, Vol. I. Washington, DC: U.S. Government Printing Office, 1975, pp. 912–916.
10. Baritz L. Backfire. New York: Ballantine Books, 1985, p. 146.
11. Bannister J. The Population of Vietnam. (International Population Reports, Series P-95, No. 77.) Washington, DC: U.S. Department of Commerce, Bureau of the Census, October 1985.
12. Vietnam Population, 1979. Hanoi: Central Census Steering Committee, 1983.
13. Westing AH. The environmental aftermath of warfare in Viet Nam. Nat Res J 1983; 23:372–387.
14. Cima RJ. Vietnam: A Country Study. Federal Research Division, Library of Congress, Washington, DC: U.S. Government Printing Office, 1989.
15. Vessey JW. The problem of the disabled in Vietnam. U.S. Department of State, Washington, DC, October 13, 1987.
16. Relief and Rehabilitation of War Victims in Indochina. IV: South Vietnam and Regional Problems. Hearing before Subcommittee to Investigate Problems Connected with Refugees and Escapees. Committee on the Judiciary, U.S. Senate, 93rd Congress, 1st session, Washington, DC: U.S. Government Printing Office, August 1, 1973.
17. Bonacci MA. The Legacy of Colonialism in Southeast Asia. Washington, DC: The Asia Resource Center, 1990.
18. Muller R. Personal communication with the Peoples' Committee on War Crimes, Hanoi, 1993. Vietnam Veterans of America Foundation, November 1994.
19. Monan J. Landmines and underdevelopment: A case study of Quang Tri Province. Hong Kong: Oxfam, 1995.
20. Civilian Casualty and Refugee Problems in South Vietnam. Findings and recommendations, Subcommittee to Investigate Problems Connected with Refugees and Escapees. Committee on the Judiciary, U.S. Senate, 90th Congress, 2nd session, Washington, DC: U.S. Government Printing Office. May 9, 1968.
21. Cavanaugh DC, Dangerfield HG, Hunter DH, et al. Some observations of the current plague outbreak in the Republic of Vietnam. Am J Public Health 1968;58: 742–752.
22. Craddock WL. United States medical programs in South Vietnam. Mil Med 1970; 135:186–191.
23. Camp E. A retrospective report: Health care in South Vietnam—Hospitals. J Am Hosp Assoc 1975;50:55–58.
24. Revsin ME. Vietnam dental education project: A five year report. J Am Dental Assoc 1972;84:1049–1062.
25. Shellard EJ. Health services in Vietnam. Med War 1992;8:169–174.
26. Ladinsky J, Levine RE. The organization of health services in Vietnam. J Public Health Policy 1985;6:255–268.

27. Quinn JS. Shortages confront Vietnam's health care. Indochina issues. Washington, DC: Center for International Policy, Indochina Project, April 1986.

28. World Health Organization, Report on the Democratic Republic of Vietnam, February 26, 1976.

29. Relief and rehabilitation of war victims in Indochina: III. North Vietnam and Laos. Hearing before Subcommittee to Investigate Problems Connected with Refugees and Escapees. Committee on the Judiciary, U.S. Senate, 93rd Congress, 1st session. Washington, DC: U.S. Government Printing Office, July 31, 1973.

30. Westing AH (ed.). Herbicides in War: The Long-term Ecological and Human Consequences. London: Taylor and Francis, 1984, p. 5.

31. Sidel VW. Farewell to arms: Impact of the arms race on the human condition. PSR Q 1993;3:18–26.

32. Cecil PF. Herbicide Warfare: The Ranch Hand Project in Vietnam. New York: Praeger, 1986.

33. Boffey PM. Herbicides in Vietnam: AAAS study finds widespread devastation. Science 1971;171:43–47.

34. Sterling TD, Arundel A. Review of recent Vietnamese studies on the carcinogenic and teratogenic effects of phenoxy herbicide exposure. Int J Health Serv 1986;16: 265–278.

35. Hardell L, Eriksson M, Lenner P, Lundgren E. Malignant lymphoma and exposure to chemical substances, especially organic solvents, chlorophenols, and phenoxy acids. Br J Cancer 1981;43:169–176.

36. Hoar SK, Blair A, Holmes FF, et al. Agricultural herbicide use and risk of lymphoma and soft-tissue sarcoma. JAMA 1986;255:1141–1147.

37. Constable JD, Hatch MC. Reproductive effects of herbicide exposure in Vietnam: Recent studies by the Vietnamese and others. Teratogenesis Carcinogenesis Mutagenesis 1985;5:231–250.

38. Hatch MC. Dioxin, teratogenicity and reproductive function. In Atwood PL (ed.). Agent Orange: Medical, Scientific, Legal, Political and Psychological Issues. Boston: The William Joiner Center for the Study of War and Social Consequences, 1993, pp. 30–34.

39. Nguyen C. Reproductive epidemiology: Symposium summary. In Westing AH (ed.). Herbicides in War. London: Taylor & Francis, 1984. pp. 133–134.

40. Centers for Disease Control. Health status of Vietnam veterans: III. Reproductive outcomes and child health. JAMA 1988;259:2715–2717.

41. Air Force Health Study. An Epidemiologic Investigation of Health Effects in Air Force Personnel Following Exposure to Herbicides: Reproductive Outcomes. A1-TR-1992–0090. Brooks AFB: USAF School of Aerospace Medicine.

42. Institute of Medicine: National Academy of Science. Veterans and Agent Orange: Health Effects of Herbicides Used in Vietnam. Washington, DC: National Academy Press, 1994, p. 6.

43. Schecter A, Dai LC, Thuy LT, et al. Agent Orange and the Vietnamese: The persistence of elevated dioxin levels in human tissues. Am J Public Health 1995;85: 516–522.

44. Dwyer JH, Flesh-Janys D. Editorial: Agent Orange in Vietnam. Am J Public Health 1995;85:476–478.

45. Institute of Medicine, National Academy of Sciences. Veterans and Agent Orange: Update 1996. Washington, DC: National Academy Press, 1996 [pre-publication copy], pp. 1–5.

46. Atwood PL (ed.). Agent Orange: Medical, Scientific, Legal, Political and Psychological Issues. Boston: The William Joiner Center for the Study of War and Social Consequences, University of Massachusetts–Boston, 1990.
47. Nass M. Monsanto's Agent Orange: The Persistent Ghost from Vietnam. Available at: http://www.organicconsumers.org/monsanto/agentorange032102.cfm (accessed June 19, 2007).
48. Vietnam Agent Orange Relief and Responsibility Campaign, New York. Agent Orange and the Vietnam War: Magnitude and Consequences. Available at: http://www .vn-agentorange.org (accessed June 19, 2007).
49. Weinstein, Judge Jack. For the United States District Court, Eastern District of New York. Memorandum, order and judgment, MDL N0.381, in re "Agent Orange" Product Liability Litigation, March 10, 2005.
50. Schecter A, Gasiewicz TA. Dioxin and Health (2nd ed.). Hoboken, NJ: John Wiley & Sons, 2003.
51. Stellman JM, Stellman SD, Christian R, et al. The extent and patterns of usage of Agent Orange and other herbicides in Vietnam. Nature 2003;422:681–687.
52. Dwernychuk LW, Cau HD, Hatfield CT, et al. Dioxin reservoirs in southern Vietnam: A legacy of Agent Orange. Chemosphere 2002;47:117–137.
53. Ngo AD, Taylor R, Roberts CL, Nguyen TV. Association between Agent Orange and birth defects: Systematic review and metaanalysis. Int J Epidemiol 2006;35:1220–1230.
54. Hitchens C. The Vietnam syndrome. Vanity Fair, August 2006, pp. 106–111.
55. U.N. Fund for Population Activity. Program Review and Strategy Development Report: Vietnam, 1993.
56. U.N. Population Fund. Vietnam: Program Review and Strategy Development Report, New York, 1991.
57. Branigan W. U.S. recovers MIA remains in Vietnam: Hopes for more fade. Washington Post, February 9, 1993.
58. Department of Defense, Vietnam-Era Unaccounted for Statistical Report, current as of October 10, 2006. Available at: http://www.dtic.mil/dpmo/pmsea/Stats20061010 .pdf (accessed June 19, 2007).
59. Charny J, Spragens J. Obstacles to Recovery in Vietnam and Kampuchea: U.S. Embargo of Humanitarian Aid. Boston: Oxfam America, 1985, pp. 30–31.
60. Khanh Hoa DT. Vietnam Population Profile and Transition [unpublished conference paper]. Presented at: Implications of Vietnam's Economic Reform for the Health Sector, Harvard University, November 18–19, 1994.
61. Info Please, Vietnam. Available at: http://infoplease.com/ipa/A0108144.html (accessed June 19, 2007).
62. Kaufman M. Vietnam, 1978: Crisis in food, nutrition and health. J Am Diet Assoc 1979;74:310–316.
63. Hiebert LG. Malnutrition among children. Indochina Issues 65. Washington, DC: Center For International Policy, 1965.
64. World Bank. Social Indicators of Development, 1994. Baltimore: Johns Hopkins University Press, 1994.
65. Phong NK. The Changing Structure of Health Care [unpublished conference paper]. Presented at: Implications of Vietnam's Reform for the Health Care Sector, Harvard University, November 18–19, 1994.
66. Gellert GA. The influence of market economics on primary health care in Vietnam. Letter from Ho Chi Minh City. JAMA 1995;273:1497–1502.

67. Chen LC, Hiebert LG. From socialism to private markets: Vietnam's health in rapid transition. (Working Paper Series, No. 94.11.) Cambridge, MA: Center For Population and Development Studies, Harvard University School of Public Health, October 1994.

68. Charny J, Spragens J. Obstacles to Recovery in Vietnam and Kampuchea: U.S. Embargo of Humanitarian Aid. Boston: Oxfam America, 1985.

69. Twining C. Personal written communication to Dr. Myron Allukian, U.S. Department of State, Office of Vietnam, Laos and Cambodia, Aug. 14, 1990, p. 17.

70. Boston Globe, November 9, 1989.

71. 109th Congress expires, jockeying starts for 110th. New York Times, December 9, 2006.

72. King F. Vietnamese president defends human rights record. Boston Globe, June 23, 2007, p A4.

73. Baskir L, Strauss W. Chance and Circumstance: The Draft, the War, and the Vietnam Generation. New York: Alfred A. Knopf, 1978.

74. Hsiao L. Project 100,000: The Great Society's answer to military manpower needs in Vietnam. Vietnam Generation 1989;1:14–37.

75. Rosenheck R, Frisman L, Chung AM. The proportions of veterans among homeless men. Am J Public Health 1994;84:466–469.

76. U.S. General Accounting Office. Homelessness: Demand for Services to Homeless Veterans Exceeds VA Program Capacity. Report to the Chairman, Committee on Veterans Affairs, U.S. Senate, Washington, DC, February 1994.

77. The Vietnam Veterans Memorial, Wall Information Page. Available at: http://www .thewall-usa.com/information.asp (accessed June 19, 2007).

78. Bullman T, Kang HK. A study of suicide among Vietnam veterans. Federal Practitioner, March 1995.

79. Staff Report: Medical evaluation of the prisoners of the Vietnam War. Nutrition Today 1973, pp. 24–30.

80. Stanton MD. Drugs, Vietnam and the Vietnam veteran: An overview. Am J Drug Abuse 1976;3:557–570.

81. Decoufle P, Holmgreen P, Boyle CA, Stroup NE. Self-reported health status of Vietnam veterans in relation to exposure to herbicides and combat. Am J Epidemiol 1992;135:312–323.

82. Goldberg J, Eisen SA, True WR, Henderson WG. Health effects of military service: Lessons learned from the Vietnam experience. Ann Epidemiol 1992;2:841–853.

83. Walker JI, Cavenar JO. Vietnam veterans: Their problems continue. J Nerv Mental Dis 1982;170:174–180.

84. Centers For Disease Control. Health Status of Vietnam Veterans: Vietnam Experience Study, Vol. I: Synopsis. Atlanta: U.S. Department of Health and Human Services, Public Health Service, Centers for Disease Control and Prevention, January 1989.

85. McNamara RS. In Retrospect: The Tragedy and Lessons of Vietnam. New York: Random House, 1995.

VI

PREVENTION OF WAR AND ITS HEALTH CONSEQUENCES

20

A Public Health Approach to Preventing the Health Consequences of Armed Conflict

Avid Reza, Mark Anderson, and James A. Mercy

> We must address the roots of violence. Only then will we transform the past century's legacy from a crushing burden into a cautionary lesson.
> —Nelson Mandela, World Report on Violence and Health[1]

Public health professionals are playing an increasingly important role in responding to the health consequences of armed conflict.* These efforts have been focused primarily on mitigating the health burden of armed conflict, either while it is occurring or in its aftermath. Mitigating the health burden typically involves assessing the health impact of armed conflict to help target and guide prevention and treatment strategies, as well as implementing programs to prevent the spread of disease and malnutrition in affected populations. However, public health professionals can do much more to apply their skills and expertise to preventing the health consequences of armed conflict by giving greater attention to (1) preventing armed conflict from occuring in the first place, and (2) addressing consequences that have received relatively little attention, such as injuries and mental health problems.

The need for more effective prevention strategies arises from the devastating impact that armed conflict has on health. Armed conflict not only directly causes premature death, disability, psychological trauma, and physical injury, but it can also destroy the integrity of health care systems and public

---

*For the purposes of this chapter, armed conflict includes violent conflict between states (countries) and within states, including war, terrorism, and state-perpetrated violence, such as genocide.

health services, such as water and sanitation systems. These disruptions lead to famine, epidemics, social dislocations, and other forms of violence—all of which may persist long after armed conflict has ended.

In this chapter, we propose an agenda for expanding the role and capacity of public health in addressing the health consequences of armed conflict. We begin by describing a unified model that integrates (1) the stages of the public health approach to prevention with (2) the temporal phases of armed conflict. This model enables us to visualize points at which public health professionals can strengthen their contributions to prevention.

A Framework to Guide Public Health

The Public Health Approach to Prevention

This approach is rooted in science. It begins with defining the problem. It then (1) identifies underlying causes and associated risk and protective factors; (2) develops and tests interventions that lower the risks; and (3) broadly disseminates and implements these interventions (Figure 20-1).[2] Several of the steps used in this approach are likely to occur simultaneously. The knowledge

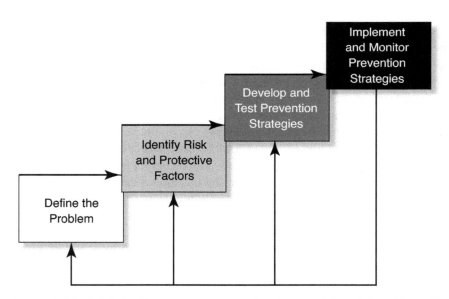

Figure 20-1. Public health approach to prevention. (Source: Adapted from Mercy JA, Rosenberg ML, Powell KE, et al. Public health policy for preventing violence. Health Affairs 1993;12:7–29.)

gained through the later steps ultimately helps to refine and clarify the knowledge gained through the earlier steps.

The first step of the public health model—defining the problem—helps us to
understand the magnitude and characteristics of a problem by collecting and
interpreting descriptive data on health events. In this step, one attempts to
describe the health events in terms of person, place, and time. Information is
collected on the demographic characteristics of the persons involved, such as
age, socioeconomic status, and whether they are refugees or internally displaced persons; the geographic characteristics of the event, such as whether it
occurs in a high-income or low-income country; and the temporal characteristics of the event, such as month and year of occurrence. Understanding the
magnitude and characteristics of the problem helps in setting public health
priorities and identifying vulnerable populations. Furthermore, this step provides the baseline data necessary to monitor progress toward achieving health
goals. Data typically are collected through point-in-time analyses or through
public health surveillance.

The second step of the model involves identifying risk and protective
factors for specific health outcomes. In this step, one attempts to determine
why certain individuals, families, communities, or even nations are at greater
or lesser risk than others for developing health problems. Public health scientists use a variety of analytical approaches to identify risk factors, including
cohort and case-control studies as well as research designs that make use of
ecological, cross-sectional, and time-series data. The second step of the model
builds on the first step by providing insights into the potential causes of health
problems that then can be used to suggest specific prevention programs and
policies.

In the third step, one uses the information obtained in the previous two steps
to develop and test prevention programs and policies. After interventions have
been developed, evaluation methods can be used to measure their effectiveness in reducing adverse health outcomes or promoting favorable health
outcomes. These evaluation methods include experimental studies, such as
randomized control trials; and quasi-experimental studies, such as time-series
analyses and ecological studies. They also include various types of economic
evaluations, such as cost-effectiveness, cost-benefit, and cost-utility studies.

In the fourth and final step in the model, one broadly disseminates and
implements those prevention strategies that were shown to be effective in the
previous step. Effectiveness should be monitored after interventions are implemented in the field. Although the third step may have shown specific prevention strategies to be effective, those strategies may not have the same
impact when implemented more broadly. Population differences or barriers to
implementation may prevent strategies identified as effective in highly controlled settings from being equally effective in the field. This last step also

includes efforts to train key people in how to implement prevention activities and communicate important information about prevention through the mass media.

The Temporal Phases of Armed Conflict

Armed conflict can be divided into three temporal phases that represent the stages through which conflict progresses: preconflict, conflict, and postconflict. Each phase offers different opportunities for prevention. Because the underlying causes of conflict often begin to emerge years before an outbreak of violence, the recognition of these causes provides an opportunity to intervene before the actual conflict takes place.[3] In addition, in countries where the potential for armed conflict is high, communities or societies can be made more resilient to potential health consequences before conflict occurs. In the conflict phase, many opportunities arise to prevent or mitigate the severity of the health consequences. The postconflict phase is important because the health consequences of armed conflict continue long after a ceasefire and because armed conflict could re-emerge if the underlying causes have not been fully resolved. However, although the distinction of these temporal phases is useful, the phases may not always be easily distinguished. For example, the start of the postconflict phase may be hard to identify because a period of unrest may exist before "normalcy" is established.

The Unified Model

The unified model provides a framework that illustrates the roles that public health can play in preventing the health consequences of armed conflict (Table 20-1). This model combines the public health approach to prevention with the temporal phases of armed conflict. The cells of this model provide both actual and potential examples of public health activities, some of which are discussed later in this chapter. The model also highlights areas where public health could expand its role and capabilities; they give direction to public health professionals for future activities.

Combining the public health approach to prevention with the three temporal phases of armed conflict enables us to more fully recognize the different types of data collection, research, and prevention strategies available during each of these phases. In addition, we must consider various logistical aspects of implementing these strategies. During the conflict phase, for example, prevention strategies need to be developed in a way that considers the challenges of implementation in the midst of political instability, social turmoil, and violence.

Table 20-1. Actual or Potential Examples of Public Health Contributions to Preventing the Health Consequences of Armed Conflict

Temporal Phase of Armed Conflict	Stage of Public Health Approach	Actual or Potential Contributions
All phases	Define the problem	• Develop standardized definitions and terminologies to guide data collection.* • Identify creative strategies to monitor the health consequences of armed conflict (such as cluster surveys).* • Modify the international classification of disease (ICD) codes to distinguish among mortality and morbidity associated with major forms of armed conflict.*
Preconflict phase	Define the problem	• Develop a surveillance system of risk factors for armed conflict.*
	Identify causes	• Identify risk and protective factors associated with the development of armed conflict.*† • Determine how preconflict societal and cultural factors influence rates of conflict-related injury, illness, and mental trauma.*†
	Develop and test interventions	• Develop strategies that can contribute to preventing armed conflict (such as conducting research to understand how best to prevent violent political transitions).* • Evaluate the efficacy and effectiveness of strategies designed to prevent armed conflict (such as economic sanctions, and United Nations [UN] peacekeeping efforts).* • Evaluate the efficacy and effectiveness of strategies to prepare communities and nations in advance of armed conflict to reduce likelihood of injury or illness (such as landmine risk education and vaccines to protect against bioterrorism).*
	Implement interventions	• Identify the most effective methods for implementing and disseminating strategies to prevent armed conflict.* • Identify the most effective methods for implementing and disseminating strategies to prepare communities and nations at risk for violence.*
Conflict phase	Define the problem	• Identify the best methods for collecting data on mental trauma and sexual violence during ongoing conflict.* • Determine the impact of ongoing conflict on nutrition, communicable diseases, injury, mental trauma, and sexual violence. • Determine key data elements for surveillance of landmine/unexploded ordnance (UXO) injuries.

(continued)

343

Table 20-1. (*continued*)

Temporal Phase of Armed Conflict	Stage of Public Health Approach	Actual or Potential Contributions
	Identify causes	• Identify risk and protective factors associated with continued armed conflict.* • Identify individual and community-level risk and protective factors for conflict-related mental trauma, sexual violence, and landmine/UXO injuries during conflict.* • Identify individual and community-level risk and protective factors for communicable diseases and malnutrition during conflict.
	Develop and test interventions	• Evaluate the efficacy and effectiveness of interventions designed to shorten the duration of armed conflict.* • Evaluate the efficacy and effectiveness of the following: – Mental health interventions implemented early in the conflict phase* – Interventions and policies designed to prevent perpetration of and victimization from sexual violence* – Mine risk education to prevent landmine/UXO injuries* • Evaluate interventions to reduce the incidence of communicable diseases and malnutrition.
	Implement interventions	• Improve effective interventions to make them more simple and affordable.* • Determine how effective interventions can be adapted for culturally diverse populations.*
Postconflict phase	Define the problem	• Determine the impact of armed conflict on postconflict rates of violence (such as suicide and intimate partner violence).* • Measure the long-term physical and mental health consequences of sexual violence and landmine/UXO injuries.* • Determine the impact of armed conflict on nutrition, communicable diseases, injury, and mental health in postconflict settings. • Determine the key data elements for surveillance of landmine/UXO injuries.
	Identify causes	• Identify risk and protective factors associated with recurring armed conflict.* • Identify risk and protective factors for other forms of violence (such as suicide and interpersonal violence) in postconflict settings.* • Identify individual and community-level risk and protective factors for mental trauma and landmine/UXO injuries in postconflict settings.*

Table 20-1. (*continued*)

Temporal Phase of Armed Conflict	Stage of Public Health Approach	Actual or Potential Contributions
	Develop and test interventions	• Identify individual and community-level risk and protective factors for communicable diseases and malnutrition in postconflict settings.
		• Evaluate the efficacy and effectiveness of interventions designed to prevent relapse into conflict.*
		• Evaluate the efficacy and effectiveness of interventions aimed at preventing the long-term consequences of mental trauma.*
		• Evaluate the cost-effectiveness of landmine/UXO injury prevention programs.*
		• Develop and evaluate interventions to reduce the incidence of communicable diseases and malnutrition.*
	Implement interventions	• Identify the most effective methods for reconstructing infrastructures and health services.*

*Activities in which public health could expand its role and capabilities.
†These research activities are placed in the preconflict phase because their intent is to identify risk and protective factors that will lead to strategies to prevent conflict from occurring, even though this research may entail comparing countries that have experienced conflict with those that have not.

Applying the Unified Model

Using this model, we broadly describe what public health workers are currently doing to prevent the health consequences of armed conflict. Through examples, we show areas in which public health could expand its role and capacity in prevention. These examples address a range of health consequences of armed conflict, including those related to mental health problems, physical injuries, and infectious diseases. The examples provided are not intended to comprise a comprehensive list, but rather to illustrate some of the ways in which public health can go beyond its traditional roles.

All Phases

Understanding the magnitude and characteristics of the health consequences of armed conflict will help to inform and track prevention efforts during all three phases. One of the major obstacles to making progress in describing this problem is the inconsistency in the definitions and terminologies used to describe the different types of armed conflict and their health outcomes. These inconsistencies limit our ability to fully interpret available data and to make comparisons over time and across communities and countries. In addition, the literature on the health outcomes of armed conflict does not consistently distinguish direct from indirect consequences, or military from civilian deaths and injuries.

Public health professionals could make a fundamental contribution to efforts to monitor and study the health consequences of armed conflict by bringing together epidemiologists and professionals in other relevant scientific disciplines to develop a set of standard definitions to guide data collection that are internationally agreed upon. This effort should include developing standardized terminologies and definitions for describing the health outcomes associated with armed conflict. First, one must distinguish among the different types of armed conflict, such as war, genocide, and terrorism, while recognizing that some overlap may exist among them. In addition, one must identify the various types of victims, including both military (armed) combatants and civilians. One must also distinguish between direct and indirect health consequences of armed conflict. Direct health outcomes include physical and psychological injury, disability, and death that results from torture, combat, or tactics of intimidation, such as sexual assault. Indirect health outcomes include communicable diseases, malnutrition, chronic diseases, and other forms of violence that result from social disruptions. These disruptions include, for example[4]:

- Destruction of clinics, hospitals, and public health programs that support safe food and clean water
- Damage to the social foundations of society, such as work, education, practice of religion, and other activities that are a part of daily life
- Forced displacement of people, making them refugees or internally displaced persons.

Other severe hindrances to the availability and quality of existing data on the health consequences of armed conflict include the following[5]:

- Most affected countries lack reliable health registration systems.
- Conflict disrupts existing surveillance systems.
- Rapid population shifts and movements make collection of data on the affected population difficult.
- Access is lacking for health services from which data are typically collected.
- Parties to a conflict may manipulate data.

Given these impediments, creative strategies are needed to improve our ability to monitor health consequences, such as the use of cluster surveys or clinic-based surveillance systems operated by nongovernmental organizations (NGOs). Rapid assessment procedures also have been suggested to provide valid information on various health outcomes, such as injury-related morbidity and mortality. These rapid assessment procedures are quicker, simpler, and less costly than standard data collection methods in settings that lack the technical and financial resources necessary for sophisticated surveillance methods.[6]

However, efforts to improve existing data collection systems also may yield benefits. Existing world health statistics on mortality, for example, do not enable distinction among deaths resulting from different forms of armed conflict, such as war and genocide.[7] After standardized definitions have been developed, the International Classification of Disease (ICD) codes could be amended so that world mortality statistics could be used to monitor the health consequences of the major categories of armed conflict. In addition to developing surveillance systems to collect information on the health outcomes of armed conflict, there are other types of surveillance systems specific to each of the temporal phases that also should be considered.

Preconflict Phase

In preconflict settings, after an adequate research base is formed, the potential exists for developing a surveillance system that monitors risk and protective factors for armed conflict. For example, countries undergoing rapid demographic or economic changes, such as sudden increases in population or unemployment, may be at greater risk for certain forms of armed conflict.[5] If these and other risk factors can be confirmed through research, they could provide the basis for a system to help forewarn global and community leaders about regions or countries at high risk for armed conflict, enabling diplomatic or other preventive measures to be implemented. In the event that armed conflict cannot be prevented, such an early warning system could help international organizations prepare more timely and efficient humanitarian aid responses to address the complex emergencies associated with armed conflict[8] (see Chapters 22 and 23).

In addition to developing and implementing surveillance systems that monitor risk and protective factors for armed conflict, public health also can become more involved in conducting research to identify these factors. Previous theoretical and empirical work has identified potential risk and protective factors (Table 20-2), but few of these factors have been confirmed through research. In addition, we do not fully understand the extent to which such factors operate alone or in combination with other factors to produce armed conflict.[3,5] One example of research in this area identified factors explaining why violent conflict between Hindus and Muslims was common in

Table 20-2. Potential Risk Factors for Armed Conflict

Demographic Factors
- High infant mortality
- Excessively high population densities
- Insufficient supply of food or access to safe water
- Disputes over territory or environmental
  resources that are claimed by distinct ethnic groups

Societal and Community Factors
- Inequality among groups
- Fueling of group fanaticism along ethnic, national, or religious lines
- Ready availability of small arms and other weapons

Political Factors*
- Lack of a democratic process
- Rapid changes in regimes
- Unequal access to power

Economic Factors*
- Grossly unequal distribution of resources
- Unequal access to resources
- Control over key natural resources

Other
- Deterioration in public services
- Cycles of violent revenge

---

*Unequal distribution of resources and unequal access to these resources and to political power—whether by geographic area, social class, religion, race, or ethnicity—have been suggested to contribute to conflict between groups.

Sources: Adapted from Zwi AB, Garfield R, Loretti A. Collective violence. In Krug EG, Dahlberg LL, Mercy JA, et al. (eds.). World Report on Violence and Health. Geneva: World Health Organization, 2002, pp. 213–239; Carnegie Commission on Preventing Deadly Conflict. Preventing Deadly Conflict: Final Report. New York: Carnegie Corporation of New York, 1998.

some Indian cities and rare in others. This study found that cities with strong associational forms of civic engagements involving both Hindus and Muslims, such as integrated business organizations, trade unions, political parties, and professional associations, were protected from outbreaks of ethnic violence, whereas communities with weaker or no associational forms of civic engagement were more likely to experience ethnic violence.[9] Policies and programs aimed at creating various types of integrated community associations may be effective in reducing some forms of armed conflict.

Public health professionals also can develop and evaluate interventions to prevent armed conflict and its health consequences. The identification of risk and protective factors in the previous step, for example, could be used with existing knowledge about the basic epidemiology of the problem to develop and test interventions designed to prevent armed conflict and its associated health consequences from occurring in the first place. For example, cross-national research suggests that countries in political transition, such as from autocratic to democratic regimes, may be at highest risk for civil war and violent political repression.[10,11] Programs and policies that assist these transitional countries in developing institutions that facilitate the peaceful transfer of power and service systems that address basic human needs may be effective in preventing violent political repression.[10] Public health professionals and other scientists can perform research to further understand how best to prevent violent transitions and bring these strategies to the attention of policy makers.[12]

In addition, public health can bring together epidemiologists and professionals in other relevant scientific disciplines to evaluate the effectiveness of existing prevention strategies. Economic sanctions, for example, may play an important role in preventing armed conflict, and several strategies have been offered to strengthen this approach.[3] Retrospective and prospective research could be conducted to evaluate the effectiveness of sanctions and the various approaches used to implement them. This information could then be provided to policy makers to help guide the development of evidence-based policies.

Public health also can participate in preparing a community or country in advance of armed conflict (such as terrorism), to reduce the likelihood and severity of illness and injury in the event that such violence occurs. For example, the Centers for Disease Control and Prevention (CDC) has implemented several strategies to prevent illness in the event of a bioterrorist attack in the United States. These activities have included, but are not limited to, improving the effectiveness and safety of the current anthrax vaccine and developing rapid diagnostic tests for detecting potential bioterrorism agents.[13] Having safe and effective vaccines and rapid diagnostic tests would be critical to controlling and containing an event. Although the effectiveness of these specific interventions remains to be seen, this concept of preparedness may be applicable to other health consequences of armed conflict, such as injuries from landmines/unexploded ordnance (UXO) and psychological trauma.

After effective interventions have been developed to prevent armed conflict or to prepare communities or countries, the challenge will be how best to implement them. Many countries at risk for armed conflict are resource-poor and potentially unstable, which could create barriers to effective implementation. Even without complete scientific knowledge of what works to prevent armed conflict, the best available information should be used to help prepare communities or nations at risk for pending armed conflict. One way in which public health professionals can assist in this preparation is by disseminating information to people in at-risk communities or countries on ways that they can protect themselves from injury and illness. For example, public health professionals could disseminate information that has been shown to be effective on landmine/UXO–related injury prevention in areas where landmines and ordinance have been used.

Conflict Phase

Public health has contributed significantly to describing the magnitude and characteristics of the health consequences of armed conflict during this phase. National and local surveys conducted during conflict have demonstrated the impact of armed conflict, ranging from injuries to malnutrition. For example, it has been shown that diarrheal diseases are a major cause of morbidity and mortality among populations affected by armed conflict.[14] After the influx of 800,000 Rwandan refugees into the Democratic Republic of Congo in 1994, diarrheal illnesses caused 85 percent of the 50,000 deaths reported during the first month.[15] Major advances also have been made in survey methodology, so that health outcomes can be more accurately described. For example, the field of emergency nutrition assessments has made significant advances during the past decade. Standard cluster survey formats are now available for conducting anthropometric surveys.[16] In addition to improving survey methodologies to more accurately describe health problems previously studied, public health professionals also have contributed to addressing the gap in knowledge about health outcomes not previously well studied, such as those related to mental health and reproductive health.[17,18]

Another way that public health can contribute during the conflict phase is to help identify risk and protective factors for illness and injury in the midst of ongoing conflict. In fact, public health professionals already have established that certain risk factors promote communicable disease transmission in complex emergencies, such as mass population movement and resettlement in temporary locations, overcrowding, economic and environmental degradation, impoverishment, scarcity of water, poor sanitation and waste management, inadequate or no shelter, poor nutrition, and poor access to health care.[14] They also have identified risk factors for malnutrition, such as poor breast-feeding practices, diarrheal and other infectious diseases among infants, and human immunodeficiency virus (HIV) infection.[19] However, further study is needed to determine risk factors for other health consequences, such as those associated with injury and mental health. For example, two studies in Afghanistan demonstrated that children were at greater risk for injuries from UXO, such as unexploded grenades and mortar shells, whereas adults were at greater risk for injuries from landmines.[20,21] Furthermore, these studies identified playing and tending animals as risk behaviors for children, and military and economic-necessity activities, such as traveling and farming, as risk behaviors for adults. More studies are needed to confirm these hypothesized risk factors and to determine whether they can be generalized to other countries. This type of information can then be used to develop and test landmine risk-education interventions that can be implemented during both the conflict and postconflict phases.

There are also few studies that describe the risk factors for psychological trauma during ongoing conflict. One study that examined psychological trauma among displaced persons during conflict in Nepal found that (1) being female, being 41 to 50 years old, and "feeling miserable" on arrival at a new place were associated with symptoms consistent with depression; and (2) experiencing greater than three traumatic events and "feeling miserable" on arrival at a new place were associated with posttraumatic stress disorder (PTSD).[22] Such studies can help identify groups at high risk for psychological trauma so that interventions can better target these populations.

Public health has contributed significantly to the development of successful interventions to address two of the leading causes of death—communicable diseases and malnutrition—in complex emergencies.[14,19] There are prevention and control interventions for the major high-mortality communicable diseases, including guidelines for on-site planning for refugee camps; clean water supply and sanitation programs to reduce fecal–oral transmission of disease; vaccines against measles, meningococcal meningitis, poliomyelitis, and yellow fever; and vector-control activities, such as indoor residual spraying and insecticide-treated nets to help prevent malaria.[14] Therapeutic feeding programs also have helped to reduce malnutrition-related mortality.[19]

However, for other health consequences, such as mental health and injury, development of better interventions depends on further research. For example, few evidence-based intervention studies of early mental health interventions have been performed during complex emergencies; such interventions include offering population-wide psychological first aid or identifying and triaging to psychiatric treatment those who have severe mental disorders.[17] Creative strategies are needed to evaluate these types of interventions, given the difficulty of performing such studies during conflict. One such study evaluated the efficacy of a counseling intervention aimed to alleviate distress in wartime Bosnia and Herzegovina and found it to be effective, demonstrating that most people who received counseling clinically recovered or experienced improved functioning.[23]

Although public health has contributed significantly to the development of proven interventions to prevent communicable diseases during armed conflict, the delivery mechanisms for these prevention strategies are often compromised in countries affected by violent conflict. This compromise of delivery mechanisms is due, in part, to insecurity, loss of health care providers, damage to infrastructure, and poor coordination.[14] These challenges are greatest in complex emergencies affecting large geographical areas or entire countries.[14] Existing interventions may be implemented more systematically with higher levels of coordination among governments, United Nations agencies, and NGOs.[14] In addition, given the logistical constraints of implementing interventions during ongoing conflict, simpler, more effective, and more affordable methods are needed to prevent communicable diseases. For example, insecticide-treated nets are very effective in preventing malaria; however, it has been challenging to make these nets widely available and usable to refugees or internally displaced persons sleeping under plastic sheeting and tents.[14] The need for more novel and convenient methods of protection has led to testing of insecticide-treated plastic sheeting and bedding.[14,24] This is an example of modifying an intervention when faced with barriers to implementation. Therefore, during the implementation step, the effectiveness of various interventions needs to be monitored so that appropriate modifications can be made as necessary.

Postconflict Phase

Because of the adverse effects of armed conflict on health care and public health systems and services, famine, spread of communicable disease, and social dislocation may persist long after armed conflict has ended. In addition, even after communities have been rebuilt and health care systems are functioning, adverse health outcomes of a preceding conflict may remain, such as mental health problems.[17] In postwar Afghanistan, the prevalence of depression, anxiety, and PTSD were extremely high; among people older than 15 years of age, the prevalence of depression was approximately 70 percent.[25] Another type of remnant of armed conflict consists of landmines/UXOs, some of which from World Wars I and II are still present in Europe and Asia.[26] Therefore, collecting data on injury-related morbidity and mortality due to landmines/UXOs should continue far beyond a ceasefire. Although some countries collect this information, it is not being collected in a comprehensive or systematic manner that would permit cross-national comparison. To address this problem, some people are attempting to develop an internationally accepted system for collecting and managing landmine casualty data on a global scale.[27] Armed conflict probably contributes to increased homicide and suicide rates after ceasefire.[28–31] Improving surveillance of injury-related morbidity and mortality during the postconflict phase could help in examining these potential consequences.

Public health can continue to contribute to understanding of the epidemiological patterns of illnesses and associated risk factors in postconflict settings. In fact, many of the illnesses that occur during armed conflict—and their underlying risk factors—often continue to occur in postconflict settings. For example, many risk factors for communicable diseases, such as economic and environmental degradation, impoverishment, poor sanitation and waste management, inadequate or no shelter, and poor access to health care, may continue to exist long after ceasefire.

Risk factors for other health outcomes have not been well studied. For example, risk factors for recurrence of armed conflict after ceasefires or periods of peace have not been adequately identified or studied. Countries that have experienced armed conflict are at high risk for relapsing into violent conflict. Approximately 40 percent of countries in the postconflict phase relapse into war within 5 years.[32] Understanding why some countries are more likely to relapse into yet another violent conflict is therefore important, because further violence is likely to exacerbate existing health problems. Studies conducted in postwar Kosovo and Afghanistan have suggested that mental illness caused by psychological trauma may be associated with feelings of hatred and the desire to take revenge.[25,33] Effective treatment for psychological trauma may therefore help prevent the recurrence of violent conflict. Public health research can be used to identify factors that contribute to recurrence of violence and thereby help develop appropriate policies and strategies to prevent such collective recidivism.

Many of the proven interventions implemented during ongoing conflict to prevent communicable diseases and malnutrition continue to be needed long after ceasefire. In addition, the lack of evidence-based interventions for mental health disorders and landmine injuries during conflict pose similar limitations in postconflict settings. However, some unique circumstances, such as the potential for relapse into armed conflict, are more specific to a postconflict setting and need to be further studied. Interventions to promote and maintain peace during this period are critical. Peacekeeping efforts of the United Nations during this crucial period have contributed significantly to the decrease in the number of conflicts since the end of the Cold War.[32] These peacekeeping efforts have gone beyond monitoring ceasefires; they are often more akin to nation-building. Two-thirds of U.N. nation-building activities have been successful, with peace and democracy being the most important measures of success.[34] Public health professionals can help further evaluate the effect that U.N. peacekeeping efforts have had on reducing the health consequences of armed conflict.

One of the greatest challenges in postconflict settings is how to best reconstruct the infrastructure and health services that existed before the armed conflict.[5] Adequate function and capacity of water and sanitation systems, clinics, hospitals, and referral systems are necessary to prevent communicable and chronic diseases. In the past, reconstruction of infrastructure and reconstitution of disease-control programs have been emphasized much more than coordination of donor responses or the establishment of effective policy frameworks.[5] Public health research can help determine how best to reconstitute and implement health services programs and policies during this reconstruction phase. In addition to determining how best to reestablish infrastructure and health services, public health needs to continue to monitor new and existing interventions that address specific health problems, such as psychological trauma, especially because logistical constraints during this phase may decrease the effectiveness of prevention strategies.

Conclusion

Public health has, for many years, contributed significantly to understanding of the impact, the underlying causes, and ways to prevent infectious disease and malnutrition associated with armed conflict during the conflict and postconflict phases. More recently, it has contributed to understanding the impact of, and risk factors for, mental health problems and landmine/UXO injuries in conflict and postconflict phases, although much work remains to be done on these issues. Despite these important contributions, however, the capabilities of public health can be expanded in other areas. In particular, public health can make significant contributions to understanding the underlying causes of armed conflict so that effective prevention strategies can be developed to prevent armed conflict and its health consequences. Public health can also contribute to understanding how to better implement prevention strategies in all three phases of conflict, especially in countries with limited resources.

These objectives can be achieved only by bringing together various perspectives, expertise, and resources. The input of multiple scientific disciplines and multiple sectors of society is necessary to fully implement a public health approach to these challenges. We need to better understand human behavior; our social, political, and physical environments; and weapons systems. Public health can provide integrative leadership by bringing together various scientific disciplines, organizations, and communities to address the complex health issues of armed conflict.

Given the enormous health consequences of armed conflict, public health professionals should play a greater role in preventing it. The concepts discussed in this chapter outline areas in which public health can make greater contributions, not only to preventing health consequences after violence occurs, but also to preventing these health consequences by understanding and addressing the roots of armed conflict. Given that public health is defined as what we, as a society, do collectively to ensure the conditions in which people can be healthy, then preventing armed conflict should be one of its highest priorities.[35]

References

1. Krug EG, Dahlberg LL, Mercy JA, et al. (eds.) World Report on Violence and Health. Geneva: World Health Organization, 2002.

2. Mercy JA, Rosenberg ML, Powell KE, et al. Public health policy for preventing violence. Health Affairs 1993;12:7–29.
3. Carnegie Commission on Preventing Deadly Conflict. Preventing Deadly Conflict: Final Report. New York: Carnegie Corporation of New York, 1998.
4. Levy BS. Health and peace. Croat Med J 2002;43:114–116.
5. Zwi AB, Garfield R, Loretti A. Collective violence. In Krug EG, Dahlberg LL, Mercy JA, et al. (eds.). World Report on Violence and Health. Geneva: World Health Organization, 2002, pp. 213–239.
6. Klevens J, Anderson M. Rapid assessment procedures in injury control. Injury Control and Safety Promotion 2004;11:9–15.
7. World Health Organization. International Statistical Classification of Diseases and Related Health Problems, 10th Revision. Available at: http://www.who.int/classifications/icd/en/ (accessed June 22, 2007).
8. Burkholder BT, Toole MJ. Evolution of complex disasters. Lancet 1995;346: 1012–1015.
9. Varshney A. Ethnic Conflict and Civic Life: Hindus and Muslims in India. New Haven, CT: Yale University Press, 2002.
10. Regan PM, Henderson EA. Democracy, threats and political repression in developing countries: Are democracies internally less violent? Third World Q 2002;23:119–139.
11. Hegre H, Ellingsen T, Gates S, Gleditsch NP. Toward a democratic civil peace? Democracy, political change, and civil war, 1816–1992. Am Polit Sci Rev 2001;95:33–48.
12. Mercy JA. Assaultive violence and war. In Levy BS, Sidel VW (eds.). Social Injustice and Public Health. New York: Oxford University Press, 2006, pp. 294–317.
13. Centers for Disease Control and Prevention. Coordinating Office of Terrorism Preparedness and Emergency Response (COTPER): CDC Key Accomplishments. Atlanta, CDC, 2006.
14. Connolly MA, Gayer M, Ryan MJ, et al. Communicable diseases in complex emergencies: Impact and challenges. Lancet 2004;364:1974–1983.
15. Goma Epidemiology Group. Public health impact of Rwandan refugee crisis: What happened in Goma, Zaire, in July, 1994? Lancet 1995;345:339–344.
16. Salama P, Spiegel P, Talley L, Waldman R. Lessons learned from complex emergencies over past decade. Lancet 2004;364:1801–1813.
17. Mollica RF, Cardozo BL, Osofsky HJ, et al. Mental health in complex emergencies. Lancet 2004;364:2058–2067.
18. Bartlett LA, Jamieson DJ, Kahn T, et al. Maternal mortality among Afghan refugees in Pakistan, 1999–2000. Lancet 2002;359:643.
19. Young H, Borrel A, Holland D, Salama P. Public nutrition in complex emergencies. Lancet 2004;356:1899–1909.
20. Bilukha OO, Brennan M. Injuries and deaths caused by unexploded ordnance in Afghanistan: Review of surveillance data, 1997–2002. BMJ 2005;330:127–128.
21. Bilukha OO, Brennan M, Woodruff BA. Death and injury from landmines and unexploded ordnance in Afghanistan. JAMA 2003;290:650–653.
22. Thapa SB, Hauff E. Psychological distress among displaced persons during an armed conflict in Nepal. Soc Psychiatry Psychiatr Epidemiol 2005;40:672–679.
23. Mooren TT, de Jong K, Kleber RJ, Ruvic J. The efficacy of a mental health program in Bosnia-Herzegovina: Impact on coping and general health. J Clin Psychol 2003;59: 57–69.
24. Graham K, Mohammad N, Rehman H, et al. Insecticide-treated plastic tarpaulins for control of malaria vectors in refugee camps. Med Vet Entomol 2002;16:404–408.

25. Lopes Cardozo B, Bilukha OO, Gotway CA, et al. Mental health, social functioning, and disability in postwar Afghanistan. JAMA 2004;292:575–584.

26. Buse M. WWII ordnance still haunts Europe and the Asia Pacific rim. J Mine Action 2000;4:2.

27. Fiederlein SL. Managing Landmine Casualty Data: Designing and Developing the Data Structures and Models Necessary to Track and Manage Landmine Casualty Data. Harrisonburg, VA: Mine Action Information Center, 2001.

28. Ember CR, Ember M. War, socialization, and interpersonal violence: A cross-cultural study. J Conflict Resolution 1994;38:620–646.

29. Reza A, Mercy JA, Krug E. Epidemiology of violent deaths in the world. Injury Prevention 2001;7:104–111.

30. Meddings DR. Weapons injuries during and after periods of conflict: Retrospective analyses. BMJ 1997;315:1417–1419.

31. Ugalde A, Selva-Sutter E, Castillo C, et al. Conflict and health. The health costs of war: Can they be measured? Lessons from El Salvador. BMJ 2000;321:169–172.

32. Human Security Centre. Human Security Report: War and Peace in the 21st Century. New York: Oxford University Press, 2005.

33. Lopes Cardozo B, Kaiser R, Gotway CA, Agani F. Mental health, social functioning, and feelings of hatred and revenge of Kosovar Albanians one year after the war in Kosovo. J Traumatic Stress 2003;16:351–360.

34. Dobbins J, Jones SG, Crane K, et al. The UN's Role in Nation-Building: From the Congo to Iraq. Santa Monica, CA: RAND Corporation, 2005.

35. Institute of Medicine. The Future of Public Health. Washington, DC: National Academy of Sciences 1988.

21

International Law

Peter Weiss

Jus ad Bellum: Is This War Legal?

Speaking of "The Great War," Sigmund Freud, writing in 1915, said: "We are constrained to believe that never has any event been destructive of so much that is valuable in the commonwealth of humanity, nor so misleading to many of the clearest intelligence, nor so debasing to the highest that we know."[1] However, as a realist about the human psyche and an idealist about the future of humanity, he added: "One need not be a sentimentalist; one may perceive the biological and psychological necessity of suffering in the economics of human life, and yet condemn war both in its means and in its aims, and devoutly look forward to the cessation of all wars."[1]

This interplay between the perceived inevitability of war—whether rooted in human nature, economics, or power politics—and the paradoxical desire to arrive at a world without war has been one of the great persistent themes of human history. In Jonathan Swift's *Gulliver's Travels,* the Yahoos were a vile, belligerent tribe, in contrast to the rational Houyhnhnms, who could see no sense in war.[2] Even Immanuel Kant, the author of *Perpetual Peace,* admitted that, until there is a world state, war is inevitable.[3]

It was not until the end of the 19th century that the first attempt was made to enlist law in the search for perpetual peace. In 1899, Czar Nicholas II of Russia, then age 30, convened in The Hague an international peace conference with the object of ensuring to all peoples the benefit of a real and lasting peace. Neither this conference nor a second one held in 1907, also in The Hague, achieved this objective. These conferences did, however, lead to the creation of the Permanent Court of Arbitration, the international institution devoted to the peaceful settlement of international disputes. In addition, they produced the Hague Conventions on the Laws and Customs of War. Thus, although the project did not achieve its goal of permanent peace, it made war less painful.

The next attempt at eliminating war occurred in 1920 with the adoption of the Covenant of the League of Nations.[4] Conventional wisdom has it that, because of its failure to attract the membership of the United States and to stop Italy's invasion of Ethiopia in 1935 (not to mention World War II), the League was a colossal failure. Largely forgotten are its successes in peacefully settling several disputes that could have erupted into war, including those between Sweden and Finland in 1921 and between Greece and Bulgaria in 1925.

The Covenant contains many good and noble provisions, some of which foreshadowed the United Nations Charter. The first objective stated in the Covenant's preamble is "the acceptance of obligations not to resort to war."[4] The members of the League recognized that the maintenance of peace required reduction of national armaments to the lowest point "consistent with national safety and the enforcement by common action of international obligations" and agreed that the manufacture of munitions and implements of war by private enterprise was open to grave objections."[4] Any war or threat of war was declared to be a matter of concern to the whole League, and the League was mandated to "take any action that may be deemed wise and effectual to safeguard the peace of nations."[4] Resort to war by any member was to be deemed an act of war against all other members and would trigger economic and financial sanctions against the warring member. Several articles of the Covenant dealt with arbitral and judicial procedures designed to supplant war with peaceful settlement, but the use of armed forces "to protect the covenants of the League" was also envisaged.[4]

One final attempt was made to lay to rest "the dogs of war" before the start of World War II. In 1928, in Paris, 11 countries, including the United States, signed "A Treaty Providing for the Renunciation of War as an Instrument of National Policy," better known as the Kellogg-Briand Pact, named for Frank B. Kellogg, the U.S. Secretary of State, and Aristide Briand, the Foreign Minister of France. In language that sounds archaic today, it began with the following words[5]:

Deeply sensible of their solemn duty to promote the welfare of mankind;

Persuaded that the time has come when a frank renunciation of war as an instrument of national policy should be made to the end that the peaceful and friendly relations now existing between their peoples may be perpetuated;

Convinced that all changes in their relations with one another should be sought only by pacific means and be the result of a peaceful and orderly process, and that any signatory Power which shall hereafter seek to promote its national interests by resort to war should be denied the benefits furnished by this Treaty;

Hopeful that, encouraged by their example, all the other nations of the world will join in this humane endeavor and by adhering to the present Treaty as soon as it comes into force bring their peoples within the scope of its beneficent provisions, thus uniting the civilized nations of the world in a common renunciation of war as an instrument of their national policy; [the undersigned]

Have decided to conclude a Treaty.

In due course, 66 countries, including all of the major ones, acceded to the Pact. It came into force in 1929 and remains in force, but only as a reminder of a dim past when dreams of peace were not regarded as quixotic. Its operative part is short and to the point: In Article 1, the "The High Contracting Parties ... condemn recourse to war ... and renounce it as an instrument of national policy." In Article 2, they agree that any disputes between them, of whatever nature, shall never be resolved "except by pacific means." What is missing is a mechanism for enforcement of these exalted aims.

On June 26, 1945, less than 2 months after the end of the second "war to end all wars," the United Nations Charter was adopted in San Francisco. It entered into force for the United States as a binding treaty on October 24, 1945. The Charter, which is the closest thing we have to a constitution for the world, begins as follows[6]:

WE THE PEOPLES OF THE UNITED NATIONS DETERMINED

To save future generations from the scourge of war, which twice in our lifetime has brought untold sorrow to mankind.

Note that the opening words are not "we the nations" or "we the states" or "we the governments," but "we the peoples." Thus, "the peoples"—what we today call "civil society"—are made the owners of the Charter and are given the responsibility of saving it from its falsifiers, its detractors, and its destroyers. Consider also these other words which define the core purpose of the United Nations, as envisaged by its founders: To save, not ourselves, but selflessly "To save future generations." From what? From "the scourge of war." Nothing is said here about the glory of war, which has cluttered so many plazas with statues of saber-wielding men on horseback.

After reciting other purposes of the United Nations, including faith in fundamental human rights and respect for the obligations arising from treaties and other sources of international law, the Charter continues[6]:

AND FOR THESE ENDS...
To ensure, by the acceptance of principles and the institution of methods, that armed force shall not be used, save in the common interest.

This call to use armed force only in the common interest represents an obligation that is contrary to today's doctrine of national interest as the supreme value, trumping all others.

We come then to the cornerstone of the Charter's definition of that part of the laws of war called *jus ad bellum* by jurists—the law governing when armed force may be used[6]:

Article 2(4): All Members shall refrain in their international relations from the threat or use of force against the territorial integrity or political independence of any state, or in any other manner inconsistent with the Purposes of the United Nations.

Then, lest anyone think that the Charter was drafted by a group of pacifists, Chapter VII introduces a note of reality[6]:

Article 39: The Security Council shall determine the existence of any threat to the peace, breach of the peace, or act of aggression and shall make recommendations, or decide what measures shall be taken in accordance with Articles 41 and 42, to maintain or restore international peace and security....
Article 41: The Security Council may decide what measures not involving the use of armed force are to be employed to give effect to its decisions...
Article 42: Should the Security Council consider that measures provided for in Article 41 would be inadequate or have proved to be inadequate, it may take such action by air, sea, or land forces as may be necessary to maintain or restore international peace and security. Such action may include demonstrations, blockade, and other operations by land, sea or air forces of the United Nations.

These three articles describe the conditions under which the Security Council may authorize the use of armed force. The following article describes the condition under which member states, individually or collectively, may use armed force in self-defense[6]:

Article 51: Nothing in the present Charter shall impair the inherent right of individual or collective self-defense if an armed attack occurs against a Member of the United Nations, until the Security Council has taken measures to secure international peace and security. Measures taken by Members in the exercise of this right of self-defense shall be immediately reported to the Security Council and shall not in any way affect the authority and responsibility of the Security Council under the present Charter to take at any time such action as it deems necessary in order to maintain or restore international peace and security.

These articles constitute all of the conditions under which the use of armed force is permitted in current international law. Hence, the United States had to invent—and persuade some of its allies to adopt—the pernicious doctrine of "preventive war," which completely undermines the central purpose of the United Nations Charter.

There is some provision in international law for *preemptive,* as opposed to *preventive,* war. Preemptive war would be justified in a situation of imminent armed attack, such as (1) a nuclear-armed bomber has taken off for a city in another country but has not yet entered that country's air space; or (2) a large body of troops is massing on the border of another country and has given the country an ultimatum with a 24-hour deadline. Such situations would be so close to satisfying the armed-attack requirement of Article 51 that it would be unreasonable to insist on waiting until the armed attack occurred. These situations would also satisfy the classic definition of justifiable self-defense in international law, based on the Caroline Incident between the United States and the United Kingdom in 1841, which requires the necessity of self-defense to be "instant, overwhelming and leaving no choice of means, and no moment for deliberation." (The U.S. brig Caroline, which had lent some support to the Canadian rebellion, was cut adrift in 1837 by British troops on the U.S. side of the Niagara River, sending it over the falls and resulting in the death of two U.S. citizens. Delicate diplomatic negotiations between the United States and the United Kingdom ensued, resulting in recognition by the United Kingdom that the definition of self-defense formulated by U.S. Secretary of State Daniel Webster was correct and did not, in retrospect, justify the British attack.)[7]

There is a great difference, however, between (1) the use of armed force to prevent or counter an imminent attack and (2) invasion of or aerial attack on another country based on speculation about what that country might do in the distant future. The former would be preemptive and justified; the latter, preventive and illegal. Calling a preventive war "preemptive," as was done by the Bush administration in the case of the United States invasion of Iraq in 2003, changes nothing. Word play does not justify armed aggression.

Jus in Bello: Is This War Being Fought in Accordance with Law?

Having failed from the outset to reach agreement on the outlawing of war, the first Hague Peace Conference turned its attention to minimizing the brutality of war. (As one contemporary observer noted: "The Emperor of Russia might have said . . . , 'I labor for peace, but when I speak to them thereof, they make them ready for battle.' "[8]) The delegates to the Conference had a long tradition of restrictions on the brutality of war on which to base their principles, including the Book of Manu, the Bible, the Koran, and the writings of Greek and Roman philosophers, medieval Catholic scholars (the Second Lateran Council of 1139 prohibited the use of crossbows as "hateful to God and unfit for Christians") and Hugo Grotius in his magisterial work, *The Law of War and Peace,* written in 1622.[9]

The Geneva Conventions prescribe the rules of conduct of armies engaged in warfare. The Conventions arose from the work of Henri Dunant, a citizen of Geneva who, in 1859, witnessed the Battle of Solferino, in which thousands of wounded soldiers died without care; had sufficient medical services been available, they could have been saved.[10] Dunant's book, *Un Souvenir de Solferino,* proposed the establishment of relief societies in every country for the care of the wounded in time of war, under a uniform distinctive sign. Dunant founded the International Society of the Red Cross in Geneva in 1863, which led to the adoption, in 1864, of the first Geneva Convention: "The Convention for the Amelioration of the Condition of the Wounded in Armies in the Field." By 1900, 57 countries had acceded to the Convention.

In 1863, Francis Lieber, a law professor at Columbia University who had immigrated to the United States from Germany, drafted, and President Abraham Lincoln promulgated, "Instructions for the Government of Armies of the United States in the Field." This germinal document, which became known as the Lieber Code,[11] was the foundation for all subsequent codes of humanitarian law, including the Hague Conventions of 1899 and 1907 and the Geneva Conventions of 1906, 1929, and 1949. The Code contains within its 157 articles virtually all the basic principles governing *jus in bello,* including the following[11]:

1. Military oppression is not martial law: it is the abuse of the power which martial law confers.
2. The law of war disclaims all cruelty and bad faith; offenses shall be severely punished, and especially so if committed by officers.
3. Military necessity admits of all direct destruction of life or limb of *armed* enemies, and of other persons whose destruction is incidentally *unavoidable* [original emphasis], but military necessity does not admit of cruelty.
4. The United States acknowledges and protects, in hostile countries occupied by them, religion and morality; strictly private property; the people or inhabitants, especially women; and the sacredness of domestic relations. Offenses to the contrary shall be rigorously punished.
5. Civilized nations look with horror upon offers of reward for the assassination of enemies as relapses into barbarism.

In 1863, yet another significant event in the history of humanitarian law occurred: the invention, in Russia, of bullets that explode on contact with their targets, later known as "dum-dum bullets." In 1868, in the Declaration of St. Petersburg, such bullets became the first weapons to be outlawed by an international convention, thus beginning to add specificity to the moral generalizations of the Lieber Code.

In 1899, the "Convention with Respect to the Laws and Customs of War on Land," adopted at the Hague Peace Conference, became the first major international humanitarian law treaty. In 5 main articles and 60 articles contained in annexed regulations, it dealt with such diverse issues as the following:[12]

- The definition of belligerents
- Treatment of spies and prisoners of war
- Prohibition of poisoned weapons and arms or material "of a nature to cause superfluous injury"
- The obligation to issue a warning prior to commencing bombardment
- The duty to spare, "as far as possible," hospitals and buildings devoted to religion, art, science, and charity
- The administration of occupied territory.

The Second Hague Peace Conference of 1907 reaffirmed the 1899 Convention with very few changes, the most significant being a new article providing for compensation to be paid by belligerents for violations of the provisions of the regulations. Both conferences produced additional declarations dealing with specific subjects, including the prescient 1899 declaration prohibiting—but only for a period of 5 years—"the launching of projectiles and explosives from balloons and other new methods of similar nature." One wonders what modern warfare would be like had this declaration been widely accepted without a term limit of 5 years.

In 1938, the League of Nations unanimously adopted a resolution proposed by the Prime Minister of the United Kingdom, Neville Chamberlain, that stated that any aerial attack on legitimate military objectives "must be carried out in such a way that civilian populations in the neighborhood are not bombed through negligence."[10]

One of the most intriguing clauses of both the 1899 and 1907 conventions was the so-called Martens Clause, named after Professor Feodor de Martens, the legal advisor to the Czar of Russia. It provides:[10]

> Until a more complete code of the laws of war is issued, the high contracting parties think it right to declare that in cases not included in the Regulations adopted by them, populations and belligerents remain under the protection and empire of the principles of international law, as they result from the usages established between civilized nations, from the laws of humanity and the requirements of the public conscience.

Given the difficulty of defining precisely what is permitted and what is prohibited in the conduct of war, it is not surprising that the Martens Clause continues to survive, not only in the Hague conventions, but also in subsequent conventions. It leads, however, a shadow existence, passionately invoked by those who use it as a basis for asserting that certain new weapons are illegal and ignored by others (mostly government officials) who rely on the dubious maxim that whatever is not specifically prohibited is legal. For example, in the Nuclear Weapons Case before the International Court of Justice, a statement bearing more than a million signatures and alleging that such weapons are incompatible with "the public conscience" was submitted to the Court, while the Russian Federation argued that the Martens Clause had outlived its usefulness.

A third Hague Conference was to be held in 1914 to elaborate "a more complete code of the laws of war." But World War I prevented it from taking place. No major binding international instrument of humanitarian law was enacted until 1949, except for (1) the 1925 Geneva Protocol "for the prohibition of the use in war of asphyxiating, poisonous or other gases, and of bacteriological methods of warfare," and (2) two 1929 conventions, one dealing with the sick and wounded and the other with the treatment of prisoners of war. In 1949, on the initiative of the International Committee of the Red Cross (ICRC) and the government of Switzerland, representatives of 64 countries met in Geneva to adopt the following four conventions:[10]

- Geneva Convention for the Amelioration of the Condition of the Wounded and Sick in Armed Forces in the Field
- Geneva Convention for the Amelioration of the Condition of Wounded, Sick and Shipwrecked Members of Armed Forces at Sea
- Geneva Convention relative to the Treatment of Prisoners of War
- Geneva Convention relative to the Protection of Civilian Persons in Time of War.

The first three built on and expanded on previous treaties; the fourth was new.

Regarding the content of the third of these four conventions, the earlier prisoner of war convention, from 1929, stated that prisoners of war shall at all times be humanely treated and protected, particularly against acts of violence, insults, and public curiosity. The 1949 convention repeated this language but added that any unlawful act by a detaining power that causes death or serious injury to the health of a prisoner of war is prohibited, as is physical mutilation, medical or scientific experimentation, and intimidation. The 1929 convention stated that women shall be treated with all consideration due to their gender; the 1949 convention added that women shall benefit by treatment as favorable as that granted to men. The definition of prisoners of war in the 1949 convention made no reference to unlawful combatants; it provided, however, that, should any doubt arise as to the status of captured persons, they "shall enjoy the benefits of the present Convention until such time as their status has been determined by a competent tribunal."

Common to all four of the 1949 conventions was an article that stated that, in the case of armed conflict that was not international, persons not taking active part in the hostilities shall be protected against violence to life and person, cruel treatment, torture, humiliation, degrading treatment, and summary execution.

In 1977, two protocols were added to the 1949 Geneva Conventions relating to the protection of victims of international conflict (Protocol I) and non-international conflict (Protocol II). Protocol I further elaborated on the definition of combatants and stated that even a combatant not qualifying as a prisoner of war "shall, nevertheless, be given protections equivalent in all respects to those accorded to prisoners of war." The United States, while a party to all of the previous conventions, has never ratified these two protocols but has stated that, to the extent that the protocols codify customary law, it believes that it is bound by them.

In 1987, the Convention against Torture and other Cruel, Inhuman or Degrading Treatment entered into force. The United States has ratified it, but the Bush administration claims that neither this convention nor the International Convention on Civil and Political Rights, which also prohibits torture, apply outside the United States—a position vigorously denied by politically progressive academics (see Chapter 14).

Participation by health professionals in interrogating detainees has been strongly criticized. The American Medical Association and the American Psychological Association (APA) oppose this practice. But the APA allows its members to participate in interrogating "enemy combatants" if they do not knowingly plan, design, and assist in the use of torture or any form of cruel, inhuman, or degrading treatment or punishment.[12a]

Weapons of Mass Destruction

Weapons of mass destruction (WMDs) are commonly described as chemical, biological, and nuclear weapons (see Chapters 8, 9, and 10). This grouping ignores several important factors:

1. Nuclear weapons, some of which today represent a destructive potential 100 or more times greater than that of the bombs dropped on Hiroshima and Nagasaki, should be regarded differently from chemical and biological weapons.
2. The massive use of conventional weapons, as in the carpet bombing of cities during World War II and in the bombing of parts of Vietnam

during the Vietnam War, should be regarded as conventional weapons raised to the level of WMDs.
3. Some of today's conventional weapons approach the yield of small nuclear weapons.

Furthermore, the line between nuclear and conventional weapons is threatening to disappear in the strategic doctrines of nuclear weapons states. For example, the United States[13] and France[14] have threatened to use nuclear weapons in response to attacks by chemical or biological weapons. The irony of the classifying of chemical, biological, and nuclear weapons as WMDs is that, whereas chemical and biological weapons have been outlawed by treaty, the legal status of nuclear weapons remains a matter of dispute—a dispute primarily between those countries that possess nuclear weapons and those that do not.

The use, but not the possession, of chemical and biological weapons was first banned by the Geneva Protocol of 1925. The Biological Weapons Convention (BWC) of 1972 went further and bound states parties "never in any circumstances to develop, produce, stockpile or otherwise acquire or retain microbial or other biological agents, or toxins whatever their origin or method of production, of types and in quantities that have no justification for prophylactic, protective or other peaceful purposes" as well as weapons for their delivery.[15] The Chemical Weapons Convention, which entered into force in 1997, contains similar provisions with respect to chemical weapons. It also provides for an enforcement structure far superior to that of the BWC.[16]

Nuclear weapons were developed by the United States during World War II as a response to the fear that an atomic bomb program was being undertaken by Nazi Germany, but the presence of nuclear weapons continued long after the German program was abandoned. The countries that possessed nuclear weapons perceived them as being too valuable to take seriously their commitment to eliminate these weapons. In the Nuclear Non-Proliferation Treaty (NPT) of 1968, the five countries then possessing nuclear weapons—the United States, the United Kingdom, France, the Soviet Union and China—promised to negotiate in good faith for nuclear disarmament, in return for the pledge by virtually every other country to refrain from acquiring nuclear weapons.

In 1993, the World Health Organization (WHO), at the initiative of the International Physicians for the Prevention of Nuclear War (IPPNW) and other groups, requested an advisory opinion from the International Court of Justice (the World Court) concerning the legality under international law, including the WHO Constitution, of the use of nuclear weapons in war or other armed conflict. In 1994, the General Assembly of the United Nations, at the initiative of the World Court Project and the International Association of

Lawyers Against Nuclear Arms (IALANA), requested an opinion on a broader question: "Is the threat or use of nuclear weapons in any circumstance permitted under international law?" In 1995, the World Court held three weeks of hearings in which 45 countries participated in writing and/or orally. In addition, for the first time in the history of the World Court, millions of declarations from all over the world, collected by the World Court Project, were submitted to and accepted by the Court. These declarations stated that nuclear weapons do not meet the requirements of the public conscience and are therefore in violation of the Hague and Geneva Conventions. In 1996, the Court dismissed the WHO petition as being beyond its mandate. However, in response to the General Assembly petition it held, by a divided vote, that the use and threat of use of nuclear weapons is generally illegal under international law. The Court also stated unanimously that "There exists an obligation to pursue in good faith and bring to a conclusion negotiations leading to nuclear disarmament in all its aspects under strict and effective international control."[17]

The practice of the countries possessing nuclear weapons has made a mockery of the term "good faith." The original five countries and the three "latecomer" countries—Israel, India, and Pakistan, who are among the very few countries not party to the NPT—have shown no inclination to eliminate their nuclear arsenals. This failure of compliance is conclusively demonstrated by the authoritative, but unofficial, Commission on Weapons of Mass Destruction, which was presented to U.N. Secretary General Kofi Annan in June 2006.[18] At a conference in 2006, several civil-society organizations, on the 10th anniversary of the World Court opinion, discussed the possibility of returning to the Court for an opinion on how long the "good faith" obligation of the countries possessing nuclear weapons to pursue and bring to a conclusion negotiations for complete nuclear disarmament could be deferred.

The justification of countries possessing nuclear weapons for retaining them has always been that they are not for use, but rather for deterrence. However, the risk that nuclear weapons will be used is being increased by changes in national policies that would permit use of nuclear weapons in a greater variety of circumstances, including, for the United States, "in the event of surprising military developments."[19]

In addition, the alleged desire of "rogue states" to acquire nuclear weapons is becoming a prime rationale for so-called preemptive war, which is really preventive war. Today Iraq. Tomorrow Iran? And North Korea? And any country perceived as inimical by another country? In his commencement address at Johns Hopkins University in 2006, Mohammed El Baradei, the recipient of the 2005 Nobel Prize for Peace and Director General of the International Atomic Energy Agency, warned that "Nukes breed nukes."[20] He might have added that "nukes" also breed war.

References

1. Freud S. *Thoughts for the Times on War and Death* (Collected Papers IV). Reprinted in Britannica Great Books 1915;53:755.
2. Swift J. Gulliver's Travels. New York: Signet Classics, 1999.
3. Kant I. Perpetual Peace. New York: Cosimo Classics, 2005.
4. Covenant of the League of Nations. The Avalon Project. Available at: http://www.yale.edu/lawweb/avalon/leagcov.htm (accessed June 22, 2007).
5. The Kellogg-Briand Pact. Available at: http://www.yale.edu/lawweb/avalon/kbpact/kbpact.htm (accessed June 22, 2007).
6. United Nations Charter. Available at: http://www.un.org/aboutun/charter/ (accessed July 13, 2007).
7. History News Network. Would Daniel Webster approve of an attack on Iraq? Available at: http://www.hnn.us/articles/1024.html (accessed June 22, 2007).
8. Greenwood C. International humanitarian law. In The Centennial of the First International Peace Conference. The Hague: Kluwer Law International, 2000, p. 173.
9. Weiss P, Weston B, Falk R, Mendlovitz S. Draft memorial in support of the application by the World Health Organization for an advisory opinion by the International Court of Justice on the legality of the use of nuclear weapons. Transnat Law Contemp Prob 1994;4:739–750.
10. Schindler D, Toman J. The Laws of War. Dordrecht: Martinus Nijhoff Publishers, 1988.
11. Lieber Code. Available at: http://www.civilwarhome.com/liebercode.htm (accessed June 22, 2007).
12. The Avalon Project at Yale Law School. Available at: http://www/yale.edu/lawweb/avaolon/lawofwar/hague02.htm (accessed July 13, 2007).
12a. http://www.apa.org/governance/resolutions/councilres0807.html (accessed September 11, 2007).
13. Pentagon revises nuclear strike plan. The Washington Post, September 11, 2005.
14. Chirac: Nuclear response to terrorism is possible. The Washington Post, January 20, 2006.
15. Biological and Toxin Weapons Convention. Available at: http://www.opbw.org (accessed June 22, 2007).
16. Organization for the Prohibition of Chemical Weapons. Chemical Weapons Convention. Available at: http://www.opcw.org (accessed June 22, 2007).
17. International Court of Justice. Legality of the Threat or Use of Nuclear Weapons, General List No. 95 (Advisory Opinion of July 8, 1996). Available at: http://www.icj-cij.org/docket/files/95/7495.pdf#view=FitH&pagemode=none&search=%22 General List No. 95% 22 (accessed July 13, 2007).
18. Weapons of Mass Destruction Commission. Weapons of Terror: Freeing the World of Nuclear, Biological, and Chemical Arms, 2006. Available at: http://www.wmd commission.org (accessed July 13, 2007).
19. Classification Department of Defense 2001 Nuclear Posture Review. Cited in Nuclear Disorder or Cooperative Security. New York: Lawyers Committee on Nuclear Policy; Oakland, CA: Western States Legal Foundation; and New York: Reaching Critical Will of the Women's International League for Peace and Freedom, 2007.
20. "Nukes Breed Nukes," El Baradei Warns. CommonDreams.org Newscenter. Available at: http://www.commondreams.org/headlines06/0526–03.htm (accessed July 13, 2007).

22

The Roles of Humanitarian Assistance Organizations

Ronald J. Waldman

The provision of health services to people affected by complex emergencies is a combination of art and science that has changed considerably over the years. Until relatively recently, humanitarian assistance was characterized by the unregulated, uncoordinated efforts of individuals working for small voluntary organizations, usually clinicians caring for individual patients, motivated by a generosity of spirit and an irrepressible idealism. Over the past 25 years, a discipline of health care in conflict settings has emerged that is characterized by an evidence-based approach that adheres to the fundamental utilitarian principle that forms the basis of public health: To do the most good for the most people.

The epidemiology of complex emergencies began to be described in 1979, in the wake of the Cambodian genocide perpetrated by the murderous Pol Pot regime. Hundreds of thousands of Cambodians, out of a well-founded fear of persecution and death, fled to Thailand, where they were settled initially in the huge Sakeo and Khao-I-Dang "holding centers." (They were not granted refugee status.) There, a team of epidemiologists from the Centers for Disease Control and Prevention (CDC) monitored mortality over the early course of the relief effort (Figure 22-1).[1] The data helped to establish health program priorities and to successfully resolve a major health crisis.

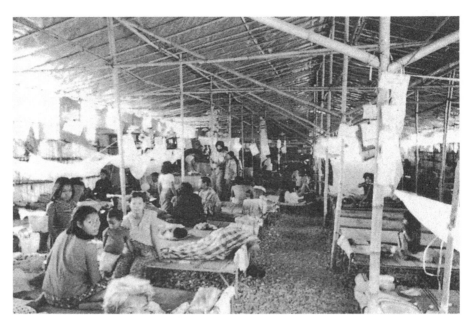

Figure 22-1. This pediatric ward operated by a nongovernmental organization at the Khao-I-Dang camp for Cambodians in Thailand and other health care facilities in the camp provided much useful epidemiological data that was used for disease prevention. (Photograph by Barry S. Levy.)

At about the same time, one of the first of a series of major movements of large populations was occurring on the Horn of Africa. More than 500,000 refugees fled a combination of political oppression and drought in the Ogaden Desert of Ethiopia, seeking shelter in more than 30 refugee camps in Somalia. As had been the case in Thailand, the capacity of the government to provide appropriate public health services was overwhelmed. Agreements were therefore established among the government, the Office of the United Nations High Commissioner for Refugees (UNHCR), and many nongovernmental humanitarian assistance organizations, mostly from Europe and North America, by which the organizations agreed to provide and manage health services in the refugee camps (see Chapter 13). The Ministry of Health established a Refugee Health Unit and prepared, with expatriate assistance, guidelines for refugee health services (including surveillance—ongoing systematic collection, analysis, and dissemination of basic health information), which provided data that were used to help prioritize and coordinate health programs.[2] Incidence rates of the major causes of morbidity and mortality were tracked. As the basic elements of surveillance, field epidemiology, and investigation began to be regularly practiced in subsequent emergency settings, patterns of disease occurrence began to emerge.

The collection and use of data by humanitarian assistance organizations in conflict settings is crucial to their ability to minimize what have been called the indirect consequences of war: the increase in the occurrence of problems of public health significance that results from a combination of a breakdown of the health infrastructure, greatly restricted access to remaining health services, and deterioration of living conditions with difficulty finding adequate food, water, sanitation facilities, and shelter.[3] Accurate measurement of all these parameters can provide information about the magnitude of the disaster affecting the civilian population that is essential to determining the specific level and nature of an appropriate response. The ability of humanitarian assistance organizations to appreciate the importance of measuring and monitoring the impact of their efforts to provide assistance to war-affected populations varies considerably. It is an area that remains underemphasized in many voluntary agencies.[4] Measures are being implemented to improve the situation.[5,6]

Figure 22-2, which depicts changes in mortality over time in four different refugee operations during the 1980s, illustrates the importance of monitoring trends during emergency situations. In three of these settings (Thailand, Somalia, and Sudan), mortality was initially at very high levels: between 10 and 25 deaths per 1,000 population per month. However, over the course of the

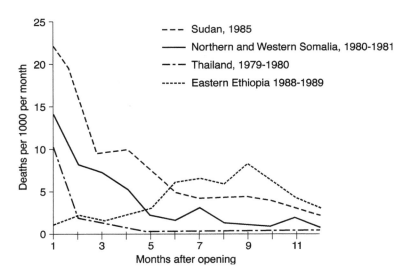

Figure 22-2. Crude mortality rates in selected refugee camps, 1979–1989. (Source: Centers for Disease Control and Prevention. Famine-affected, refugee, and displaced populations: Recommendations for public health issues. MMWR Morb Mort Wkly Rep 1992;41 [RR-13]:7.)

first year of the relief effort, at least partially due to work of the humanitarian assistance organizations, mortality declined precipitously. Although the fall in mortality rates was less dramatic in Somalia and Sudan than it had been among Cambodian refugees in Thailand, and although baseline levels had not been achieved by the end of the first year, the data indicate that all three of these relief operations should be considered at least qualified successes. However, in Hartisheik B camp in Eastern Ethiopia, where the recorded mortality was quite low at first, the rate at which people died *increased* for 9 consecutive months, which was remarkable because the population was entirely dependent on external relief. Careful and competent measurement and regular monitoring are required to prevent disasters like this, and humanitarian assistance organizations should be prepared to take on this role.

Another way in which humanitarian relief in conflict settings has changed concerns the environment in which humanitarian assistance organizations are called upon to provide assistance. Well-ordered refugee camps administered by international agencies, such as those in the Thailand and Somalia situations, have become the exception; they have been replaced by situations in which internally displaced persons are difficult to reach or beleaguered villagers face rampant violence and widespread human rights abuses in situations of gene-

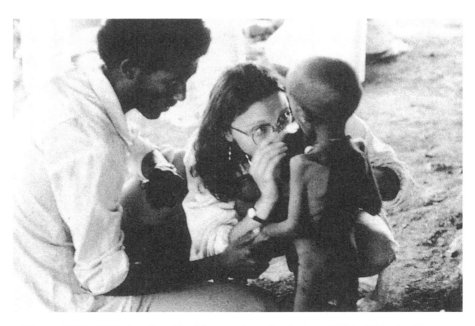

Figure 22-3. Médecins Sans Frontières worker attends to a child in Ethiopia. (Source: Médecins Sans Frontières.)

ralized insecurity. In these and similar situations, health care workers need to work with limited equipment and supplies (Figure 22-3).

Even in these settings, however, it is the breakdown of health services and the vicissitudes of the environment that contribute most to increased levels of morbidity and mortality. Violence, while common, is rarely the most important cause of death, with some exceptions; for example, in Bosnia and Kosovo,[7] during the Rwandan genocide, in Iraq (see Chapter 15),[8] and in Darfur (see Box 13-1 in Chapter 13), violence was reported to be the major contributor to elevated mortality.[9] In addition, violence that does not result in death, such as the rape of women, is a common feature of modern warfare[10,11] (see Chapter 12). In these cases, humanitarian assistance organizations should be strong advocates for international intervention, even military intervention if necessary, and many have developed programs devoted to the protection and security of vulnerable populations.

A watershed event in the modern history of humanitarian assistance occurred during and after the Rwandan genocide that took place in 1994.[12–15] The humanitarian community was helpless in preventing the deaths of more than 500,000 Rwandans but played a major role in the provision of relief to those who were able to flee. The population fled during the period of rampant violence and, to an even greater extent, after the Rwanda Patriotic Front (the Tutsi militia) was able to wrest control of the country from the Hutu leadership that had been responsible for the perpetration of the genocide. This takeover resulted in the sudden, massive exodus of up to 1 million people to hastily assembled refugee camps in Tanzania and to the north and south ends of Lake Kivu in the Democratic Republic of Congo (DRC, then Zaire).

In the camps near Goma, Zaire, the situation quickly got out of hand. Local officials were unable to provide for the many refugees, and the humanitarian assistance organizations—hundreds of which gathered on or near the site over the ensuing weeks—seemed similarly unprepared, unequipped, and unable to deal with what transpired. Of the estimated 500,000 refugees gathered in the area, almost 10 percent (up to 45,000 people) died during the first 4 weeks of the relief operation.[16]

Three aspects of this disaster merit further discussion. First, the determination of the number of deaths was more accurate than is usually the case. The volcanic soil of which the area was composed precluded the digging of graves, and the organizing relief authority—in this case the UNHCR—hired trucks to carry corpses off to sites where they were buried in mass graves.

Second, although bodies were counted, mortality rates could not be determined accurately because the population was never properly enumerated. Estimates of the number of people in the area ranged between 500,000 and 800,000, and the failure to know more precisely how many people required assistance hampered relief efforts considerably. This failure highlighted the need for humanitarian assistance organizations to pay more attention to and develop more effective techniques for determining population size. Best estimates suggested that mortality ranged from about 30 to 45 deaths per 10,000 per day over the first few weeks of the disaster.

Finally, and perhaps most tellingly, surveys revealed that the vast majority of deaths occurred beyond the reach of the international relief community. Almost all of the deaths during the first month of this emergency were caused by cholera, a disease for which treatment is readily available. Yet, of the 45,435 bodies collected by UNHCR, only 4,335 were reported by the humanitarian assistance organizations working in the health sector. Common practice at the time was for relief agencies, when arriving in an area, to establish health facilities, such as hospitals and outpatient clinics; to stock them with supplies and drugs; and to help those who were able to reach them. In large refugee camps or in areas where the local population feels too insecure to move around freely, this practice leads to limited access and low rates of utilization of the newly available services. Because of the documentation of experiences in Goma and similar disasters, humanitarian assistance organizations must make every effort to penetrate communities as rapidly and as deeply as possible, in order to determine and competently address the principal health needs of the population.

The failure of the relief effort in Goma led to several formal and informal reviews of the performance of humanitarian assistance organizations. The most comprehensive of these was an evaluation, funded by multiple donors, that sharply condemned the manner in which the situation had been handled and made a series of strong recommendations.[17] The most important consequence of the Goma experience for organizations that regularly engage in humanitarian assistance efforts in areas affected by conflict has been the Sphere Project, a series of declarations, guidelines, and training courses that were developed by more than 100 humanitarian assistance organizations in an effort to bring order, discipline, and professional performance standards to the field.[18]

The Sphere Project handbook focuses on two sets of issues that may be difficult for humanitarian agencies to address at the same time: (1) the protection of human rights and the desire to denounce those who violate them, and (2) the humanitarian imperative of providing assistance to those in need. Accordingly, a "Humanitarian Charter" was promulgated that calls upon all agencies to respect the right to life with dignity, the distinction between combatants and noncombatants, and the principle of non-refoulement.* These principles are central to the Sphere Project. Each is based on aspects of international humanitarian law, embodied in the Geneva Conventions of 1949

---

*Protection of refugees from being returned to places where their lives or freedoms could be threatened.

and their Additional Protocols of 1977. In addition, these principles draw heavily from a set of principles of humanitarian assistance that are not legally binding, the Code of Conduct for the International Red Cross and Crescent Movement and Non-Governmental Organizations in Disaster Relief.[18]

In addition, the Humanitarian Charter spells out roles and responsibilities of the humanitarian assistance organizations, recognizing that the primary obligation to provide for civilians affected by conflict lies with the state but also noting, realistically, that states are frequently unwilling, or unable, to fulfill that obligation. When this occurs, humanitarian assistance organizations, to the extent that they are capable, are frequently called upon to fill the gap. The Charter recognizes that intervention by humanitarian assistance organizations has, at times, had a harmful impact on those it sought to help; for example, intervention has sometimes made civilians more vulnerable to attack or provided goods and services that have allowed fighting factions to prolong conflict. The Charter calls on humanitarian assistance organizations to be more aware of all of the consequences of their well-intended actions, especially those that might backfire.[19–20]

Finally, at the heart of the Sphere Project is a series of minimum standards, and indicators of their achievement, which the humanitarian assistance organizations commit themselves to strive to achieve. Following a set of elements common to all of the technical areas addressed, standards are presented in the areas of water and sanitation; food security, nutrition, and food aid; shelter, settlement, and nonfood items; and health services. Through a series of consultations held around the world that brought together knowledgeable individuals from hundreds of humanitarian assistance organizations, technical experts, and those concerned with field-level operations, the Sphere Project was able to assemble, in one compendium, what exists of the "science" of humanitarian assistance. However, its fundamental assertion is that, important as it is to know the minimum amount of water to provide to every individual receiving assistance (15 liters per day) or how much space should be provided when building temporary settlements (45 m^2 per person), the provision of assistance at these levels is not simply a generous act by those donors who provide funding or those humanitarian assistance organizations who implement programs but also a legal right of those affected. The standards it establishes and the indicators it codifies exist, according to the Sphere Project, to support a rights-based approach to humanitarian assistance.

In essence, then, the standards and their accompanying indicators are a partial quantification of the principles enunciated by the Humanitarian Charter, especially of what it means to assist an individual or a population to be able to live "a life with dignity." Very few of the standards and indicators delineated in the Sphere Project are original. Most are drawn from previous descriptions of the epidemiology of complex emergencies or previously established guidelines, whether published widely or contained in the "gray literature" (operations manuals and other internal publications of the donor agencies, United Nations organizations, or humanitarian assistance organizations).

The Sphere Project recognizes that it addresses only part of the overall scope of humanitarian assistance. Standards for education, for example, are not presented; neither are recommendations regarding the physical protection of those affected by conflict. Similarly, it explicitly recognizes that humanitarian assistance organizations are frequently constrained by external factors, such as insecurity and, importantly, funding levels,[21] which they cannot control. Nevertheless, in those areas that the Sphere Project addresses, the standards that it has established are considered by most donors and humanitarian assistance organizations to be those that define the contemporary objectives of humanitarian assistance.

The first general health standard to which humanitarian assistance organizations are asked to adhere is to provide access to all conflict-affected individuals to a prioritized set of health services—those that address the major causes of mortality and morbidity.[22] A principal indicator of whether this standard is attained is a reduction of both the overall crude mortality rate and the mortality rate of children younger than 5 years of age to less than double the rates that prevailed before the emergency

The second general health standard calls for health services to be delivered in a manner that supports existing health systems in the area, including their facilities and personnel. It anticipates that the need for emergency relief will be relatively short in duration. It calls on humanitarian assistance organizations to facilitate the transition from relief to renewed development. Wherever local authorities are available and capable, they should be in leadership positions and external relief agencies should provide support to them. Wherever national guidelines exist for the treatment of priority conditions, they should prevail (assuming that they are technically sound). External structures staffed by foreign experts, such as temporary field hospitals, should be erected and used only when the magnitude of the problem exceeds the ability of the local system to cope (an all-too-frequent occurrence). Other standards relating to local health systems are written in the same vein, stressing organizational and technical coordination.

Finally, the Sphere Project emphasizes the importance of collecting, analyzing, and disseminating appropriate data and using those data for (1) continuously reassessing priorities, and (2) designing, monitoring, and evaluating relief interventions.

Another set of standards deals with the control of communicable diseases.[3,23,24] An early public health intervention in emergencies, including those involving armed conflict, should be mass vaccination of all children against measles. Emphasis is also given to prevention and treatment of diarrhea, pneumonia, and malaria, which are also common leading causes of morbidity and mortality in many emergency relief operations.

Given that humanitarian assistance organizations may be in an area for only a relatively short period, their role in initiating treatment for more chronic communicable diseases has been somewhat controversial. Specifically, before initiating programs for the management of tuberculosis and HIV/AIDS, for which interruption of treatment, once begun, can have disastrous long-term consequences, relief agencies should proceed with due deliberation. For both of these diseases, relief agencies should ensure that they (1) will be in the area and capable of operating effective intervention programs for a minimum of 12 months; (2) will be reasonably assured of effective access to patients begun on treatment for at least the same period of time; and (3) have funding for both pharmaceuticals and operations before initiating programs.[25] Because of the possibility, especially in unstable areas, that personnel of nongovernmental organizations may have to be evacuated or that patients may be suddenly displaced, agencies might consider providing patients who are being treated for tuberculosis or HIV/AIDS (with antiretroviral drugs) with at least a 30-day reserve supply of medications.

Noncommunicable chronic conditions, some of which are also addressed by the Sphere Project, may require more specialized care. The trauma of war—involving at best the near-total disruption of normal life and, at worst, the loss of livelihood, home, and loved ones—is an experience that leaves many with stress-related conditions that require assistance. Although a minority of those affected require psychotropic medication, the provision of other psychosocial services by trained experts, from nurses to social workers, is often an important role for humanitarian assistance organizations.

These organizations need to address the physical protection of those to whom they are providing assistance. In recent years, there have been repeated occurrences of ethnic cleansing (such as in the former Yugoslavia), genocide (Rwanda and Darfur), and wanton violence (such as in East Timor and the DRC) that have had serious and widespread physical threats to the lives of civilians. Increasingly, countries have been unable or unwilling to provide adequate protection to their residents, and humanitarian assistance organizations have been called upon to do so. It is reasonable to consider as the fundamental interventions of humanitarian assistance the protection of vulnerable populations from widespread human rights abuses and the provision of a secure environment. Without these interventions, the provision of other services would be ineffectual or impossible. Guidelines can help humanitarian assistance organizations implement protection and security programs.[26–28]

Women are especially vulnerable during armed conflicts (see Chapter 12). Cultural inequalities and the unfair exercise of power that occurs when resources are scarce frequently result in less access for women than for men to food, water, shelter, and health services. Unless humanitarian assistance organizations pay particular attention to their situation, women are likely to suffer worse health outcomes than men. Humanitarian assistance organizations should be careful to design programs in a gender-balanced manner and to carefully monitor access to and use of health services by and for women. The provision of reproductive health programs should be made a high, early priority.[29] Although there may be a tendency to minimize data collection and reporting requirements, all health sector–related data should be disaggregated by gender, and appropriate gender-specific analyses should be performed in order to report with basic principles of fairness and equity.

Gender-based violence occurs frequently in emergency situations, especially when societies are affected by armed conflict. The specific kinds of violence directed toward women range from sexual exploitation to forced prostitution and rape. Humanitarian assistance organizations should carefully coordinate their reporting and their interventions aimed at preventing and mitigating the consequences of gender-based violence. The likelihood of violence against women should be considered in all aspects of a relief operation, including planning of temporary settlements, siting of water points and latrines, times and places of food and commodity distribution, and content of health programs. Procedures for reporting and management of sexual abuses should consider cultural and individual sensitivities. Legal and other disciplinary measures for perpetrators of gender-based violence should be implemented.[30]

Most emergency relief operations represent, at best, the equivalent of public health first aid. The leading cause of morbidity and mortality in war settings may be neither direct violence nor commonly occurring diseases, but rather the setting itself. A recent survey in the DRC attributed large differentials in mortality simply to the existence of violence in a health service area[31] (see Chapter 17). In health zones reporting violence, the crude mortality rate was 3.0 per 1,000 population per month, whereas in those not reporting violence, it was 1.7 per 1,000 per month. Similarly, the mortality rate for children younger than 5 years of age in the zones reporting violence was 6.4 per 1,000 per month, compared with 3.1 per 1,000 per month in the zones not reporting violence.

Addressing the armed conflict that is the root cause of excess preventable mortality would have a large impact on the health status of the affected civilian population. Humanitarian assistance organizations may be able to exert some influence simply by being witnesses and reporters to appropriate authorities of violence and atrocities. They can be strong and forceful advocates on behalf of the civilian populations with which they live and to which they provide humanitarian assistance. But humanitarian assistance organizations that are organized to provide health services aimed at mitigating the consequences of conflict have only played a small role in bringing about a resolution to conflict. The prevention and resolution of war remain largely in the domain of diplomats, politicians, and armed forces. Until those working in these areas do their jobs competently and successfully to bring about a cessation to hostilities, the health of affected civilians is likely to remain perilous. The waging of war and the practice of public health are, to a large degree, incompatible pursuits.[32]

References

1. Glass RI, Cates W Jr, Nieburg P, et al. Rapid assessment of health status and preventive-medicine needs of newly arrived Kampuchean refugees, Sa Kaeo, Thailand. Lancet 1980;1:868–872.
2. Follow-up on refugees—Somalia. MMWR Morb Mortal Wkly Rep 1981;30:85–88.
3. Toole MJ, Waldman RJ, Zwi A. Complex emergencies. In Merson MH, Black RE, Mills AJ (eds.). International Public Health: Diseases, Programs, Systems, and Policies, 2nd ed. Sudbury, MA: Jones and Bartlett Publishers, 2006, pp. 445–511.
4. Boss LP, Toole MJ, Yip R. Assessments of mortality, morbidity, and nutritional status in Somalia during the 1991–1992 famine. JAMA 1994;272:371–376.
5. Checchi F, Roberts L. Interpreting and using mortality data in humanitarian emergencies: A primer for non-epidemiologists. (HPN Network Paper 52.) London: Overseas Development Institute, 2005.
6. Spiegel PB, Salama P, Maloney S, van der Veen A. Quality of malnutrition assessment surveys conducted during famine in Ethiopia. JAMA 2004;292:613–618.
7. Spiegel PB, Salama P. War and mortality in Kosovo, 1998–99: An epidemiological testimony. Lancet 2000;355:2204–2209.
8. Roberts L, Lafta R, Garfield R, et al. Mortality before and after the 2003 invasion of Iraq: Cluster sample survey. Lancet 2004;364:1857–1864.
9. Depoortere E, Checchi F, Broillet F, et al. Violence and mortality in West Darfur, Sudan (2003–2004): Epidemiological evidence from four surveys. Lancet 2004;364: 1315–1320.
10. Hynes M, Robertson K, Ward J, Crouse C. A determination of the prevalence of gender-based violence among conflict-affected populations in East Timor. Disasters 2004;28:294–321.
11. Our Bodies, Their Battle Ground: Gender-Based Violence in Conflict Zones. IRIN Web special. September 2004. Available at: http://www.irinnews.org/IndepthMain .aspx?IndepthId=20&ReportId=62814 (accessed July 10, 2007).
12. Uvin P. Aiding Violence: The Development Enterprise in Rwanda. West Hartford, CT: Kumarian Press, 1998.
13. Power S. Bystanders to genocide. Atlantic Monthly, September 2001.
14. Gourevitch P. We Wish to Inform You That Tomorrow We Will Be Killed with Our Families. New York: Picador USA, 1998.
15. Courtemanche G. A Sunday by the Pool in Kigali. Canada: Vintage, 2004.
16. Goma Epidemiology Group. Public health impact of Rwandan refugee crisis: What happened in Goma, Zaire, in July, 1994? Lancet 1995;345:339–344.
17. Steering Committee of the Joint Evaluation of Emergency Assistance to Rwanda. The International Response to Conflict and Genocide: Lessons from the Rwanda Experience. Synthesis Report. Odense, Denmark, 1996.

18. Sphere Project. Humanitarian Charter and Minimum Standards in Disaster Response, 2nd ed. Geneva: The Sphere Project, 2004.
19. Terry F. Condemned to Repeat? The Paradox of Humanitarian Action. Ithaca, NY: Cornell University Press, 2002.
20. Anderson M. Do No Harm: How Aid Can Support Peace—or War. Boulder, CO: Lynne Rienne Publishers, 1999.
21. Salama P, Laurence B, Nolan ML. Health and human rights in contemporary humanitarian crises: Is Kosovo more important than Sierra Leone? BMJ 1999;319:1569–1571.
22. Waldman RJ. Prioritising health care in complex emergencies. Lancet 2001;357:1427.
23. Médecins Sans Frontières. Refugee Health: An Approach to Emergency Situations. London: MacMillan, 1997.
24. Connolly MA, Gayer M, Ryan M. Communicable diseases in complex emergencies. Lancet 2004;364:1974–1983.
25. World Health Organization. Tuberculosis Control in Refugee Situations—An Interagency Field Manual. Geneva: WHO, 1997.
26. Protecting Refugees: A Field Guide for NGOs. Geneva: UNHCR, 1999.
27. International Committee of the Red Cross. Strengthening Protection in War: A Search for Professional Standards. Geneva: ICRC, 2001.
28. Slim H, Bonwick W. Protection: An ALNAP Guide for Humanitarian Agencies. London: ALNAP and the Overseas Development Institute, 2006.
29. United Nations High Commissioner for Refugees. An Inter-agency Field Manual for Reproductive Health in Refugee Situations. Geneva: UNHCR, 1999.
30. United Nations High Commissioner for Refugees. Sexual and Gender-based Violence against Refugees, Returnees and Internally Displaced Persons: Guidelines for Prevention and Response. Geneva: UNHCR, 2003.
31. Coghlan B, Brennan RJ, Ngoy P. Mortality in Democratic Republic of Congo: A nation-wide survey. Lancet 2006;367:44–51.
32. Toole MJ, Galson S, Brady W. Are war and public health compatible? Lancet 1993; 341:1193–1196.

23

The Roles of Nongovernmental Organizations

John Loretz

Nongovernmental organizations (NGOs), which are increasingly being called "civil-society organizations," focus on war from a medical and public health perspective in a variety of ways:

- They intervene to mitigate the consequences of armed conflict (see Chapter 22).
- They research the effects of war.
- They educate the public and decision makers about the impact of war on health and the environment.
- They advocate for changes in global attitudes and policies toward war and the most dangerous weapons and practices of war.

This chapter illustrates the research, education, advocacy, and victim assistance functions that some NGOs and their supporters have performed in order to demonstrate the connections between the public health dimensions of war and appropriate policy goals (Figures 23-1 and 23-2).

The Red Cross, founded in the 1860s, was the first NGO to be based on a framework of neutrality—adopted subsequently by many others—that emphasizes (1) medical access to both sides of a conflict; (2) rights to cross over lines of confrontation without harm and without payment to import

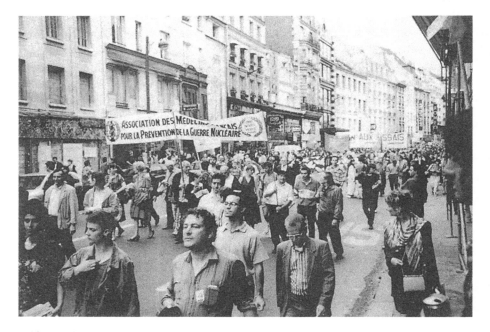

Figure 23-1. Members of International Physicians for the Prevention of Nuclear War (IPPNW) march in Paris in 1995 to protest French nuclear testing. (Source: Dr. Jacques Mongnet and Dr. Abraham Behar, IPPNW/France.)

supplies and equipment that are necessary for sustaining life and to distribute them only on the basis of need; and (3) guarantees of protection from aggression while carrying out its work. In addition to providing humanitarian assistance in the midst of armed conflict, hundreds of NGOs worldwide today play many other active roles, ranging from education to advocacy.

Mitigating the Effects of War

Medical and public health NGOs have frequently intervened during armed conflicts to treat the victims and to protect the rights of civilian populations under international law. A brief, but incomplete, survey of some of the more prominent groups, with examples of their work, follows.

Médecins Sans Frontières

Médecins Sans Frontières (MSF), also known as Doctors Without Borders, was founded in 1971 by a group of French physicians. From its Geneva

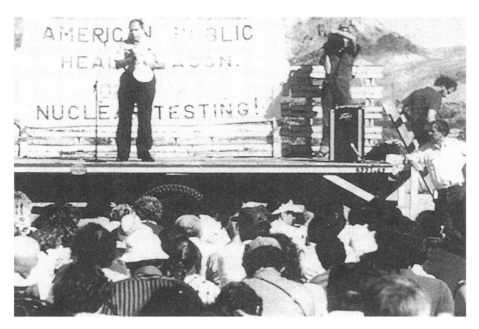

Figure 23-2. Members of the American Public Health Association demonstrate at a nuclear weapons underground test site in Nevada in 1986. (Reprinted with permission from the American Public Health Association.)

headquarters and 19 national sections, MSF organizes thousands of volunteer physicians, nurses, and other health workers to provide humanitarian aid in war-torn countries. Largely funded by private donations, with some governmental and corporate support, MSF has an annual budget of approximately US$400 million.[1]

Physicians, nurses, and paramedics in MSF have set up field hospitals, trauma centers, feeding centers, and other treatment facilities within war zones in Central America, Africa, Asia, and elsewhere. Like their counterparts at the International Committee of the Red Cross (ICRC) and United Nations relief agencies, MSF operates under strict principles of medical neutrality. Unlike the ICRC and United Nations relief agencies, however, some MSF chapters have occasionally criticized governments and military authorities in public for allegedly violating the Geneva Conventions, failing to protect medical personnel while they are treating victims of war, and using or permitting the use of weapons such as landmines, cluster bombs, and fragmenting bullets.

MSF teams have, for example, treated rape victims in the Democratic Republic of Congo (DRC); operated a district hospital in Nepal; provided medical and psychological care to Palestinians in the West Bank and Gaza

Strip; and opened and maintained primary health care centers in Somalia. A willingness to risk their own lives in order to help endangered populations, which was a factor in the awarding of the Nobel Peace Prize to MSF in 1999, has gone hand in hand with a refusal to be co-opted or to have its mission undermined by abusive governments. In 2001, for example, the French section of MSF (MSF France) established malaria treatment programs in Myanmar (Burma), primarily in areas where poor access to health care due to the armed conflict between government and rebel forces was resulting in large numbers of malaria deaths. After 4 years of frustration over travel restrictions imposed by Burmese authorities, MSF France withdrew from Myanmar, declaring that "the Burmese authorities do not want anyone to witness the abuses they are committing against their own population."[2]

MSF made Darfur a priority in 2005, treating rape victims, injured civilians, and more than 50,000 children suffering from malnutrition. In 2006, MSF sent 27 international volunteers to support almost 600 Sudanese health workers and increased its budget for programs in Darfur by 20 percent, to $4.5 million.

Physicians for Human Rights

Physicians for Human Rights (PHR), founded in 1987 by U.S. physicians and others and based in Cambridge, Massachusetts, has focused on war-related abuses of fundamental human rights. PHR has sent forensic investigators into war zones to uncover evidence of atrocities, pinpoint responsibility, and demand accountability to international humanitarian law and the Universal Declaration of Human Rights. PHR publicizes the results of its investigations and condemns governments and military forces that commit or tolerate atrocities.

Over two decades, PHR has documented (1) the use of chemical weapons by Iraq against Kurdish villagers, human rights abuses resulting from the Persian Gulf War, and sanctions on Iraq to import food and medicine; (2) the use of rape as a weapon of war in Liberia; (3) the devastating medical and social consequences of the civil war in Somalia; and (4) wartime attacks on hospitals and patients in the former Yugoslavia. PHR investigators have uncovered mass graves in Croatia, Bosnia, Rwanda, and Iraq, setting the stage for charges of genocide and other war crimes that have been brought before the international war crimes tribunals.

PHR was one of the first NGOs to call for a ban on landmines. In 1991, it was one of six founding organizations of the International Campaign to Ban Landmines (ICBL), which, in 1997, received the Nobel Peace Prize. In 2005, PHR produced evidence that U.S. interrogators at Guantanamo Bay and in Afghanistan and Iraq had engaged in systematic psychological torture of detainees.[3]

Like MSF, PHR has committed substantial organizational resources to addressing the human tragedy of the genocidal armed conflict in Sudan. Between May 2004 and July 2005, PHR representatives went to the region three times, compiling irrefutable evidence that the Sudanese government and its proxy militia had engaged in a "scorched-earth" campaign designed not only to kill the non-Arab people of Darfur but also to destroy their way of life. Invoking the Genocide Convention, PHR called for the establishment of a Compensation Commission "to redress the rights of the Darfurian victims."[4] (See Box 13-1 in Chapter 13.)

International Medical Corps

The International Medical Corps (IMC) is a humanitarian NGO established by a group of U.S. physicians and nurses in 1984. It has provided primary health care, mental health care, nutritional services, and emergency relief and has engaged in health care training and capacity-building activities in more than 40 countries affected by war, poverty, and disaster.

As one of several NGOs providing emergency health services to internally displaced persons in Darfur, IMC has operated primary health care centers and mobile clinics and has undertaken studies of the health needs of internally displaced women. A grant of more than $500,000 from the Bill and Melinda Gates Foundation in 2005 enabled IMC to establish and operate similar health care services in eastern Chad, which has seen large influxes of Sudanese refugees, compounding the effects of war-related suffering on both displaced and host populations.

In the DRC, where entrenched armed conflict between government forces and rebel militias has devastated the country's health infrastructure, IMC has sent volunteers into Katanga Province to establish therapeutic feeding centers, immunization programs, and water and sanitation systems and to address problems of gender-based violence in camps for internally displaced persons. Working with local NGOs, it has developed programs to help former child soldiers re-enter civil society.

CARE

One of the world's largest humanitarian relief organizations, CARE was founded in 1945 to provide relief after World War II and has continued to deliver emergency aid to survivors of war as part of its mission to alleviate global poverty. Emergency relief efforts are complemented by post-conflict rehabilitation and capacity-building programs that often focus on basic infrastructure for health, nutrition, and sanitation.

In both southern and eastern Chad, for example, CARE has supported tens of thousands of refugees from conflicts in the Central African Republic and

Sudan. By closely observing and evaluating changing conditions in refugee camps and among other war-affected populations, CARE has frequently been able to alert the international community to impending armed violence or an intensification of ongoing conflicts. The arrival of almost 3,500 people within 3 months at the Dadaab refugee camp in Kenya, for example, led CARE to warn, in June 2006, that the conflict in Somalia was causing growing instability in both Kenya and Chad. The influx of new refugees, CARE noted, consisted mostly of women and children but also included young men fleeing forced conscription.

Sometimes the disaster relief and war-related activities of NGOs converge. After the 2004 tsunami, which killed more than 30,000 Sri Lankans, CARE noted an escalation in violence between the government and the Liberation Tigers of Tamil Eelam (LTTE), which not only made its relief efforts in the country more difficult but also led to killings and abductions of humanitarian workers as well as civilians. (See Chapter 26.)

Oxfam

Although Oxfam International (Oxfam) now focuses mainly on systemic causes of human suffering, primarily poverty and economic and social injustice, its historical roots can be traced back to 1942, when the British-based Oxford Committee for Famine Relief campaigned for grain shipments to be sent to German-occupied Greece. That concern for the civilian victims of war has found contemporary expression in an emphasis on "protection of the most vulnerable people, particularly women and children in conflict situations."[5]

A confederation of 12 national Oxfam organizations (rather than a single organization), Oxfam International works at the community level on issues such as trade, conflict, and debt. In 2003, Oxfam joined with Amnesty International and the International Action Network on Small Arms (IANSA) to launch a global "control arms" campaign to slow the proliferation of small arms and light weapons and to lobby for an international arms trade treaty.

Save the Children

Save the Children is a global federation of 27 organizations that operate in more than 100 countries, some of which are entrenched in armed conflicts or have just emerged from civil wars. As a contribution to the Millennium Development Goals, it has launched a global campaign to provide education for 8 million war-affected children. In addition to working with ministries of education in Afghanistan, Angola, the DRC, Nepal, Sudan, and Uganda to improve basic curricula, establish functioning classrooms, and guarantee access to primary education for girls and vulnerable children, Save the Children promotes the concept of schools as "zones of peace," reintegrating demobilized child soldiers into society and preventing new instances of forced recruitment.

International Physicians for the Prevention of Nuclear War

The International Physicians for the Prevention of Nuclear War (IPPNW) was founded in 1980 to educate leaders of the United States and the Soviet Union about the medical consequences of nuclear war, and to inform the public and policymakers that health care workers would be helpless to respond to the unimaginable catastrophe of a nuclear war between the Cold War superpowers—a mission for which the organization was awarded the Nobel Peace Prize in 1985.

IPPNW now comprises medical groups in approximately 60 countries that address the public health dimensions of all aspects of armed conflict. Each IPPNW affiliate is an autonomous NGO, setting its own national priorities and developing its own programs consistent with the overall goals of the federation. Affiliates range in size from relatively few active members, in countries such as Kenya or Spain, to several thousand members in the United States and Germany, with varying budgets and varying fundraising activities. Although grants account for a small portion of its funding at the international level, most of the core budget of IPPNW is raised from appeals to individual donors, primarily in the United States. Although the abolition of nuclear weapons remains the federation's top priority in the post–Cold War world, IPPNW expanded its mission in the 1990s to include the prevention of all war.

Eliminating Nuclear Weapons

Preventing nuclear war—the almost unimaginable extreme on the continuum of armed violence—requires the elimination of nuclear weapons from arsenals worldwide. The call for nuclear abolition that has been adopted by thousands of peace and disarmament NGOs[6] is morally analogous to the calls for the abolition of slavery and torture and medically analogous to the campaigns to eradicate smallpox, polio, and HIV/AIDS.

NGO campaigns for nuclear disarmament can be traced back to the 1955 Russell–Einstein Manifesto[7] and the beginnings of the Pugwash Movement. The public understanding of the nature of nuclear weapons began a few years later. In 1962, a groundbreaking collection of research studies on the medical effects of nuclear war was published by the Physicians for Social Responsibility (PSR) Study Group.[8,9] At about the same time, a campaign for a nuclear test ban began, led by the National Committee for a Sane Nuclear

Policy (SANE) and by pediatrician Benjamin Spock, based on evidence that strontium-90 from atmospheric testing fallout was present in the deciduous teeth of children[10] and that iodine-131 was concentrated in the thyroid gland after ingestion of milk from cows that had grazed in fields where the radio-isotope was deposited.

With the founding of IPPNW in 1980 by U.S. and Soviet physicians, knowledge about the burn, blast, and radiation injuries of nuclear weapons became a cornerstone of global nuclear disarmament campaigning, informing civil-society arguments in favor of the Comprehensive Test Ban Treaty, the Nuclear Weapons Freeze, and, more recently, a Nuclear Weapons Convention. The 1985 Nobel Peace Prize given to IPPNW lent additional authority to projects throughout the 1980s and the 1990s that documented the health and environmental effects of the production, testing, and use of nuclear weapons.[11,12]

As the Cold War ended in the early 1990s and the public perceived that the nuclear threat appeared to diminish, the task of advocating for the abolition of nuclear weapons became more difficult. IPPNW organized the International Citizens' Congress for a Nuclear Test Ban in Kazakhstan in 1990, an event that helped convince Russian officials to close the principal Soviet nuclear test site at Semipalatinsk in 1991. IPPNW joined with the International Association of Lawyers Against Nuclear Arms (IALANA) and the International Peace Bureau in 1994 to seek an advisory opinion from the International Court of Justice on the legality of nuclear weapons. The medical brief submitted to the Court helped persuade it to make its historic 1996 advisory opinion[13] that the use—and even the threatened use—of nuclear weapons was illegal under the norms of international humanitarian law. Following this opinion, IPPNW helped draft the Model Nuclear Weapons Convention.[14] When India and Pakistan tested nuclear weapons in 1998 and subsequently declared themselves to be nuclear weapons states, IPPNW published a report documenting the effects of a regional nuclear war in South Asia.[15] Toward the end of the 1990s, as fears of nuclear terrorism began to enter public consciousness, IPPNW produced an early assessment of the effects of "crude" nuclear weapons that might be acquired by non-state actors, repeating the call for abolition as the only permanent means of preventing a nuclear catastrophe.[16] After September 11, 2001, IPPNW and other NGOs emphasized concern over the proliferation of fissile materials and the possibility that commercial nuclear power plants could become terrorist targets.[17]

As a response to the failure of the 2005 Nuclear Non-Proliferation Treaty (NPT) Review Conference and the apparent inability of the United Nations First Committee to make any progress toward nuclear disarmament, IPPNW launched at its 2006 World Congress in Helsinki, the International Campaign to Abolish Nuclear Weapons (ICAN). The goals of ICAN are to create public outrage about the continued presence of nuclear weapons and to advocate for a convention that would prohibit the possession of nuclear weapons (see Chapter 10).

Documenting the Consequences of War

Before the U.S. invasion of Iraq in March 2003, hundreds of NGOs and other civil-society groups in much of the world helped to inform millions of people about the situation and questioned the need for war. Much collection and analysis of data after the Persian Gulf War had been performed by researchers at universities, NGOs, and United Nations agencies. With war looming again in 2002, a new Canadian-led team of experts backed by more than 20 NGOs returned to Iraq to assess the likely consequences of war on an already vulnerable civilian population. They warned that war in Iraq could lead to hundreds of thousands of children's deaths.[18] A parallel fact-finding mission by the Center for Economic and Social Rights predicted that military intervention in Iraq would trigger the collapse of an already fragile Iraqi public health system.[19]

NGOs working under the banner of IPPNW mobilized physicians, medical students, and other health workers to participate in massive antiwar demonstrations in many countries. Representatives of IPPNW and IALANA delivered an international physicians petition against the war to U.N. Secretary-General Kofi Annan and to U.N. missions. PSR, the U.S. affiliate of IPPNW, argued against the idea of preemptive war in Iraq in advertisements in the *New York Times* and *The Nation*.

Medact, the IPPNW affiliate in the United Kingdom, warned that the U.S. "shock and awe" strategy could cause up to 261,000 military and civilian deaths and that postwar health impacts could result in another 200,000 civilian deaths.[20] It stressed that a projected war cost of $100 billion could address the health needs of the world's poorest people for 4 years. (See Chapter 15.)

Reducing Small Arms Violence

NGO campaigns against gun violence have generally focused on supply and demand issues—the global arms trade and illicit trafficking—and on national and international policies to restrict the flow of the more than 6 million small arms in global markets. This work has been performed largely by the London-based IANSA, a coalition of more than 500 civil-society organizations in almost 100 countries (see Chapter 6).

A public health perspective that could quantify the human costs of small arms violence and put faces on the victims of armed conflict was missing from these arms control strategies. To redress this gap, IPPNW began in 2001 its Aiming For Prevention campaign to document the health and humanitarian consequences of small arms and to mobilize physicians and other health professionals to support preventive programs and policies. The tools of this campaign are credible public health research, physician participation in international conferences addressing small arms and light weapons and other aspects of armed violence and injury, and the development of evidence-based policy proposals and their dissemination through a global public health network. In El Salvador, for example, doctors and medical students working with the NGO Médicos Salvadoreños para la Responsabilidad Social (MESARES) have compiled research on firearms injuries from hospital records and interviews showing that the treatment of gunshot wounds was expending more than 7 percent of the public hospital system's budget.[21] A coalition of groups presented this research to President Elias Antonio Saca in 2005 and persuaded him to create a national commission to review and strengthen El Salvador's gun laws. Later that year, IPPNW commissioned a six-country, hospital-based pilot research study on firearm injuries in Africa and Latin America. Standardized, contextual data on victims of gun violence will be used to promote local, national, and international policy reforms.

The educational centerpiece of the Aiming For Prevention campaign is the "One Bullet Story," which traces—in words and graphic images—the impact of a single firearm injury on the life of the victim, the victim's family, and the local community, documenting the costs of treatment, rehabilitation, and lost productivity. Moving stories of survivors focus attention on the human tragedy of war and other forms of armed violence.

Conclusion

Nongovernmental organizations play vital roles in mitigating the consequences of war and in research, education, and advocacy. Health professionals play important roles in participating in and supporting the work of these organizations.

References

1. Médecins Sans Frontières. Available at: http://en.wikipedia.org/wiki/Medecins_Sans _Frontieres (accessed June 22, 2007).

2. Médecins Sans Frontières. Prevented from working, the French section of MSF leaves Myanmar. Press release. March 29, 2006.
3. Physicians for Human Rights. Break them down: The systematic use of psychological torture by U.S. forces. Cambridge, MA: PHR. May 2005. Available at: http://www.physiciansforhumanrights.org/library/documents/reports/break-them-down-the.pdf (accessed June 22, 2007).
4. Physicians for Human Rights. Darfur—Assault on survival: A call for security, justice and restitution. Cambridge, MA: PHR. January 2006. Available at http://www.physiciansforhumanrights.org/library/documents/reports/darfur-assault-on-survival.pdf (accessed June 22, 2007).
5. Oxfam International. Towards Global Equity: Strategic Plan, 2001–2004. Oxford: Oxfam International, 2001.
6. Abolition 2000. Abolition 2000 Founding Statement. Available at: http://www.abolition2000.org/site/c.cdJIKKNpFqG/b.1316717/k.8870/The_Abolition_2000_Statement_English.htm (accessed July 5, 2007).
7. Russell B, Einstein A. Russell Einstein Manifesto. London. July 9, 1955. Available at Pugwash Online: www.pugwash.org/about/manifesto.htm (Accessed July 5, 2007).
8. Nathan DG, Geiger HJ, Sidel VW, Lown B. The medical consequences of thermonuclear war: Introduction. N Engl J Med 1962;266:1126–1127.
9. Sidel VW, Geiger HJ, Lown B. The medical consequences of thermonuclear war: II. The physician's role in the postattack period. N Engl J Med 1962;266:1137–1145.
10. Wittner LS. The Struggle against the Bomb: Resisting the Bomb—A History of the World Nuclear Disarmament Movement, 1954–1970. Palo Alto, CA: Stanford University Press, 1997.
11. International Physicians for the Prevention of Nuclear War and Institute for Energy and Environmental Research. Radioactive Heaven and Earth: The Health and Environmental Effects of Nuclear Weapons Testing In, On, and Above the Earth. New York: Apex Press/Zed Books, 1991.
12. International Physicians for the Prevention of Nuclear War and Institute for Energy and Environmental Research. Nuclear Wastelands: Nuclear Weapons Production Worldwide and Its Environmental and Health Effects. Cambridge, MA: MIT Press, 1995.
13. International Court of Justice. Legality of the Threat or Use of Nuclear Weapons: Advisory Opinion. General List, No. 95. The Hague: July 8, 1996. Available at: http://prop1.org/2000/icjop1.htm (accessed June 22, 2007).
14. International Physicians for the Prevention of Nuclear War, International Network of Engineers and Scientists Against Proliferation, and International Association of Lawyers Against Nuclear Arms. Security and Survival: The Case for a Nuclear Weapons Convention. Cambridge, MA: IPPNW, 1999.
15. Ramana MV. Bombing Bombay? Effects of Nuclear Weapons and a Case Study of a Hypothetical Explosion. Cambridge, MA: IPPNW, 1999.
16. International Physicians for the Prevention of Nuclear War. Crude Nuclear Weapons: Proliferation and the Terrorist Threat. Cambridge, MA: IPPNW, 1997.
17. International Physicians for the Prevention of Nuclear War. Rethinking Nuclear Energy and Democracy after September 11, 2001. Cambridge, MA: IPPNW, 2004.
18. International Study Team. Our Common Responsibility: The Impact of a New War on Iraqi Children. Toronto: War Child Canada, January 2003.

19. Center for Economic and Social Rights. The human costs of war in Iraq. New York: CESR. 2003. Available online at www.cesr.org/iraq (accessed July 20, 2007).
20. Medact. Collateral Damage: The Health and Environmental Costs of War on Iraq. London: Medact, 2002. Available at: http://www.medact.org (accessed June 22, 2007).
21. International Action Network on Small Arms. El Salvador: President persuaded to review gun laws (www.iansa.org/regions/camerica/el-salvador-commission.htm) (accessed July 5, 2007).

24

The Roles and Ethical Dilemmas for Military Medical Care Workers

Victor W. Sidel and Barry S. Levy

The essence of ethical behavior is the ability to make appropriate choices between possible courses of action. For medical care workers (MCWs)—physicians, nurses, physical therapists, physicians' assistants, nurse practitioners, and others—engaged in treating or counseling patients, the ethical choice is usually clear: The action should serve the best interests of the patient as the MCW and patient perceive those interests. In the infrequent instances when the patient's and the MCW's perceptions of the best interests of the patient differ, the MCW is expected to act as the patient wishes or, if the MCW for some reason cannot do so, to withdraw and refer the patient to other medical care.

In some circumstances in which the MCW has obligations to others in addition to obligations to the patient, a situation known as "mixed agency," the ethical choice may be more complex and more difficult. There are many examples of mixed agency in civilian medical care. Some of these are caused by the legal requirement to report certain health situations to appropriate agencies, such as reporting a case of hepatitis or syphilis to public health officials or a gunshot wound to law enforcement authorities. There are also requirements imposed by employers on MCWs practicing occupational medicine or prison medicine, and requirements are imposed by managed care organizations. Clinical research may also lead to mixed-agency ethical conflicts. In all of these situations of mixed-agency ethical conflict in civilian practice, however, there are usually ways to resolve them. If necessary, MCWs in civilian practice can withdraw from such situations by referring patients to other MCWs or other sources of health care, or by resigning positions that create the conflict situations.

There may be quite different mixed-agency dilemmas for MCWs working under a military command structure. These include obligations to promote the fighting strength of the military force and national security as it is defined by the military command and to perform specific duties for fixed periods of military service, precluding options that civilian MCWs have for resolving role conflict.

We believe that the overriding ethical principles of medical practice are "concern for the welfare of the patient" and "primarily, do no harm (*primum non nocere*)," and that, in contrast, the overriding principles of military service are "concern for the effective function of the fighting force" and "obedience to the command structure." We believe that the ethical principles of medical practice make medical practice under military control fundamentally dysfunctional and unethical. Medical practice under military control may be harmful to the personnel being cared for, to the overall mission of the armed forces, and to the practice of medicine.

There is a long history of MCW involvement with military forces. Homer praised the efforts of two sons of Asklepios who provided surgical care during the siege of Troy.[1] Hippocrates, recognizing the battleground as an important training ground for surgeons, urged that "he who would become a surgeon should join an army and follow it."[2] To the armies of the Czar in Russia, Peter the Great brought the feldsher, modeled on the *feldscherer* (field barber-surgeon) of the Prussian armies. During the American Revolution, deplorable medical care caused bitter political conflicts over the management of hospitals and health care for military personnel. The increase in military deaths during wars in the 19th century and the extraordinary increase in both military and civilian deaths during wars of the 20th century, together with dramatic improvements in the ability to treat the wounded successfully and to prevent illness, led to changes in the ethical dilemmas that may arise and an increase in their number. These dilemmas are described in the following five sections.

1. Obligations to Enhance Military Strength versus Obligations to Meet the Needs of Individual Military Personnel

Setting Medical Priorities for Military Purposes

Because the primary role of the military MCW is to conserve the fighting strength of the force,[3] the military's needs may override medical needs, requiring military MCWs to accept different priorities than their civilian counterparts. Attention to military needs and to patient-centered medical care may not involve ethical conflict. But if it does, the military MCW is usually expected to give higher priority to the military's needs, possibly subordinating the best interests of the patient to the good of the fighting force or the completion of the mission.[4]

Performing Medical Research on Military Personnel without Informed Consent

Another example of treating individuals as military personnel rather than as patients is using them as subjects in medical research for military purposes without their free and informed consent. The Nuremberg Code and accepted practice in the United States require the free and informed consent of human subjects. Because they cannot simply "quit their jobs" or "file a grievance" with a union, government agency, or professional organization, military personnel may not believe that they have the right to refuse to participate in these experiments. Also, they may not be fully informed of the risks. Examples include U.S. troops who were required to be present at atmospheric tests of nuclear weapons in the 1940s and 1950s[5] and troops who participated in chemical weapons experiments in the 1950s and 1960s.[6] More recent examples include administration of pyridostigmine during the Persian Gulf War as an experimental protection against nerve agents.[7,8]

Violating Patient Confidentiality

Patient confidentiality may be breached in military medicine in the name of military or national security.[9–10] Violation of patient privacy would also be unacceptable in civilian practice except under circumstances strictly defined by law. But a commanding officer may request disclosure by the MCW of all medical information relevant to the military performance of an individual in the officer's unit.

Failing to Keep Adequate Records

Military personnel who have been treated or given immunizations according to military guidelines or have been subjected to medical research may develop problems much later in life that can best be treated by full disclosure of all procedures or agents to which they were exposed. However, the military does not always keep adequate or accurate records, or see the need to do so.[11]

2. Ability to Override the Patient's Wishes for "The Patient's Benefit"

Overriding Patients' Wishes

Military MCWs have more coercive capabilities than do most of their civilian counterparts. They may have enormous power to override the wishes of individual patients "for the patient's own good." This powerful paternalism is permitted and may be fostered by the power and self-image of the individual military MCW and by the power and wishes of the command structure. The power of the military MCW over the patient has potential for clouding judgment and for corruption, similar to the ways in which MCWs in other "total institutions," such as prisons and mental hospitals, have the power to substitute their values and their judgments for those of the patient and the patient's family.[12]

Addressing Psychiatric Problems from a Military Perspective

Difficult issues arise in dealing with work performance by military personnel, especially in relation to psychiatric problems. Is "battle fatigue" or a severe stress reaction simply a normal reaction to an abnormal situation, to be treated by rest and prompt return to the battlefield, or are these symptoms of illness that require more treatment? The practice of "over-evacuation" (the presumed excessive transfer of ill or injured personnel to a safe area rather than back to the frontlines of the military operation) has been cited as "one of the cardinal sins of military medicine."[1] We believe the military MCW must be free to make such decisions in the best interest of the patient.

Performing Battlefield Triage

How far can a military MCW go in the course of making decisions in the best interest of the patient? If a wounded soldier is in agony, with no hope of effective treatment, evacuation, or reasonable pain relief, is it ethical for the military MCW to use large doses of analgesia for the "dual purpose" of relieving pain and hastening death? Although the "double effect" is well recognized and well accepted ethically when informed consent is possible, "mercy euthanasia" in military situations may be ethically questionable. Even more troubling is the scenario in which there is no way to help a suffering soldier whose cries are likely to give away the position of the rest of the unit, thus jeopardizing others. Is it ethical for the MCW to use large doses of analgesics in such a situation? How might the MCW's identification with the unit affect such decision-making? Would the MCW even be aware of the influence of the well-being of others on this decision-making? In military practice, an MCW might assume the authority to make such decisions, either to protect the fighting force or "for the service member's own good."[13]

Imposing Immunization or Treatment for the Good of the Patient

The ability of the military MCW to make decisions for the "good of the patient" can also be seen in the immunization of military personnel. The military may ethically require some immunizations, both to protect the fighting force and for the soldier's own good. Some specific immunizations are needed to protect the fighting force, especially in those instances where troops are deploying to an area with a known incidence of a specific disease and there is an effective, safe, Food and Drug Administration–approved vaccine for the disease to which the troops would most likely be exposed.

Communities have the need and the right to protect themselves from the spread of known preventable diseases. When immunization is required in civilian public health practice to protect others beyond the individuals immunized, as in the case of an infectious disease spread from person to person, few would argue against immunization for community protection. We have no argument with that position being taken by the military. But we would disagree with the military if it ordered, without informed consent, immunization of questionable effectiveness or with potential adverse effects, either to "protect the fighting force" or to protect the individual patient.[14–21]

3. Obligations of MCWs to Serve Those in Need of Care

Under the Geneva Conventions, MCWs are given certain specific protections by an explicit separation of their medical role from the combatant role. MCWs and treatment facilities are designated as immune from attack, and captured MCWs are to be promptly repatriated. In return, MCWs must[22–24]

1. Not engage in or be parties to acts of war
2. Respect, protect, and humanely treat the wounded and sick soldiers and civilians and care for belligerents
3. Not leave the wounded and sick without medical assistance, and only for urgent medical reasons authorize setting any priorities in the order of their treatment
4. Provide medical aid solely on medical grounds, "without distinctions founded on sex, race, nationality, religion, political opinions, or any other similar criteria"

5. Exercise no physical or moral coercion against protected persons (civilians), especially to obtain information from them or from third parties.

We believe that military medical training gives insufficient attention to the requirements of the Geneva Conventions and too much attention to the coherence and interdependence of the various components and missions of the military force.

Failing to Provide Care to Enemy Military Personnel

Despite obligations under the Geneva Conventions to provide care to enemy soldiers, there are reasons why military MCWs may be unwilling or unable to accept these obligations. For example, refusal to treat the "enemy" for reasons of "patriotism" or "national security" may be seen by some MCWs as so important that it supersedes the MCW's ethical responsibilities to "enemies." Ethical conflicts arise for military MCWs because they are a part of the armed forces. They wear the uniform, they observe the regulations and formalities, and they bond with their fellow military personnel. It is easy for these medical workers to see themselves as "us" and enemy soldiers as "them." The Geneva Conventions forbid military services to require that their health care personnel give preference in care to their own troops or deny care to others, even members of the "enemy" force in times of war. The Law of Land Warfare specifically reinforces this duty of medical impartiality.[25] Neither document, however, addresses the human tendency to bond and identify with one's "own type" and to turn against those seen as "others."

Failing to Provide Care to Civilians

Civilians are increasingly being injured or killed during the conduct of contemporary war (see Chapter 1). Civilian homes are also damaged or destroyed, and their occupants are forced to move on, becoming internally displaced persons or refugees who often need health services, not only for war-related injuries and psychological trauma but also for ongoing health needs.

Except in very special circumstances in which military MCWs are specifically assigned to provide medical care for civilian populations, military MCWs may not be officially permitted to provide such care even for those whose need is greater than that of military personnel. Unless the command structure for military MCWs specifically requires them to base priorities for medical care on medical need, no matter whose need is involved, care for civilians may have low priority or none at all.

Failing to Provide Optimal Care to U.S. Military Personnel

MCWs may become very closely identified with the command structure in which they serve. This happens because the MCW who trains or works closely with a unit, particularly with an elite unit, over a long period becomes dependent on the unit, just as the unit becomes dependent on the MCW. MCWs who are members of military units feel "bonded" to "their own" and may feel pressure from their commanders and peers to give preference to the medical needs of their own troops, even if they are less urgent than the needs of others. It may then be impossible for the MCW to set priorities based solely on medical need, even among military personnel in their own forces.

4. Blurring Combatant and Noncombatant Roles

If one describes a scene in which MCWs appear with weapons in hand, it is natural to assume that they are defending themselves or their patients from an attack. That may be the most frequent circumstance under which MCWs take up arms and inflict injury or death upon the enemy. However, that is not the blurring of roles that we are addressing here. When we offer the image of the MCW, "weapon in hand," we refer instead to that most troubling of images, in which the MCW is actively participating in combat, or perhaps less actively participating but nonetheless subverting the aim and intent of medical care.

Participating in Combatant Roles

The Geneva Conventions require strict separation of the military and medical care functions, but this has not always been the case. In the 19th century in the United States, there were instances in which medical officers were combatants without any apparent immediate need to protect those under their medical care. The most prominent of these medical combatants was Leonard Wood, who, as a recent graduate of the Harvard Medical School and a civilian contract surgeon in the U.S. Army in the Southwest in 1886, carried dispatches through a region populated with hostile Indians. For several weeks, while in close pursuit of Geronimo's forces and constantly expecting an encounter, he commanded a detachment of infantry, which was then without an officer, and to the command of which he was assigned upon his own request."[26] In his defense, one might say that he had requested the infantry assignment that allowed him to pursue Geronimo, and therefore he ceased to be an MCW during that time. Should it be ethically permissible for a medical officer to quit his medical role for a combatant role, either temporarily or for a longer period?

Using Medical Care as a Weapon

The U.S. Army Special Forces in Vietnam were given the mission of "winning the hearts and minds" of indigenous populations to further the military mission. The primary task of Special Forces aidmen was "to seek and destroy the enemy" and only incidentally to care for the medical needs of others on the patrol.[27] These aidmen were not considered protected medical personnel but were classified as combatants. Although their primary task was as combatants, aidmen also administered medical assistance to their own forces and could do the same for other persons deemed to need assistance. The military, by combining combat capabilities with medical skills, had perverted medical care into a "weapon." The aidmen could offer care to indigenous populations, especially if it served the need of the Special Forces mission. Just because aidmen were not considered medical personnel by the U.S. Army does not mean that the indigenous population did not see them as medical personnel who could choose to help or not. Even though Special Forces aidmen did not wear a medical emblem, once they opened their bags and offered medicine, they become helpers in the eyes of patients—a clearly unethical deception. The cross-training of aidmen in combat and medical techniques was the reason given by Dr. Howard Levy for refusing to train them, for which he was convicted at court martial and imprisoned at Fort Leavenworth.[27–29]

Participating in Militarily Useful Research and Development

Weapons systems are designed to render the enemy ineffective, usually by causing destruction, maiming, and killing, or the fear of these, that the enemy is unable or unwilling to fight. These offensive systems must consider physical and medical factors, such as the amount of force necessary to penetrate structures and disable or kill their inhabitants. Inside or outside the armed forces, some MCWs are involved in militarily useful research and development, such as work on biological weapons or on the radiation effects of nuclear weapons. In such work, it is said to have been common practice to concentrate physicians into "principally or primarily defensive operations."[30] But work on weapons and their effects can never be exclusively defensive, and at times the distinction is quite arbitrary. The question arises whether there is a special ethical duty for MCWs (because of their obligation to "do no harm") to refuse to participate in such work, or whether in non–patient care situations MCWs simply share the ethical duties of all human beings.[31] We believe that MCWs are always MCWs and therefore should adhere to their ethical duty to "do no harm."

Participating in, or Failing to Report, Torture

Egregiously, medical knowledge is sometimes used in the development of offensive weapons and defensive strategies for dealing with such weapons. More egregious is the use of medical knowledge in participating in, or failing to report, torture. MCWs have been given the privilege by society to learn about the human body, including what can be endured and what cannot (see Chapter 14). Using such knowledge to facilitate torture is indeed an abhorrent activity.[32–37]

Preventing Moral Actions by Medical Care Workers in Military Operations

In "total institutions," such as prisons and mental hospitals, the role of the individual to make independent decisions is severely limited.[12] The impact of the total institution on medical ethics is particularly seen in the field situation. The field commander may not understand the perspective or the needs of the health professional or may not have time to evaluate the ethical dilemmas that health professionals face. Response to psychiatric conditions may pose special problems in the field. The health professional's inability to refuse to obey orders, even when the orders conflict with ethical judgments, is an example of the effect of the military institution on medical ethics.

Preventing Moral Protest Actions by Medical Care Workers

When MCWs don military uniforms and raise their hands to take the oath of induction into the armed forces, they do more than join an organization. They also leave behind their civilian lives and, with them, many of the basic rights they enjoyed as civilians. Chief among these rights is that of actively participating in the political process, including the right to publicly protest as members of their profession. Like all members of the armed forces, military MCWs are limited by threat of military discipline in the extent to which they can publicly protest what they believe to be unjust or harmful acts. Military personnel cannot publicly make contemptuous statements about the President or other officials, nor can they make statements held to be disloyal. We believe that MCWs should have the right of moral protest, but within the military major sanctions may be imposed for protesting acts deemed by the protesters to be unjust or harmful.[38,39]

Just as military personnel cannot publicly protest what they believe to be unjust acts, they are also limited in the extent to which they can publicly protest what they believe to be an unjust war. (The issue of what is a "just war"[40,41] has been debated for more than two millennia.)

Membership in the armed forces, even in a noncombatant role such as that of a MCW, may require self-censorship of public doubts about the justness of a war in which the armed forces are engaged. However, many MCWs consider themselves pacifists. "Absolute pacifists" oppose the use of any force against another human being, even in self-defense against direct, personal attack. They believe that the use of force can be ended only when all humans refuse to use it, and that acceptance of one's own injury or even death is preferable to use of force against another. More limited forms of pacifism hold, for example, that the use of certain weapons of mass destruction in war is never justified, no matter how great the provocation or how terrible the consequences of failure to use them.

One pacifist-type response was suggested in the late 1930s by John A. Ryle, then Regius Professor of Physic at the University of Cambridge[42]:

> By withholding service from the Armed Forces before and during war, by declining to examine and inoculate recruits, by refusing sanitary advice and the training and command of ambulances, clearing stations, medical transport, and hospitals, the doctors could so cripple the efficiency of the staff and aggravate the difficulties of campaign and so damage the morale of the troops that war would become almost unthinkable.

It is, of course, unlikely that wars would cease if no medical care support were provided. In addition, refusal to provide military medical care is not a viable option for MCWs in countries where dissent of this type is not permitted. But it is important to encourage such opposition by MCWs, because it can foster discussion of these ethical dilemmas.

An MCW's right to refuse to serve in the military at all, on the basis of conscientious objection, is complicated by the status of the MCW as a noncombatant. When military service by MCWs is required, such as by a draft, the MCW may not be able to avoid the ethical problems caused by mixed agency and may not be permitted to resign from military service as a conscientious objector. When military service by MCWs is voluntary, the so-called noncombatant status of health workers may also prevent the MCW who has volunteered for military service from resigning as a conscientious objector when ethical conflict arises.

There is considerable debate whether MCWs, because of a special dedication to preservation of life and health, have a special obligation to serve or to refuse to serve in a military effort. That position is made more complex by a role as a military noncombatant. Many military forces nonetheless permit health workers, like other military personnel, to claim conscientious objector status. In the United States, conscientious objection is defined as "[a] firm, fixed and sincere objection to participation in war in any form or the bearing of arms because of religious training or belief."[43] Religious training and belief is defined as "belief in an external power or being or deeply held moral or ethical belief, to which all else is subordinate . . . and which has the power or force to affect moral well-being."[44] The person claiming conscientious objector status must convince a military hearing officer that the objection is sincere.[45] Those who can convince the hearing officers that they oppose war in all forms can be released from military service. MCWs who are situational pacifists—that is, those who have refused to support a specific war effort rather than war in general—have great difficulty in the military.[46] An example is the refusal of Dr. Yolanda Huet-Vaughn, a physician in the U.S. Army Reserve, to report for duty during the Persian Gulf War; she was convicted at court martial for "refusing to obey a lawful order" and was imprisoned at Fort Leavenworth.[47]

5. Enhancing the Ability of Medical Care Workers to Serve as Moral Agents

We believe MCWs have a special ethical responsibility to refuse to support a war that they believe will cause major destruction to health and environment.[48] We also believe that the military and the civilian society it protects will be more ethical if these issues are discussed and resolved. Because we believe MCWs cannot act as moral agents within the military, we propose the following two alternatives.

Restructuring Medical Service in the Military

An important reason for a health professional to become or remain a member of the armed forces of a nation is to use the position as an opportunity to insist on behavior that is consistent with ethical values and international humanitarian law. If military MCWs were always people of exceptional moral character and moral will, military MCWs might exert more influence on the command structure to consider both the tactical considerations and the humanitarian aspects of military decisions.

    If the nature of the roles of those serving in the medical care services of the armed forces is sufficiently changed, and if those serving have the strength of character to avoid ethical compromise, they can make an important contribution to the moral level of the military.[49–51] One of the most important responsibilities that military MCWs have is to make certain that they and all other military personnel do not commit unethical acts. We believe that there are extremely limited opportunities under a structure of military control of the medical system for military MCWs to contribute effectively to military ethics.

It is possible, but unlikely, that the structure could be changed sufficiently to permit ethical service and ethical contributions by MCWs.

Selecting Alternatives to Military Service

These alternatives may take the form of overt dissent, seeking conscientious objector status, or serving in a nonmilitary health organization. With civilians accounting for a large fraction of those killed in war and with threats of the use of weapons of mass destruction continuing, is any form of military service appropriate for the ethical health professional? Other MCWs may wish to accept a service alternative that is consistent with an ethical obligation to protect health and prevent illness or to care for those wounded or maimed, without simultaneously supporting a war effort. Although opportunities for service in an international corps, such as Médecins du Monde or Médecins Sans Frontières, are limited, MCWs may have opportunities to work with such organizations (see Chapters 22 and 23).

We believe that at some point in the future (even though it clearly has not been that way in the past) the world will truly evolve into a "global community" in which individuals as well as nations will understand that what people have in common is far greater than their areas of difference. At that point, we believe that a global perspective on medical care will help ensure that all humans have equal and competent care. Until this is achieved, we believe that MCWs have a special responsibility to attempt to prevent injury and death to military personnel and civilians. Therefore, they may wish to help prevent war wherever it may occur. MCWs should do so by contributing to public and professional understanding of the nature of war, the risks of weapons of mass destruction, and the nature and effectiveness of alternatives to war.

What form of service is appropriate for ethical MCWs? Some MCWs have refused to support war by refusing to serve in the armed forces. Do MCWs have a special ethical responsibility, in view of their obligation to protect the health and the lives of their patients and the people of their communities, to refuse to support a war they believe will cause major destruction to the health and environment of both combatants and noncombatants? If an MCW considers service in support of a particular war unethical, may (or, indeed, must) that person refuse to serve, even if the objection does not qualify the MCW for formal conscientious objector status? Is there an ethical difference if the service is required by the society, as in a "doctor draft," or if the service obligation has been entered into voluntarily to fulfill an obligation in return for military support of medical training or for other reasons? And is military service indeed a "voluntary obligation" if enlistment is prodded, as it is for many poor people and members of minority groups, by lack of educational and employment opportunities or, as for many MCWs, by the cost of education or training that in other societies would be provided at public expense?

MCWs may wish, as individuals and particularly in groups, to help to prevent war by contributing to public and professional understanding of the nature of modem war, the risks of weapons of mass destruction, and the nature and effectiveness of alternatives to war. Among the groups organized for this purpose are the national affiliates of the International Physicians for the Prevention of Nuclear War (see Chapter 23). In the interest of public health, MCWs may need to consider new forms of national service and contribute in a broader sense to their nation and the world.[52]

Opposition to war does not permit ethical MCWs to refuse care to victims of war whom they are able to serve. Such care, in appropriate organized settings, does not presume support by MCWs of the war being fought. The ethical dilemmas arise when MCWs actively support the war effort by membership in a military medical service or by assigning priority to patient care based on military demands rather than patient needs. These issues and those associated with the role of the MCW in peacemaking and peacekeeping, often grotesquely distorted by the fervor that may accompany war and preparation for war, require dispassionate analysis and action in times of peace.

Acknowledgments: The authors are grateful to Tod Ensign, H. Jack Geiger, John C. Moskop, and Edmund Pellegrino for their suggestions, in which earlier discussions of these issues were presented.

Additional background readings on the material covered in this chapter include the following:

Sidel VW. Aesculapius and Mars. The Lancet 1968;1(7549):966–967.

Sidel VW. Quid est amor patriae? PSR Quarterly 1991;1:96–104.

Sidel VW. Warfare 1: Medicine and War. In Reich WT (ed.). Encyclopedia of Bioethics, 2nd ed. New York: Macmillan, 1995, pp. 2533–2588.

Sidel VW. The role and ethics of health professionals in war. In Levy BS, Sidel VW (eds.). War and Public Health. New York: Oxford University Press, 1997.

Sidel VW, Levy BS. Physician-Soldier: A Moral Dilemma. In Beam TE, Sparacino LR, (eds.). Military Medical Ethics. Washington, DC: TMM Publications, Office of the Surgeon General, Department of the Army, 2004.

References

1. Homer. The Iliad. Translated by Robert Fagles. New York: Viking Penguin, 1990.
2. Vastyan EA. Warriors in white: Some questions about the nature and mission of military medicine. Tex Rep Biol Med 1974;32:327–342.

3. Bellamy RF. Conserve the fighting strength. Mil Med 1988;153:185–187.
4. Swan KG, Swan KG Jr. Triage: The past revisited. Mil Med 1996;161:448–452.
5. Advisory Committee on Human Radiation Experiments. Final Report. Washington, DC: Government Printing Office, 1995.
6. Pechura CM, Rall DM. Veterans at Risk: The Health Effects of Mustard Gas and Lewisite. Washington, DC: National Academy Press, 1993.
7. Annas GJ. Changing the consent rules for Desert Storm. N Engl J Med 1992;326: 770–773.
8. Annas GJ. Protecting soldiers from friendly fire: The consent requirement for using investigational drugs and vaccines in combat. Am J Law Med 1998;24:245–260.
9. Auster SL. Confidentiality in military medicine. Mil Med 1985;150:341–346.
10. Steinfels MO, Levin C (eds.). In the service of the state. The psychiatrist as double agent [Conference transcript]. Hastings Cent Rep 1978;8(2 Suppl):8.
11. Presidential Advisory Committee on Gulf War Veterans' Illnesses. Special Report. October 31, 1997. Available at: http://www.gulflink.osd.mil/gwvi/ (accessed June 22, 2007).
12. Goffman E. Asylums: Essays on the Social Situation of Mental Patients and Other Inmates. New York: Doubleday, 1961.
13. Swann SW. Euthanasia on the battlefield. Mil Med 1987;152:545–549.
14. Cohen HW, Gould RM, Sidel VW. The pitfalls of bioterrorism preparedness: The anthrax and smallpox experiences. Am J Public Health 2004;94:1667–1671.
15. Myers SL. US armed forces to be vaccinated against anthrax. New York Times, December 16, 1997.
16. Ivins B, Fellows P, Pitt L, et al. Experimental anthrax vaccines: Efficacy of adjuvants combined with protective antigen against an aerosol *Bacillus anthracis* spore challenge in guinea pigs. Vaccine 1995;13:1779–1784.
17. United States Senate. Is Military Research Hazardous to Veterans' Health? Lessons Spanning Half a Century. Washington, DC: Government Printing Office, 1994.
18. Sloat B, Epstein K. Army misled troops who got vaccine in Bosnia. Plain Dealer (Cleveland, Ohio). January 25, 1998, pp. 1A, 18A.
19. Committee on Health Effects Associated with Exposures during the Gulf War. An Assessment of the Safety of the Anthrax Vaccine [Electronic resource]. A Letter Report. Washington, DC: Institute of Medicine, 2000.
20. Ginburg Y. Sailors refuse vaccine. Navy Times, April 20, 1998, p. 3.
21. Subcommittee on National Security, Veterans Affairs and International Relations, House Committee on Government Reform. The Department of Defense Anthrax Vaccine Immunization Program; Unproven Force Protection. Washington DC: Government Printing Office, 2000.
22. Geneva Conventions of 1949. In Human Rights Documents: Compilation of Documents Pertaining to Human Rights. Washington, DC: Government Printing Office, 1983.
23. Vastyan EA. Warfare: 1. Medicine and war. In Reich WT (ed.). Encyclopedia of Bioethics. New York: Macmillan, 1978, pp. 1695–1699.
24. U.S. Department of the Army. Treaties Governing Land Warfare. (DA Pamphlet PAM 27–1). Washington, DC: Department of the Army, 1956.
25. U.S. Department of the Army. The Law of Land Warfare. (Field Manual 27–10). Washington, DC: Department of the Army, 1956.
26. U.S. Department of the Army. The Medal of Honor of the United States Army. Washington, DC: Government Printing Office, 1948.
27. Bourne PG. Men, Stress, and Vietnam. Boston: Little, Brown, 1970.

28. Langer E. The court-martial of Captain Levy: Medical ethics v. military law. Science 1967;56:1346,1349.
29. Glasser I. Judgment at Fort Jackson: The court-martial of Captain Howard B. Levy. Law Transition Q 1967;4:123–156.
30. Rosebury T. Medical ethics and biological warfare. Perspect Biol Med 1963;6: 312–323.
31. Sidel VW. Biological weapons research and physicians: Historical and ethical analysis. PSR Quarterly 1991;1:31–42.
32. Cilasun U. Torture and the participation of doctors. J Med Ethics 1991;17(Suppl):21– 22. (Cited in Moskop JC. A moral analysis of military medicine. Mil Med 1998; 163:76–79.)
33. Bleche MG. Uruguay's military physicians: Cogs in a system of state terror. JAMA 1986;225:2788–2793.
34. Iacopino V, Heisler M, Pishevar S, Kirschner RH. Physician complicity in misrepresentation and omission of evidence of torture in postdetention medical examinations in Turkey. JAMA 1996;276:396–402.
35. British Medical Association. Medicine Betrayed: The Participation of Doctors in Human Rights Abuses. London: Zed Books, 1992.
36. Amnesty International. Prescription for Change: Health Professionals and the Exposure of Human Rights Violations. London: Amnesty International, 1996.
37. Westermeyer J. Compromise, complicity, and torture [Editorial]. JAMA 1996; 276:416–417.
38. Moskop JC. A moral analysis of military medicine. Mil Med 1998;163:76–79.
39. Pellegrino ED. Societal duty and moral complicity: The physician's dilemma of divided loyalty. Int J Law Psychiatry 1993;6:371–391.
40. Walzer M. Just and Unjust Wars: A Moral Argument with Historical Illustrations. New York: Basic Books, 1977.
41. Seabury P, Codevilla A. War: Ends and Means. New York: Basic Books, 1989.
42. Ryle JA. Foreword. In Joules E (ed.). The Doctor's View of War. London: George Allen & Unwin Ltd, 1938, pp. 7–10.
43. U.S. Department of Defense. Directive 1300.6—Conscientious Objectors. Available at: Central Committee for Conscientious Objectors. Advice for Conscientious Objectors in the Armed Forces: Conscientious Objection and the Law. http://www.objector.org/ advice/conscientious_objector-12.html#pgfId-119 (accessed July 20, 2007).
44. U.S. Department of Defense. Directive 1300.6—Conscientious Objectors. Available at: Central Committee for Conscientious Objectors. Advice for Conscientious Objectors in the Armed Forces: Religious Training and Belief. Available at: http:// www.objector.org/advice/conscientious_objector-15.html#pgfId-145 (accessed July 20, 2007).
45. U.S. Department of the Army. Conscientious Objection. (Army Regulation 600–43). Washington, DC: Department of the Army, 1998.
46. Blaustein M, Procter WC. The active duty conscientious objector: A psychiatric-psychological evaluation. Mil Med 1977;142:619–621.
47. Clemency for army doctor who refused war service. New York Times, April 8, 1992.
48. Levy BS, Sidel VW. Preventing war and its health consequences: Roles of public health professionals. In Levy BS, Sidel VW (eds.). War and Public Health. New York: Oxford University Press, 1997, pp. 388–393.
49. Wakin MM. Wanted: Moral virtues in the military. Hastings Cent Rep 1985;15: 25–26.

50. Farrar JT. Medicine needs a code of ethics. Mil Med 1986;151:130.
51. Platoni KT. The quest for ethical leadership in military medicine. Mil Med 1994;159: 169–171.
52. Lown B. Nobel Peace Prize lecture: A prescription for hope. N Engl J Med 1986;314: 985–987.

25

The Roles of Health Professionals in Postconflict Situations

Susannah Sirkin, Susanna Facci Calì, and Mary Ellen Keough

When the bombing stops and the guns fall silent,[1] a new battle begins for war victims. While the world's attention may move to the next acute crisis or the most dramatic headline, devastated people and societies begin to pick up the pieces of their ruptured lives and fragmented nations. All too frequently, their hopes for peace and justice are met with broken promises from leaders and an international community that has forgotten them and their war and has failed to invest in their future.

What Is Postconflict?

The cessation of a conflict could be the result of an international or domestic peace agreement between warring factions or nations. Grievances of an armed group may be addressed. Or a government waging war on insurgents may end hostilities as priorities shift or the balance of power alters. Military dictatorships may be overthrown by violence or through peaceful transitions to more participatory governments. Whether the end of a conflict involves great bloodshed or comes about through peaceful transition affects, to a large extent, the needs and abilities to restore health, rebuild systems, and reconstruct a society that promotes and respects the rights of all people to health and dignity.

Immediate challenges facing societies in the aftermath of war include massive displacement within and across borders, family separation, excessive mortality, untreated infectious disease and chronic noninfectious disease (including mental disorders), injuries, missing loved ones, economic collapse, and destruction of infrastructure. Survivors experience fear, hatred of those who waged the war or anger at those who stood by, and, often, desire for revenge. Their physical environment may be polluted by the detritus of war: unexploded ordnance, landmines, and the remains of those who died. Post-conflict societies are usually torn between dependence on international assistance and the need to restore self-sufficiency.[2]

The goal for these communities and individuals is to move from despair to hope. Physical and psychological recovery is essential and must take place at the individual, community, and national levels, often with international support and engagement (Figure 25-1). In addition to all of the material exigencies, nations and societies emerging from war need to establish structures that will begin to address the root causes of the war and implement measures to prevent its recurrence.

While leaders instinctively look forward, they must also look back. A society cannot begin to build the future without confronting its past.[3] In the quest for lasting peace, there is a need for truth, acknowledgment, justice, reha-

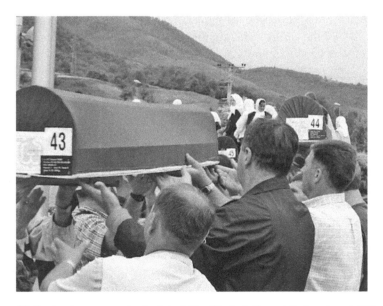

Figure 25-1. Anniversary and reburial of identified victims at Srebrenica at 10th anniversary event, during which more than 600 caskets were passed to graves by family members of the deceased. (Photograph by Mary Ellen Keough.)

bilitation (in the form of reparations), and, ultimately, reconciliation. Health professionals play specific and vital roles in every aspect of this process— and, in the course of this work, they must also preserve their own health (Box 25-1).

The Return of the Displaced

Both refugees and internally displaced persons endure similar psychological and physical consequences that persist after armed conflict (see Chapter 13). These include physical dislocation, separation from everyday practices, social disruption, and material dispossession.[4]

Conflict and mass atrocity in the 1990s and during the first years of this century in Bosnia, Liberia, Rwanda, Sierra Leone, Democratic Republic of Congo, Uganda, and Sudan were also marked by the systematic use of rape as an instrument of war and terror, posing a unique challenge to health professionals who must address the physical and psychological trauma as well as the social isolation of the victims.[5] Children may have witnessed mass killings, suffered violent acts, or participated in combat themselves. In all such cases, displacement prolongs trauma and hinders a natural healing process.[5]

Even after a conflict is officially over, the displaced frequently experience ongoing violence and abuse. Whereas some groups languish in displaced limbo for years, others are too quickly forced back into insecure environments. It is critical that health professionals advocate for prompt return and restoration of lives and livelihoods whenever possible but oppose forced relocation or return into insecure environments.

Although health professionals play important roles during refugee crises in war, they may overlook the longer-term consequences of war and displacement, especially those affecting mental health. High rates of psychological morbidity are debilitating to those displaced in war, not only during the emergency phase but also in postconflict reconstruction. Failure to address symptoms affecting as many as 50 percent of persons displaced by war who may suffer depression and posttraumatic stress disorder (PTSD), personal insufficiency, and loss of self-esteem[6,7] opens the door to long-term unemployment and poverty, as well as transmission of trauma to the next generation.

New programs established in many locations in the 1990s to serve populations traumatized by war and human rights violations are still far from adequate.[8] The current challenge is to develop community programs that respect local practices of healing and reconciliation and can thrive in countries where conflicts have occurred and where most survivors reside.[9,10] All health professionals in postconflict settings have a responsibility to protect human rights, especially when populations have been so harmed. Women in

Box 25-1 The Impact of Postconflict Situations on Health Workers
Susannah Sirkin, Susanna Facci Cali, and Mary Ellen Keough

As health professionals respond to victims in the aftermath of armed conflict, relatively little attention is paid to the impact of crises on those who provide humanitarian assistance or conduct human rights investigations or advocacy, including health professionals. Humanitarian and human rights workers are all too often assumed to be strong enough and well enough trained to withstand stressful conditions. However, the reality has been quite different. Understanding and responding to the physical and psychological consequences of working in postconflict situations is a duty of all agencies that send workers into war zones, and helping health professionals to function efficiently and effectively in postconflict environments is finally becoming an essential part of providing humanitarian assistance.[1]

People generally assume that, for the health professionals who work in postconflict situations, the risk goes with the job. Health workers entering a former war zone will find its residues, including landmines and unexploded ordnance; poor sanitation; weak infrastructure; damaged homes, offices, and hospitals; disruptions in agriculture and commerce; collapse of schools, community networks, police, and judicial systems; political uncertainty; and psychosocial trauma at the individual and community levels. Sometimes the safety of health workers is at risk because they may be perceived as serving the interests of a particular government or group.[2] Even after wars end, health worker safety and access can be threatened by unchecked violence, kidnapping, and harassment at checkpoints.[1]

However, the risks for health professionals are not only physical but also psychological. Health workers may fail to acknowledge the psychological stress that their work produces, denying feelings and carrying on with the task at hand.[1] Eventually, psychological symptoms may affect even the most experienced health workers and first responders. Even toughened forensic scientists who are used to death investigations are not immune. Many months after collecting evidence of large-scale atrocities in Rwanda and the former Yugoslavia, professionals experienced sudden onsets of crying, sadness, and guilt. A pediatrician who worked in a hospital for unaccompanied children in Rwanda in the aftermath of the genocide of 1994 stated that, after returning to her own country, she was unable to work for more than a year.[3]

Typical symptoms affecting health workers include "burnout," a state of emotional and physical exhaustion. Physical or somatic symptoms may occur, such as rapid heartbeat, stomach pain, trembling, and headaches, but also psychological symptoms, such as difficulty concentrating, poor memory, and feeling overwhelmed or fearful.[4] Health workers may also experience countertransference, which generally occurs when the professional takes on the emotional reactions of the victims and overidentifies with their suffering.

(continued)

Compassion fatigue—the convergence of primary traumatic stress, secondary traumatic stress, and cumulative stress/burnout—is widely reported. Secondary trauma usually affects people who are indirectly exposed to traumatic events of others, such as in conducting interviews with victims of human rights abuses or receiving case material. Common emotional reactions include disillusionment, fear, avoidance, helplessness over identification, anger, guilt, and depression. [5]

Although some health professionals try to avoid any emotional involvement in order to do their work[4] and others seek psychological support in interpersonal relationships with local communities, the psychological impact may incapacitate workers and compromise their efforts,[6] or even the capacity to make the right choices for their own security.

Adequate preparation enables professionals to cope with the consequences of postconflict work.[7] Increasingly, aid organizations provide services to prevent and respond to the most severe reactions.[1]

The World Health Organization has recently established a group to deal with the occupational health of humanitarian workers, assessing risks and ensuring risk management; performing predeparture and field-based prevention activities; providing a minimal operational safety net in the field; and monitoring and reporting on health security measures and incidents.[4]

Organizations can also assist staff by reducing bureaucracy and paperwork; promoting a sense of support among colleagues; intervening to reduce conflicts among workers; maintaining communication; supporting their adequate food and rest; recognizing and appreciating the sacrifices that staff are making; and organizing regular debriefings so that workers can share their thoughts and experiences.[2,4]

References

1. Leous X, Bower H. Health workers on the front line. In Yael D (ed.). Sharing the Front Line and the Back Hills. Amityville, NY: Baywood Publishing Company, 2002.
2. Ehrenreich JH. A Guide for Humanitarian, Health Care, and Human Rights Workers. Center for Psychology and Society, State University of New York, College at Old Westbury, July 2002.
3. Cardozo BL, Salama P. Mental health of humanitarian aid workers in complex emergencies. In Yael D (ed.). Sharing the Front Line and the Back Hills. Amityville, NY: Baywood Publishing Company,2002.
4. Physicians for Human Rights. PHR Investigation Manual. PHR Research Department in-house document for investigation teams. 2005.
5. MacLean E. Food Aid Monitor. We cannot allow emotional involvement. In Yael D (ed.). Sharing the Front Line and the Back Hills. Amityville, NY: Baywood Publishing Company,2002.
6. Smith B. The dangers of aid work. In Yael D (ed.). Sharing the Front Line and the Back Hills. Amityville, NY: Baywood Publishing Company,2002.
7. Haglund WD, Sirkin SM. Surviving with the dead: Forensic investigations in the service of human rights. In Yael D (ed.). Sharing the Front Line and the Back Hills. Amityville, NY: Baywood Publishing Company, 2002.

particular, including widows, who may have few legal rights, and the many who survive sexual assault, need advocates to defend and promote their rights to health, dignity, and economic opportunity, not to mention basic security. (See Chapter 12.)

Restoration of Health and Health Care

Since World War II, more than 85 percent of armed conflicts have occurred in developing countries. War has exacerbated the decline of health systems that were weak or virtually nonexistent before the conflicts. Postconflict health workers must contend with the most vulnerable of the victims—not only those most traumatized by violence and atrocities but also those who suffered from chronic diseases and/or nutritional deficiencies before the beginning of the conflict. They must restore disrupted essential medical services, deal with damaged or destroyed equipment and facilities, and restore empty pharmacies. They must rely on partner organizations and agencies to rebuild or create infrastructure, such as water treatment and supply, waste management, transport, and communication systems. They must contend with a surge in HIV/AIDS and other sexually transmitted infections. But they also must help in the treatment and recovery of those wounded by war and those who continue to be injured by the remains of war. Confronting the stark data is daunting: At the purported end of the conflict in Sierra Leone in 1999, health workers faced an infant mortality rate of 170 per 1,000 live births and a maternal mortality ratio of 1,800 per 100,000 live births.[11]

A major impediment to post-conflict reconstruction of health care is "brain drain." During wars, health professionals exit their countries in search of better and safer working conditions abroad, leaving behind an impoverished and demoralized workforce.[12] In Iraq, low salaries and poor working conditions have also discouraged the entry of new personnel into the health professions. In East Timor, no more than 30 of the 160 physicians who were there before the beginning of the conflict remained when it had ended in 1999. The horrific war in Liberia during the 1990s reduced the number of physicians from 300 to 24, all working with nongovernmental organizations (NGOs).[13] Recruiting and training a new health workforce in the shortest possible time is a key priority for postconflict reconstruction. This requires adequate salaries, technical assistance, equipment, infection control, an efficient drug supply, and decent working conditions.[14]

Limited access to health care in postconflict settings is compounded for women due to inequality, discrimination, and insecurity. Years of war in Afghanistan have contributed to the decline in women's physical and mental health by personal isolation, financial hardship, and family losses.[15]

Political and Humanitarian Decision-making
in Transitional Societies and Public Health

As postwar nations make the transition to peace from dictatorship or political instability and chaos, a new socioeconomic framework for the society is vital. But who has the right to set priorities and control resources? During post-conflict reconstruction, decisions about revenue, sector expenditures, and prioritization of programs may be made outside of the country by international agencies. The absence of a legitimate and credible national authority can create problems both for gaining funds from potential donors and for the coordination of international assistance, especially if there are illegitimate or corrupt leaders or residuals of criminal regimes.

Generally, postconflict rehabilitation programs for the health sector are structured into three main phases:

- Phase I: Provision of immediate and basic health needs
- Phase II: Installation of basic health services
- Phase III: Long-term rehabilitation of the health system.

These programs may also include a process to vet health professionals who may have previously colluded in violations of medical neutrality, war crimes and human rights violations, or violations of medical ethics before and during the conflict. Ideally, they also include a process to create a health professional cadre trained in ethics and human rights. A rights approach to restoration of health systems must guard against discrimination, ensure access to prevention and care with affordable services of adequate quality, protect vulnerable groups, and promote participation by stakeholders in decision-making regarding health and health services.[16] In coordinating the work of civil-society organizations, international NGOs, United Nations agencies, and local government units can maximize scarce human and financial resources.[11]

Sometimes, even the best planning strategies are compromised by the complexity of the transition process from war to peace. In the 1990s in Mozambique, the Ministry of Health, envisaging peace in the near future, developed a health care plan for the 1996–2001 period with a budget of $355 million and detailed plans for all three phases, including rebuilding of infrastructure, development of new human resources through training and wage increases, and the creation of management capacity with decentralization. In reality, the transition from war to peace was much more complex, and progress was slower and more expensive than had been foreseen.[11]

In postwar settings, lack of financial resources poses a huge obstacle to restoration of health and a healthy population, which in turn diminishes the investment capability of affected countries.[17] In a cruel cycle, compromised economic development hinders development of a health care system, but good health is essential for economic development.

A report by Physicians for Human Rights (PHR) on El Salvador after 6 years of an internationally brokered peace settlement revealed that the socioeconomic provisions of such an agreement must be adhered to if basic human rights to food, education, and health care are to be guaranteed to vulnerable populations or repatriated refugees. Using child nutrition as a general indicator of the effectiveness of reconstruction, a team of epidemiologists found a prevalence of stunting among children younger than 5 years of age and linked it to the failures of land reform measures.[18]

To guarantee adherence to peace settlements as a prerequisite for the respect for basic human rights to food, education, and health care, the United Nations has implemented programs of complex peacekeeping operations, known as Disarmament, Demobilization, and Reintegration (DDR) Programs to address the needs of civilians, including the right to health care in war-affected areas. The approach is comprehensive and aims at demilitarization and reconstruction of basic infrastructure.[19]

The United Nations Development Program (UNDP) has implemented several programs in postconflict countries. In 2000, UNDP established its Bureau for Crisis Prevention and Recovery (BCPR), and in 2001, it created the Thematic Fund for Crisis Prevention and Recovery to prevent conflicts and to meet postconflict needs. In Sierra Leone, for example, the UNDP established a national recovery strategy and a district recovery committee to assist in the reconstruction of all infrastructures.[20]

Humanitarian organizations historically move their emergency response teams from crisis to crisis, and the strength of their presence during postconflict situations is far too often determined by the priorities and whims of donors and the governments on whose funding most of them depend. NGOs specializing in short-term interventions have been taken to task for failing to conduct their work in a manner that supports future development or capacity-building for the postconflict environment. Some analysts urge spending "more time [in] being strategic, cunning, as effective as we can."[21] Humanitarian responders are recognizing that they must support a gradual transition from dependence on international aid to self-sufficient local health systems. Some maintain focused war recovery programs, such as the ICRC and Handicap International, which provide prostheses, rehabilitation, and training for those disabled in wars.

The commitment of postconflict national governments ultimately determines the success of recovery, but the creation of partnerships can hasten and strengthen success. Public health workers are critical agents for change in these contexts and can forge new and creative initiatives to restore health and rights to societies emerging from war.

Truth, Justice, and Reconciliation

> We present it . . . as a mandate from those no longer here and those
> who have been forgotten, to the Nation as a whole. The history that
> is told here speaks about us, of what we were and what we must cease
> to be. This history speaks of our work ahead. This history begins
> today.
>
> —S. Lerner, Preface of the Peru Truth
> and Reconciliation Commission[22]

In order for a society to move forward and to meet the needs of survivors in the aftermath of mass atrocity, processes must be developed for arriving at the truth regarding the crimes, acknowledgment of the crimes by officials and society, accountability in the form of trials and punishment, restitution toward making people more whole or compensating them for losses, and memorials to commemorate the crimes and the victims. Each step of this process is fraught with complexities.

Memory can be manipulated for political ends. Memory exists individually and collectively. It can be used in a manner that promotes healing or perpetuates conflict. It can be used to feed nationalism or even incite revenge. But many experts believe that individual reckoning with the past is essential to true reconciliation at the national level.[23]

For many years, the human rights movement rightly focused on criminal justice in the aftermath of atrocities. Until the 1990s, there was enormous dismay that for 50 years since the Nuremberg and Tokyo war crimes trials, no international mechanism for prosecuting crimes against humanity and genocide existed. Then, in the early 1990s, the era of impunity in the aftermath of atrocity came to an end with the establishment of the International Criminal Tribunals for the former Yugoslavia and Rwanda. In the new millennium, the International Criminal Court in The Hague, established by the Rome Treaty of 1998, which entered into force in 2002[24], will test the world's commitment to prosecuting the most heinous of war crimes.

At the same time, truth commissions in several Latin American countries and in postapartheid South Africa have produced massive accounts of torture, disappearances, extrajudicial executions, and the dumping of bodies in unmarked graves. A few countries, such as Sierra Leone, now have the experience of both truth and reconciliation commissions and prosecutions in parallel or seriatim. With two decades of experience with these mechanisms now being assessed in the relevant countries and by expert observers, each of the processes is being studied and scrutinized and their assumptions tested or re-examined.

Often, health professionals are the first to hear and document stories of severe violation. Many victims of war, including victims of human-rights and humanitarian-law violations, are primarily accessing health care for the purpose of treatment and rehabilitation, but many also seek to tell their stories, looking for acknowledgment, validation, truth, or justice. Organizations such as Amnesty International, Human Rights Watch, and PHR formally document incidents and violations in armed conflict on an individual basis, and occasionally on a population basis. Human rights groups obtain information and data from a variety of sources, including relatives of victims, lawyers, domestic human rights groups, the news media, and testimony of refugees. The United Nations High Commissioner for Human Rights (UNHCHR) also usually establishes a presence, during and after conflict, with specific human rights monitoring and reporting capacities. Increasingly, courageous indigenous human rights groups compile such information during and after conflicts for the purpose of local, regional, or international truth and justice processes.

A "one-size-fits-all" approach to truth, justice, and reconciliation is neither possible nor desirable. In countries emerging from a situation of mass violations of human rights in war, the balance of power is still critical and the peace fragile. Often, as in Argentina in the 1980s, residuals of the old regime are still in positions of authority, or are granted amnesty, preventing citizens from coming forward to reveal crimes for fear of retaliation, and thus thwarting accountability and the pursuit of justice.[25] Or, as in the case of northern Uganda in 2005–2006, a peace negotiation can run headlong into international prosecution efforts, forcing questions about perplexing tradeoffs between accountability and ending of hostilities.

Truth and reconciliation commissions—nonjudicial truth-seeking mechanisms that serve as official inquiries into patterns of past abuse and attempt to establish an accurate record of historical events—have been established in more than 25 countries since 1974.[26] They are based on the conviction that the truth-telling process will help reconciliation among people of troubled societies, facilitating the rebuilding of broken relationships.

Many have come to see that, because truth commissions are not based on an adversarial legal process, they are more likely than a trial to reveal the "truth." They also provide a forum for a great number of victims who will never have access to individual trials. In 2003, the Peruvian Truth Commission submitted its report, having collected more than 17,000 statements from witnesses. In East Timor, a process begun in 2002 involved hundreds of hearings and statements from thousands of victims of violence between 1974 and 1999. The Sierra Leone Truth and Reconciliation Commission received more than 7,000 statements. A Sierra Leonean lawyer described the importance of this process: "We need to hear that these atrocities are condemned to at least relieve some of the shame and the grief. It is not just a legal issue. It is about people's lives. Something must be done so the society that was affected by the conflict can invest in peace."[27]

These processes require certain preconditions for success. The relative effectiveness of the Truth and Reconciliation Commission in South Africa can be attributed to its starting point, a democratic referendum that implied broad consensus. In Argentina in the 1980s, on the other hand, the effort to search for truth with a subsequent application of amnesty for military leaders was nothing less than an attempt by the former regime to escape punishment for its campaign of torture, killings, and disappearances. A secure environment is essential for people to come forward and tell their truth without fearing retaliation; this can happen, for example, through a witness protection program, as was established in South Africa.[28] The reconstruction of truth was accomplished by both witnesses and perpetrators, allowing victims to have abuses acknowledged as a precursor to a healing process, with amnesties for perpetrators who revealed and admitted their own crimes.[29]

Although truth-telling processes serve important purposes, prosecution for the most severe crimes is essential to reestablish the rule of law and end a climate of impunity for war crimes. As one expert remarked, "Truth commissions may serve to vindicate the sufferings of victims and their families and to de-legitimate the actions of perpetrators; but without effective efforts to punish the worst violence and restore the fortunes of those affected, they may leave open the wounds of the past."[30] Certainly some victims and witnesses of the crimes that took place under South African apartheid felt betrayed in the end by a process that failed to punish many perpetrators of gross violations, such as killing and torture.

Many caution against outsiders presuming to know or understand what survivors require. No mechanisms can provide a quick fix to individuals or societies convulsed by bloodshed and loss. A study of the Sierra Leone commission noted, "Ideas concerning the conciliatory and therapeutic efficacy of truth telling are the product of a Western culture of memory deriving from North American and European historical processes. Nations, however, do not have psyches that can be healed. Nor can it be assumed that truth telling is healing on a personal level: truth commissions do not constitute therapy."[31]

On an even more sobering note, one expert warned, "Healing is an absurd or even obscene notion for those who have died. Survivors of mass atrocity may feel as though in fact they have died, or live among the dead. Perhaps endurance, not healing, is what survivors at best can seek."[32]

At the same time, indigenous national efforts to address the past can be effective. In a remarkable study of the peace process in Mozambique after the horrific civil war there, Carolyn Nordstrom described how traditional healers saw violence as an illness that could be cured. She cited efforts to create a "political culture of peace" that engaged the local traditions, based on grass-roots resistance to war, and involved millions who "delegitimized violence and built the basis for a lasting peace."[33] (See Chapter 28.)

Addressing "The Missing"

One of the most powerful barriers to healing, reconciliation, and rebuilding in postconflict societies is the emotionally fraught issue of missing persons. In the course of war or civil unrest, individuals "go missing"—through capture, internment, temporary displacement, forced disappearance, kidnapping, execution, ethnic cleansing, and genocide.

Surviving family members are left in a state of uncertainty as to the fate of their missing, suspended in a "no man's land" of psychological and spiritual existence.[34] The magnitude of the problem also affects local and international judicial entities and historians who need to record events accurately. Resolving the fate of the missing is a crucial political concern between former warring parties.[35]

The psychological need to mourn, to conduct rituals for the deceased, and to reach closure on the loss of a missing loved one is well recognized. As a complement to the current U.N. General Assembly Declaration on the Protection of All Persons from Enforced Disappearance,[36] the U.N. Human Rights Council in 2006 adopted the International Convention for the Protection of All Persons from Enforced Disappearance and submitted it to the General Assembly for its adoption. The Convention affirms the right of any victim to know the truth about the circumstances of an enforced disappearance and the right to seek, receive, and impart information to this end.[36]

As a practical matter, determination of living status and the issuance of death certification by a recognized authority establishes a family member's eligibility for survivor benefits, property inheritance, and health services. At the same time, some families fear to investigate the fate of missing relatives, because answers may dash hopes of finding loved ones alive. Some family members may feel that, if they accept the death of the disappeared loved one, they are actually "killing" him or her.[37]

The scientific search for missing persons may begin with the exhumation of individual or mass graves. Because the primary goal of most forensic investigations is criminal prosecution, the identification and return of remains becomes secondary, even an afterthought, for courts and tribunals. However, it is vital to create a missing persons recovery system that can serve families' needs as well as those of investigators and prosecutors. The primacy of war-crimes prosecutions cannot supplant obligations to the living. Forensic scientists must continue to advocate for the dead and the needs and rights of the survivors and their communities.[38] The ICRC has recommended the principle that "identification for the purposes of informing the family and returning the remains is just as important as providing evidence for criminal investigations and constitutes due recognition of the rights of families."[39,40] Ultimately, to ensure that victims are heard, it is imperative to generate an accurate record and a legacy to aid in the prevention of future human rights abuses.

These are compelling human rights arguments for the creation of an integrated, multidisciplinary team approach to the search for the "missing" that encompasses credible scientific forensic investigation while simultaneously providing psychosocial support to families. As work proceeds, it is critical to establish cooperation among local and international agencies, with the goal of complementing efforts. The ICRC's role, for example, is to record tracing reports of the missing but not to participate in investigations of war crimes and related exhumations of mass graves. Therefore, the process of establishing and managing antemortem and postmortem databases must be transparent to the public, must present the limitations of the forensic or identification process, and must avoid creating false expectations. Engaging local participation in developing the process lends cultural and psychological sensitivity to both content and design of projects. Support and participation of religious and community leaders is critical. Hiring and training of local staff establishes credibility, promotes goodwill, and ensures cultural sensitivity.[41]

International guidelines on best practices to address the persistent dilemma of missing persons are long overdue. In addressing the "missing," public health professionals need to be versatile, flexible, and proactive while politically neutral. They can serve as advocates while they engage with the community. There is no easy exit strategy after a forensic investigation and identification project. It is therefore vital to follow up with families to ensure transition and sustained integration with local support systems and with the authorized forensic investigative authorities.

References

1. Harroff-Tavel M. Do wars ever end? The work of the International Committee of the Red Cross when the guns fall silent. Int Rev Red Cross 2003;851:465–496.
2. Ball N. The challenge of rebuilding war-torn societies. In Crocker CA, Hampson FO, Aall P (eds.). Turbulent Peace. Washington, DC: U.S. Institute of Peace 2001, pp. 721–722.
3. Méndez JE. Opinion: Key to the future is in confronting the past. Center for Transitional Justice. Available at: http://www.ictj.org/en/news/features/896.html (accessed June 22, 2007).
4. United Nations Office for the Coordination of Humanitarian Affairs. Guiding Principles: A Tool for the Empowerment of Internally Displaced. United Nations Publication, E/CN.4/1998/53/Add.2, Geneva, Switzerland, May 2006 (reprinted).
5. Ehrenreich JH. A Guide for Humanitarian, Health Care, and Human Rights Workers. Center for Psychology and Society, State University of New York, College at Old Westbury, July 2002.

6. World Health Organization. Mental health of refugees, internally displaced persons and other populations affected by conflict. Available at: http://www.who.int (accessed June 22, 2007).

7. Carballo M, Smajkic A, Zeric D, et al. Mental Health and Coping with War Situation: The Case of Bosnia and Herzegovina. Cambridge, UK: Cambridge University Press, 2004.

8. Welsh J. Violations of human rights. Traumatic stress and the role of NGOs: The contribution of non-governmental organizations. In Yael D, Rodley NS, Weisaeth L (eds.). International Responses to Traumatic Stress. New York: Baywood Publishing Company, 1996.

9. Komproe IH. Closing the gap between psychiatric epidemiology and mental health in post-conflict situations. Lancet 2002;359:1793–1794.

10. Mollica RF. Healing Invisible Wounds: Paths to Hope and Recovery in a Violent World. Orlando, FL: Harcourt, Inc., 2006.

11. Waters H, Garrett B, Burnham G. Rehabilitating Health Systems in Post-conflict Situations. Paper prepared for the Making Peace Work conference, Helsinki, Finland, June 4–5, 2004.

12. MedAct. Challenging Barriers to Health: Enduring Effects of War—Health in Iraq 2004. London: MedAct, 2004.

13. World Health Organization. Liberia: Providing assistance and promoting preparedness. 2006 HAC Forum. Available at: http://www.who.int (accessed June 22, 2007).

14. Physicians for Human Rights. An Action Plan to Prevent Brain Drain: Building Equitable Health Systems in Africa. Boston, PHR, July 2004.

15. Physicians for Human Rights. Women's health and human rights in Afghanistan, 2001. Available at: http://www.physiciansforhumanrights.org/library/news-2001–01–01.html (accessed June 22, 2007).

16. United Nations Committee on Economic, Social, and Cultural Rights (UN CESCR). General Comment 14: The Right to the Highest Attainable Standard of Health. Geneva: UN CESCR, August 11, 2000.

17. Maiese M. The damage caused by war. Available at: http://www.beyondintractability.org/essay/reconstructive_programs/?nid=1385 (accessed June 22, 2007).

18. Physicians for Human Rights. Annual Report 1999. Available at: http://www.physicansforhumanrights.org/about/annual-report/pdf/ar99_complete.pdf (accessed June 22, 2007).

19. Disarmament, Demobilization and Reintegration (DDR). Available at: http://www.womenwarpeace.org/issues/ddr/ddr.htm (accessed June 22, 2007).

20. United Nations Development Program. Post-conflict Reconstruction of Communities and Socio-economic Development. UNDP issue paper prepared for the TICAD Conference on Consolidation of Peace, Addis Ababa, Ethiopia, February 16–17, 2006. Available at: http://www.ticad.net/documents/issuepaper.doc (accessed July 11, 2007).

21. Slim H. A Call to Arms: Humanitarian Action and the Art of War. Geneva: Center for Humanitarian Dialogue, 2004.

22. Lerner S. Excerpt from Preface of the Peru Truth and Reconciliation Commission. Available at http://www.cverdad.org.pe/ifinal/pdf/TOMO%20I/PREFACIO.pdf (in Spanish) (accessed July 18, 2007).

23. Kelman H. Social psychological dimensions of international conflict. In Zantman W, Rusmussen JL (eds.). Peacemaking in International Conflict: Methods and Techniques. Washington DC: USIP Press, 1997.

24. International Criminal Court. Rome Statute. Available at: http://www.un.org/law/icc/index.html (accessed July 11, 2007).

25. Brody R. Justice: The First Casualty of Truth? Available at: http://hrw.org/editorials/2001/justice0430.htm (accessed June 22, 2007).
26. REDRESS. Seeking reparation for torture survivors. Reparation for torture in Iraq in the context of transitional justice: Ensuring justice for victims and preventing future violations. Discussion paper. Available at: http://www.redress.org/publications/Iraq_en.pdf (accessed June 22, 2007).
27. Dyfan I. Cited in Issue Brief on Justice, U.N. Development Fund for Women (document covers obstacles to women's seeking and gaining justice that remain despite strides made by ICTY and ICTR). Available at: http://www.womenwarpeace.org/issues/justice/justice.htm (accessed June 22, 2007).
28. Steiner HJ, Alston P. International Human Rights in Context: Law, Politics, Morals. New York: Oxford University Press, 2000.
29. Mkhize H. Truth Commissions: Actors in the reconciliation process. Paper presented at the XXIX Round Table on Justice and Reconciliation: An Integrated Approach, Sanremo, Italy, September 7–9, 2006.
30. Minow M (ed.). Between Vengeance and Forgiveness: Facing History after Genocide and Mass Violence. Boston: Beacon Press, 1998.
31. Shaw R. Rethinking Truth and Reconciliation Commissions: Lessons from Sierra Leone. (USIP Special Report #130). Washington, DC: USIP, 2005.
32. Minow M, paraphrasing comments by Lawrence Wechsler. In Minow M (ed.). Between Vengeance and Forgiveness: Facing History after Genocide and Mass Violence. Boston: Beacon Press, 1998.
33. Foley MW. Memory, forgiveness and reconciliation: Confronting the violence of history: Report on a conference at the Institute on Conflict Resolution and Ethnic Conflict, Catholic University of America, April 23–26, 1999.
34. Keough ME, Simmons T, Samuels M. Missing persons in post-conflict settings: Best practices for integrating psychosocial and scientific approaches. J R Soc Health 2004;124:271–275.
35. International Commission on Missing Persons. About ICMP: Overview. Available at: http://www.ic-mp.org/home.php?act=icmp (accessed July 11, 2007).
36. U.N. General Assembly. Resolution 47/133. Declaration on the Protection of All Persons from Enforced Disappearances. Article 18(1). December 18, 1992. Available at: http://www.un.org (accessed June 22, 2007).
37. Keough ME, Kahn S, Andrejevic A. Disclosing the truth: Informed participation in the ante-mortem database project for survivors of Srebrenica. Health Hum Rights 2000;5:68–87.
38. Stover E, Shigekane R. Exhumation of mass graves: Balancing legal and humanitarian needs. In Stover E, Weinstein HM (eds.). My Neighbor, My Enemy: Justice and Community in the Aftermath of Mass Atrocity. Cambridge, UK: Cambridge University Press, 2004.
39. Stover E, Shigekane, R. The missing in the aftermath of war: When do the needs of victims' families and international war crimes tribunals clash. Int Rev Red Cross 2002; 84:845–865.
40. International Committee of the Red Cross. The Missing and their Families: Documents of Reference. Geneva, Switzerland: February, 2004.
41. Sirkin S, Kern B, Dutli MT. Panel on Resolving the Problem of People Unaccounted For As a Result of Armed Conflict or Other Situations of Violence: Important Element in an Integrated Strategy. Held at the XXIX Round Table on Justice and Reconciliation: An Integrated Approach, Sanremo, Italy, September 7–9, 2006.

26

Peacemaking in the Aftermath of Disasters

Michael Renner

The Indian Ocean tsunami of December 2004, Hurricane Katrina in August 2005, and the massive earthquake in northern Pakistan and Kashmir in October 2005 have etched into the human psyche the extraordinary destructive power that nature is capable of unleashing. These megadisasters are not aberrations, as a database maintained by the Center for Research on the Epidemiology of Disasters (CRED) in Belgium shows. Over the past 25 years, the number of natural disasters—events in which at least 10 deaths occurred, at least 100 people were affected, or the area was declared a state of emergency or required international assistance—has increased steadily, from about 1,000 in the 1987–1991 period to more than 1,900 in the 2002–2006 period. The number of people affected by natural disasters—those injured, made homeless, or otherwise requiring immediate assistance—also rose, from an average of 209 million per year in 1987–1996 to 231 million per year in 1997–2006.[1]

Powerful natural disasters impose immense human suffering and huge economic costs. But they can also have a powerful influence—positive or negative—on political developments in affected countries.

On the one hand, disasters may trigger fresh conflict or further complicate complex political situations. An inept response by the authorities may invigorate political opposition. Fault lines may deepen between rich and poor, between urban and rural areas, and among ethnic groups. If relief aid and reconstruction end up accentuating social and economic inequalities or inflaming grievances, then they may well cause fresh disputes.

On the other hand, by triggering an outpouring of sympathy and by introducing new conditions and dynamics, disasters can also generate unprecedented opportunities to bring long-running conflicts to an end. The shared grief and the need to cooperate in the face of overwhelming destruction and hardship may provide the spark necessary for overcoming distrust and political divides. Such instances might be called "disaster diplomacy"[2] or humanitarian peacemaking.

In a range of cases, disasters and conflicts have intersected, with a variety of outcomes. Consider the following examples:[3]

- In August 1970, the slow and indifferent response by Pakistan's military government to catastrophic floods in what was then the eastern province of Pakistan gave an added jolt to demands for political autonomy. Islamabad's repressive response soon provoked a war for secession that succeeded in making Bangladesh independent in December 1971.
- In December 1972, Nicaragua's capital, Managua, was devastated by an earthquake. After Dictator Anastasio Somoza Debayle embezzled international reconstruction aid, unrest grew amid deteriorating economic conditions, leading to his eventual overthrow by the Sandinista National Liberation Front in 1979.
- In 1999, a series of powerful earthquakes shook Turkey and Greece, which had long been hostile to each other. The quakes elicited a surprising degree of mutual assistance and an outpouring of goodwill between the two countries. This impromptu cooperation facilitated steps to improve overall political relations between them.

This chapter examines the long-raging civil conflicts in Sri Lanka and Aceh (Indonesia) and the changed dynamics in both locations during the aftermath of the December 2004 tsunami. Both areas suffered large numbers of dead and displaced people as a result of the disaster, rivaling or surpassing what many years of violent conflict had wrought. These two situations are instructive, in part because of the almost opposite outcomes thus far: In Aceh, a peace agreement was struck; yet in Sri Lanka, initial euphoria quickly gave way to new quarrels and, about 1 year after the tsunami, the resumption of hostilities.

Challenges and Opportunities in the Aftermath of Disasters

Natural disasters, both rapid-onset events such as storms and floods and slow-onset ones such as droughts, can undermine livelihoods and compromise human security. Such impacts occur in the form of destroyed dwellings; loss of critical physical infrastructure; severe damage to industries, fisheries, and agriculture; job loss; and epidemics of disease. Although some adverse effects are temporary, others involve long-term compromise of habitability in or economic viability of an affected area. The outcome is determined not only by the severity of the disaster but also by (1) the timeliness and adequacy of relief and rebuilding programs and (2) the degree of resilience in affected communities and societies.

Disasters often exact a heavy economic toll. In poorer countries, they may obliterate hard-won social gains and sharpen the problems of indebtedness, poverty, and unemployment. Losses of $2 billion from a 2001 earthquake in El Salvador, for example, were equivalent to 15 percent of the gross domestic product.[4]

Economic and ecological marginalization worsen the impacts on the poor and on ethnic minorities. A disproportionate number of the world's poor live on the frontline of exposure to disasters. Countries with low human development account for 53 percent of all recorded deaths from disasters, even though they are home to only 11 percent of the people exposed to natural hazards worldwide.[4] In urban areas, the poor contend with precarious housing in slums. In rural areas, inequitable land distribution means that small farmers are often forced onto steep hillsides, where they are much more vulnerable to massive erosion and landslides.

Aside from adverse impacts on livelihoods, the human response to disasters may well reinforce socioeconomic inequities and lead to societal conflicts by increasing discontent and polarization. As examples:

- Disputes may erupt over the proper compensation for land, buildings, and other property. A disaster may alter the physical landscape so fundamentally that it becomes almost impossible to identify property lines and other boundaries or to adjudicate property disputes. Where a disaster wipes out public records such as identification cards, birth and marriage certificates, and property titles, people cannot easily prove their identity or property ownership.
- In divided societies, conflict may arise if relief and reconstruction aid is wielded as a tool for dispensing favors to one community over another or for tightening the government's political control. Competitive relief efforts involving opposing forces in a civil war situation may reinforce, rather than surmount, distrust.
- Conflicts may ensue if resettlement and reconstruction are driven forward without proper consultation with affected communities and protection of their rights.

- Finally, populations displaced by disaster may not be welcome elsewhere and could be seen as competitors for scarce land, water, jobs, and social services, especially in countries that are already confronting social, economic, environmental, or political stress.

Disasters may thus generate new storm clouds. But by dramatically reshaping the societal landscape, disasters may also entail a silver lining—transforming armed conflicts in ways that generate fresh opportunities to bring them to an end. A disaster may create suffering that cuts across the divides of conflict, prompting common relief needs and interests. The destruction wrought by a disaster may be of such a large scale that reconstruction can only proceed by striking a ceasefire or negotiating a peace agreement. Cooperative relief and reconstruction can lay the basis for greater trust and aid the emergence of a new political dynamic that is able to sustain broader peacemaking efforts.

Whereas a corrupt or indifferent government response is likely to stoke popular resentment, competent and fair disaster relief can tremendously improve a government's image in the eyes of populations that are demanding greater autonomy or independence, easing existing resentments and perhaps paving the way for a more serious dialogue to address grievances.

Whether such peacemaking opportunities are realized depends strongly on the sincerity and commitment of a country's political leadership. And peacemaking, in order to succeed, needs to consider the interests and motivations of various actors. If opposition parties or other important segments of society are left out of a peacemaking stratagem, they may well see political benefit in thwarting such efforts.

The role of the military is especially critical. Post-disaster relief efforts usually rely heavily on the armed forces, due to their unparalleled manpower and logistical capacities. But this is the same institution that is typically the very instrument of oppression in countries plagued by civil wars. Indeed, a government embroiled in civil war may be tempted to turn tragedy into military advantage, subjecting a rebellious area to renewed central government control. Or the military leadership may pursue interests and agendas in contradiction to the wishes of the civilian leadership.

Large-scale natural calamities usually trigger humanitarian assistance efforts by the United Nations, donor nations' aid agencies, and many nongovernmental organizations (NGOs). The influx of many foreigners, accompanied by intense (although typically short-lived) global media interest, turns the spotlight on a war-torn area that may previously have been ignored or even off-limits to outsiders. These circumstances offer an opportunity for enhancing transparency and reducing the likelihood of continued violence and human rights abuses.

Outsiders may indeed need to play an assertive role in encouraging and cajoling the warring parties to resolve their conflict or at least adopt a ceasefire. International donors are likely to insist that the protagonists undertake concrete steps toward that end, so that emergency aid can be delivered and reconstruction efforts are not ultimately in vain. In the longer term, a key challenge is overcoming the resistance of those who benefit, politically or materially, from the continuation of conflict and who therefore might seek to torpedo efforts at conflict resolution.

Aceh: Lasting Peace within Reach

The December 2004 tsunami that devastated Aceh also kick-started negotiations to end a conflict that has lasted for almost 30 years (Table 26-1). After

Table 26-1. Impacts of the Civil War and the 2004 Tsunami on Aceh

	Numbers of People
Aceh population (2003 census)	4,200,000
Civil War Impacts	
Killed	At least 15,000
Displaced after 1999	500,000–700,000
Displaced in 2003-2004	125,000–150,000*
Tsunami Impacts	
Killed	131,000
Missing	37,000
Displaced or homeless:	
Initial estimates	500,000–1,000,000
Remaining (August 2005)	>500,000
Damaged and destroyed houses	116,800

*These official government figures do not include those displaced outside of official refugee camps or those who fled Aceh. There was considerable fluctuation in the number of people displaced over time.

Sources: Indian Ocean Earthquake and Tsunami Emergency Update. Center for Excellence in Disaster Management and Humanitarian Assistance. September 18, 2005. Available at: http://www.coe-dmha.org/tsunami.htm (accessed June 22, 2007); Global IDP Project. Indonesia: Post-tsunami assistance risks neglecting reintegration needs of conflict-induced IDPs. May 26, 2005. Available at: http://www.reliefweb.int/rw/rwb.nsf/db900SID/SODA-6CS4QH?OpenDocument (accessed July 4, 2007); Internal Displacement Monitoring Centre. Between 500,000 and 700,000 people could have been displaced from Aceh since 1999 http://www.internal-displacement.org/idmc/website/countries.nsf/(httpEnvelopes)/799F41D75CDAE7A6802570B8005A73A4?OpenDocument (accessed July 4, 2007); United Nations High Commissioner for Refugees. 2004 Global Refugee Trends. Geneva: UNHCR, June 17, 2005; Katri Merikallio. Making Peace: Ahtisaari and Aceh (Porvoo, Finland: WS Bookwell Oy, 2006).

Aceh, which is located at the northern tip of Sumatra, was incorporated into the newly established Republic of Indonesia after World War II, a fundamental clash developed between Jakarta's insistence on strong central control and Acehnese longings for independence. Promises of special autonomy for the province remained unfulfilled. Rebellion broke out as early as 1953. The current conflict dates back to 1976, when the Free Aceh Movement (Gerakan Aceh Merdeka, or GAM) was founded with the express goal of secession.[5–7]

Aceh is rich in natural resources, including oil, natural gas, timber, and minerals. It provides 15 to 20 percent of Indonesia's oil and gas output.[8] But this wealth benefited mostly multinational companies and cronies of the long-reigning Suharto dictatorship. Aceh today remains one of Indonesia's poorest provinces. Unemployment is rampant, and more than 35 percent of the population lives below the poverty line—up from about 10 percent in 1996 and 20 percent in 1999.[6,9] In 2002, 48 percent of the population had no access to clean water, 36 percent of children younger than 5 years of age were undernourished, and 38 percent of the population had no access to health facilities.[10]

Excessive political centralization and unjust exploitation of Aceh's natural resources lay at the heart of the conflict. Military repression, massive human rights violations, and a high degree of impunity enjoyed by the security forces additionally fueled Acehnese resentment. With membership surging in the late 1980s and 1990s, GAM came to pose an increasingly serious challenge to Jakarta.[6,7]

The Indonesian military had long been opposed to resolving the Aceh conflict through negotiations and had sometimes appeared to undermine the fledgling peace efforts that were undertaken between 2000 and 2003. Economic interests explain this attitude. Since the 1950s, the business dealings of the security forces had grown substantially in all of Indonesia. Profits from legal and illegal ventures supplemented the official defense budget and enriched military and police commanders. Some elements of the military in Aceh were involved in marijuana production and trafficking, prostitution, and pervasive extortion of individuals and businesses.[5] One of the most lucrative sources of income for the military and police was their involvement in illegal logging. Conflict was a convenient cover for plundering the region's natural resources, and elements of the security forces did not shy away from orchestrating violence to justify a continued military presence in Aceh.[11,12]

The humanitarian emergency triggered by the tsunami provided a critical opportunity for change in Aceh—prying the province, which was under martial law, open to international scrutiny; promising an end to the human rights violations by the security forces; and offering an avenue for ending the conflict. Although civilian and military hardliners were pressing to bar foreign relief personnel from Aceh, the huge scale of the catastrophe made the need for massive international assistance irrefutable (Figure 26-1).

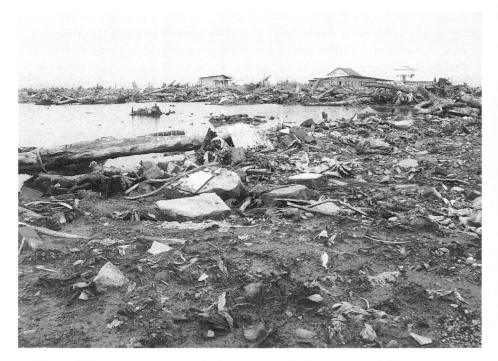

Figure 26-1. Devastation in Aceh after the tsunami. (Photograph by Michael Renner.)

The tsunami shifted the political dynamic quite decisively. As Richard Baker of the East–West Center explained: "It provided a powerful and catalyzing shock; it produced a focus on common goals of relief, recovery and reconstruction; and it brought increased international attention."[13] With the eyes of the world trained on Aceh, government officials and rebels were anxious to seize the moral high ground and not to be seen as sabotaging the peace process.

President Susilo Bambang Yudhoyono came to power in 2004 committed to resolving the Aceh conflict. His government saw an opportunity to repair Indonesia's international credibility, sullied by endemic corruption and the military's reputation for brutality. For their part, the rebels had suffered significant military setbacks during martial law, and they realized that negotiations were the only way to gain international legitimacy for their struggle.[14] While not making aid directly conditional on conflict resolution, several donors, including Germany and Japan, made it clear to both sides that they expected progress in the peace negotiations so that reconstruction could proceed unimpeded.[15]

From January to July 2005, five rounds of peace negotiations took place in Helsinki, mediated by former Finnish President Martti Ahtisaari. Low-level violence between the Indonesian army and GAM continued throughout the talks but did not derail them. Once GAM dropped its demand for Aceh independence in favor of autonomy, an agreement (officially called the Memorandum of Understanding, or MOU) was reached fairly quickly and was signed in August. Table 26-2 summarizes its major provisions.

Table 26-2. Key Provisions of the Aceh Peace Agreement and Status of Each, as of June 2007

Human rights	• A Human Rights Court and a Commission for Truth and Reconciliation will be established. *(Not implemented)*
Amnesty	• Free Aceh Movement (Gerakan Aceh Merdeka, GAM) members receive amnesty and political prisoners will be released. *(Fulfilled)*
Reintegration	• Former combatants, pardoned prisoners, and affected civilians are to receive farmland, jobs, or other compensation. *(In February 2006, Aceh Reintegration Agency BRA declared more than 20,000 people eligible for assistance, but disputes are continuing.)*
Security	• GAM is to demobilize its 3,000 fighters and relinquish 840 weapons between September 15 and December 31, 2005. *(Fulfilled)* • Simultaneously, nonlocal government military forces are to be reduced to 14,700 and nonlocal police forces to 9,100. *(Fulfilled)*
Political participation	• Free and fair elections are to be held in April 2006 (for Aceh governor) and in 2009 (for Aceh legislature). *(Gubernatorial elections were postponed to December 2006)* • The government is to facilitate the establishment of local political parties (by amending the national election law) no later than January 2007. *(New Aceh Governing Law passed in July 2006)*
Economy	• Aceh is entitled to retain 70 percent of its natural resource revenues. *(It remains to be seen how fully this will be implemented.)* • GAM representatives will participate in the post-tsunami Reconstruction and Rehabilitation Commission. *(Fulfilled)*
Monitoring	• The European Union and the Association of South East Asian Nations (ASEAN) contributing countries establish an Aceh Monitoring Mission (AMM). It will monitor human rights, demobilization, disarmament, and reintegration progress and will rule on disputes. *(Fulfilled; AMM mandate ended in December 2006)*

Sources: Crisis Management Initiative. Memorandum of Understanding between the Government of the Republic of Indonesia and the Free Aceh Movement. August 15, 2005. Available at: http://www.cmi.fi/?content=aceh_project (accessed June 22, 2007); Renner M. Unexpected Promise: Disaster Creates an Opening for Peace in a Conflict-riven Land. World Watch, November/December 2006; Renner M, Chafe Z. Beyond Disasters: Creating Opportunities for Peace. Worldwatch Institute, June 2007.

The initial phase of the peace process was implemented very smoothly. GAM fighters turned in their weapons, and the government sharply reduced its military and police forces in Aceh. The next phase, focused on democratization and the political process, was more difficult. A new governing law for Aceh was to incorporate key provisions of the MOU and lead the province to greater self-government. Contentious issues concerned the creation of provincial-level political parties (an exception from Indonesian law, which requires all parties to have offices in at least half the country's provinces), the question of whether independent candidates should be allowed to run for office, and the establishment of the Human Rights Court.[16] There is a strong need to establish accountability for past human rights violations. A March 2006 poll found that half of the Acehnese people remain worried about arbitrary arrests by security forces.[17]

Legislation submitted by the Indonesian president to parliament was much weaker than the initial draft law that emerged from public consultations within Aceh. Parliamentary deliberations, in turn, were marked by a "tug of war" between those who felt that the Acehnese needed to be given a strong stake in peace and those who were virulently opposed to anything that could be seen as a concession to Acehnese demands.[16] Parliament missed the original March 2006 deadline. When it finally passed the law in July, many Acehnese were unhappy about some of its provisions, particularly with regard to central government powers, the role of the military, and the lack of accountability for past human rights violations.[18] However, these complaints did not derail the peace process. A few months later, the December 2006 elections were a crucial next step toward consolidating peace. They swept a former GAM leader, Yusuf Irwandi, into the governor's mansion in Banda Aceh. By all accounts a capable leader, Yusuf faces a range of tough political and economic challenges.[19]

Ultimately, the peace deal will need to deliver tangible benefits to both members of GAM and anti-GAM militias, many of whom are unskilled and unemployed young men. As of May 2006, Aceh's unemployment rate stood at 27 percent. In order to provide livelihoods that can sustain peace, the economy will need to undergo a transition, not only from short-term emergency aid to long-term recovery and from demobilization to reintegration of combatants into society, but also from the unsustainable exploitation of natural resources to a broader mix of economic activities.

The needs of survivors of both the conflict and the tsunami must be addressed; already this is a source of resentment, because those displaced by the conflict feel that they have received far less support than those hurt by the tsunami. Rebuilding has progressed slowly and has been plagued by corruption and by failure, in many cases, to consult with affected communities.[20] Of 141,000 new houses needed, only 57,000 had been built 2 years after the tsunami.[21] In March 2006, some 10,000 of the new houses were revealed to be of such poor quality that they needed major additional work.[22]

Peace in Aceh is not yet irreversible, and reconstruction has a long way to go. Yet the province nevertheless has an excellent chance to emerge from the long decades of war and repression.

Sri Lanka: Back to War

Even though Sri Lanka, like Aceh, was plagued by a long civil war and was hit by the same disaster, its post-disaster experience was dramatically different. Until a fragile ceasefire was reached in February 2002, Sri Lanka had been tormented by armed conflict since 1983 (Table 26-3). The conflict had its origins in the 1950s, when assertive Sinhala nationalism translated into language and education policies that discriminated against the country's minority Tamils. Until the early 1970s, Tamil leaders responded by pressing for equal rights and autonomy in the largely Tamil-speaking regions of the north and east. But government administrations led by the main Sinhala political

Table 26-3. Impacts of the Civil War and the 2004 Tsunami on Sri Lanka

	Numbers of People
Sri Lanka Population (2004)	19,600,000
Civil War Impacts	
Killed or missing, 1983-2002	81,000
Killed, January 2006-June 2007	5,800
Displaced, at peak	800,000
Still displaced, as of January 2006	321,742*
Newly Displaced, 2006-2007	302,000
Tsunami Impacts	
Killed or missing	35,322
Displaced, May 2005	511,428
Remaining displaced, late 2006	325,000
Damaged and destroyed houses	105,000

*In addition to 124,800 refugees abroad.

Sources: United Nations High Commissioner for Refugees, Sri Lanka Office. Statistical Summaries of New Displacement. Available at: www.unhcr.lk/statistics/index.html (accessed July 4, 2007); Reconstruction and Development Agency. Progress Report of Housing. February 2007. Available at: http://www.rada.gov.lk/portal/resources/_housing/Feb%202007%20Final.pdf; Internal Displacement Monitoring Centre. Escalation of Conflict Leaves Tens of Thousands of IDPs Without Protection and Assistance. November 2006. Available at: http://www.internal-displacement.org/8025708F004CE90B/(httpCountrySummaries)/6CB0B70A99B5EA22C125721F00348545?OpenDocument&count=10000; South Asia Terrorism Portal. Casualties of Terrorist Violence in Sri Lanka since March 2000. Available at: http://www.satp.org/satporgtp/countries/shrilanka/database/annual_casualties.htm (accessed July 4, 2007).

parties—the United National Party (UNP) and the Sri Lanka Freedom Party (SLFP)—repeatedly reneged on agreements. And when either party was in the opposition, it stirred up Sinhala passions to thwart compromise. This resulted in growing radicalization among Tamils, the emergence of the hardline Liberation Tigers of Tamil Eelam (LTTE), and the outbreak of open civil war.[23–25]

By the time the 2002 ceasefire was reached with the aid of Norwegian mediation, both sides had fought each other to a standstill, suffered desertions, and faced growing public demands for peace. Still, despite initial enthusiasm, peace negotiations stalled, and the LTTE broke off the talks in April 2003 after it was excluded from an international donors meeting.[25]

The underlying factors that contributed to the conflict were left in place. Although the resulting "no war, no peace" situation ended large-scale military violence, it failed to prevent high levels of political violence, and it left human rights concerns unaddressed. [26]

Post-ceasefire economics had largely adverse effects as well. Reconstruction funding was limited in the northeast of the country, controlled by the Tamils. Meanwhile, macroeconomic reforms in the south, controlled by Sinhala, brought hardships for the poor, producing the opposite of an expected peace dividend. [26]

Another key problem inherent in the 2002 ceasefire was that it narrowly focused on a deal between the two main actors, the main governing party and the LTTE. But the dividing lines are at times blurred, and there is much dissent and even violence *within* the Sinhala and Tamil communities. Sri Lankan Muslims, meanwhile, have not only been caught in the middle of the conflict but have also been sidelined in negotiations, leading to growing radicalization among them. The Sinhala-nationalist Janatha Vimukhti Peramuna party (JVP, or People's Liberation Front) and the Buddhist clergy have repeatedly acted as spoilers against peace.[25,26] By the time the tsunami struck, the political infighting had intensified so much that resumption of war had become a dreaded expectation. It took nature's fury to give the foes a shared challenge and revive interest in peacemaking.

Indeed, the immediate aftermath of the tsunami was marked by a groundswell of solidarity, with many spontaneous acts of empathy across the conflict's dividing lines. An array of political and religious leaders called for national unity, and public opinion became strongly inclined toward reconciliation. On the ground, the disaster led to the closest cooperation since the ceasefire was signed, with soldiers from both sides working together to repair roads and distribute relief aid. There was considerable hope that the tsunami could be a catalyst for reinvigorating the peace process.[27–28]

But the basic rifts re-emerged before long. A report compiled for the British government noted: "Though the tsunami itself did bring people together, the *response* reflected and accentuated pre-existing tensions. Like the peace process itself, the tsunami response heightened the political and economic stakes."[26]

Both the government and the LTTE saw the tsunami as an opportunity to strengthen their legitimacy. Post-tsunami aid politics became increasingly ethnicized and deepened political fault lines.[26] Whereas the Tamils felt largely excluded, people in the south perceived that the northeast was receiving a disproportionate share of aid.[29]

International donors demanded a "joint mechanism" for the equitable distribution of $3 billion in international relief and reconstruction aid pledges. A deal was also regarded as a confidence-building tool that could reinvigorate the deadlocked peace process. After months of wrangling, the government and LTTE finally agreed on the Post-Tsunami Operational Management Structure (P-TOMS) in June 2005. Under the pact, a panel comprising government officials, rebels, and representatives of Muslim communities would recommend, prioritize, and monitor aid projects in six affected regions in the north and east.[30,31]

But the JVP, a partner in the coalition government and the third-largest party in parliament, vehemently opposed P-TOMS as a measure that would legitimize the LTTE and help it carve out a separate state. The JVP withdrew from the government coalition in protest.[30,32] In response to a complaint brought by the JVP, arguing that the aid-sharing deal was unconstitutional, Sri Lanka's Supreme Court temporarily suspended the deal in July 2005.[33,34] Presidential elections in November 2005 brought further complications. Promising to redraft the ceasefire agreement with the LTTE and to scrap P-TOMS, Mahinda Rajapakse won with the support of the JVP and the Buddhist hardline party Jathika Hela Urumaya (JHU). Tensions between the government and the LTTE rose immediately. In the eastern part of the country, a shadow war had already been raging ever since a renegade faction of the Tamil Tiger rebels broke away in March 2004. (The LTTE accuses the government of using the breakaway group as a proxy force.) Political killings rose sharply after the elections, giving rise to renewed worries that full-scale conflict might resume.

New talks to save the increasingly fragile 2002 ceasefire, held in February 2006 in Geneva, temporarily calmed the situation. But in an act of political brinkmanship, the LTTE refused to attend a second round of talks scheduled for late April 2006.[35] The months since then have been marked by escalating violence. Fresh peace talks were held in Geneva in late October 2006 but also ended in failure.[36] Close to 5,800 people died in the renewed fighting between January 2006 and June 2007.[37] Although both the government and the LTTE maintain that they are still honoring the 2002 ceasefire, their actions are no longer guided by such constraints. The government appears to believe that it can resolve the conflict through military victory, and the LTTE seems to welcome the renewed confrontation.

Emerging Lessons

Humanitarian action in the aftermath of natural disasters can be a powerful catalyst for transforming conflict dynamics, providing the impetus needed for overcoming deep human divides and jump-starting peace efforts. But a rush of post-disaster goodwill alone is unlikely to carry warring factions through the complexities and stumbling blocks of a peace process. In order to maintain momentum in post-disaster peacemaking initiatives, humanitarianism needs to translate into political change—addressing the root causes of the conflict at hand, putting in place confidence-building measures, and taking on the vested interests of those who benefit from a continuation of conflict.

Both war-affected and disaster-ravaged populations need comprehensive assistance. It makes sense to blend their needs into a comprehensive program. Broad, community-based reconstruction efforts benefit war-displaced individuals and ex-combatants as well as the general population if they provide housing, infrastructure, vocational skills, and jobs in a timely and nondiscriminatory manner. Conversely, measures to deal with postconflict issues are also of importance to the population at large: Weapons collection reduces the level of lawlessness, and efforts to locate and collect antipersonnel landmines enable areas that were once populated and fertile to become accessible again.

Better coordination among the various actors is needed with regard to post-disaster humanitarian, reconstruction, environmental restoration, economic development, and postconflict disarmament efforts. Such coordinated action is critical to reduce the likelihood of recurring conflict and to minimize vulnerability to future disasters. Yet, all too often, concerned agencies and organizations operate in parallel spheres, with inadequate communication or collaboration. They often have different agendas, constituencies, operational cultures, and time horizons, and they may well compete for funding, visibility, and influence.

To date, more opportunities for disaster-related peacemaking have been missed than grasped. A 2004 report by the United Nations Development Program concluded that, on a global scale, "Little or no attention has been paid to the potential of disaster management as a tool for conflict prevention initiatives."[4]

Post-disaster peacemaking requires adequate funding. Large-scale aid flows can, in principle, serve as an economic incentive for peace. Yet that very inflow also presents a tempting target for embezzlement in corrupt countries.

As developments in Sri Lanka have shown, aid flows can trigger political infighting that slows or prevents delivery of assistance to victims and may even endanger peacemaking. [26]

International donors are mistaken if they simply assume that economic incentives can override political imperatives and calculations of the parties to conflict. Although economics is undoubtedly critical to making peace, it alone is not a substitute for a politics of peace. Disaster diplomacy and humanitarian peacemaking require active, yet careful, engagement by the international community.

References

1. Center for Research on the Epidemiology of Disasters (EM-DAT): The OFDA/ CRED International Disaster Database, continuously updated. Available at: http:// www.em-dat.net (accessed June 22, 2007).

2. Disaster Diplomacy. Available at: http://www.disasterdiplomacy.org (accessed June 22, 2007).

3. Renner M, Chafe Z. Turning disasters into peacemaking opportunities. In World-watch Institute. State of the World 2006. New York: WW Norton & Co., 2006.

4. United Nations Development Program. Reducing Disaster Risk: A Challenge for Development. New York: UNDP, 2004.

5. McCulloch L. Aceh: Then and Now. London: Minority Rights Group International, May 2005.

6. Sukma R. Security Operations in Aceh: Goals, Consequences and Lessons. Washington, DC: East–West Center, 2004.

7. Schulze KE. The Free Aceh Movement (GAM): Anatomy of a Separatist Organization. Washington, DC: East–West Center, 2004.

8. Arie K. Crisis Profile: Deadlock in Indonesia's Aceh Conflict. Reuters AlertNet, February 22, 2005. Available at: http://www.alertnet.org/thenews/photoalbum/1109081433 .htm (accessed June 22, 2007).

9. World Bank, Aceh Public Expenditure Analysis. September 2006. Available at: http:// siteresources.worldbank.org/INTINDONESIA/Resources/Publication/280016–115287 0963030/APEA.pdf (accessed July 4, 2007).

10. Oxfam International. Targeting Poor People: Rebuilding Lives After the Tsunami. June 25, 2005. Available at: http://www.oxfam.org/en/files/bn050625_tsunami_targetingthe poor.pdf/download (accessed July 4, 2007).

11. Aceh: Ecological War Zone. Down to Earth, 47, November 2000.

12. Down to Earth, London. Aceh: Logging a Conflict Zone. October 2004. Available at: http://www.acheh-eye.org/data_files/english_format/ngo/ngo_eoa/ ngo_eoa_2004_10_00.html (accessed July 4, 2007).

13. Baker RW. Asian Insurgencies—Two Conflicts, Two Stories. East–West Wire, July 19, 2005. Available at: http://eastwestcenter.org/events-en-detail.asp?news_ID=290 (accessed June 22, 2007).

14. Rusli E. After Big Step Toward Aceh Peace, Still Many Hurdles to Overcome. International Herald Tribune, July 19, 2005.

15. Harvey R. Aceh Looks for a New Political Future. BBC News Online, March 21, 2005. Available at: http://news.bbc.co.uk/2/hi/asia-pacific/4368275.stm (accessed June 22, 2007).

16. International Crisis Group, Jakarta and Brussels. Aceh: Now for the Hard Part. March 29, 2006. Available at: http://www.crisisgroup.org/home/index.cfm?id=4049&1=1 (accessed June 22, 2007).

17. Aceh: Half of Acehnese Still Fear Security Arrest. Reuters, March 29, 2006. Available at: http://www.unpo.org/article.php?id=4126 (accessed July 4, 2007).

18. Perlez J. Aceh Says Indonesia Law Falls Far Short on Autonomy. International Herald Tribune, July 12, 2006.

19. International Crisis Group, Jakarta and Brussels. Indonesia: How GAM Won in Aceh. March 22, 2007. Available at: http://www.crisisgroup.org/home/index.cfm?id=4715 &l=1 (accessed July 4, 2007).

20. Eye on Aceh and Aid Watch. A People's Agenda? Post-Tsunami Aid in Aceh. February 2006. Available at: http://www.reliefweb.int/library/documents/2006/eoa-idn-28feb .pdf (accessed July 4, 2007).

21. Mydans S. Tsunami-Tossed City's Survivors Struggle to Carry On. New York Times, December 26, 2006.

22. Renner M. Unexpected promise: Disaster creates an opening for peace in a conflict-riven land. World Watch, November/December 2006.

23. Sri Lanka. In Human Rights Watch. Slaughter Among Neighbors: The Political Origins of Communal Violence. New Haven and London: Yale University Press, 1995.

24. Nissan E. Historical context. In Armon J, Philipson L (eds.). Accord Issue 4. Demanding Sacrifice: War and Negotiation in Sri Lanka. London: Conciliation Resources, August 1998. Available at: http:/www.c-r.org/our-work/accord/sri-lanka/index.php (accessed June 22, 2007).

25. Keenan A. No Peace, No War. Boston Review, Summer 2005. Available at: http://bostonreview.net/BR30.3/keenan.html (accessed June 22, 2007).

26. Goodhand J, et al. Aid, Conflict and Peacebuilding in Sri Lanka, 2000—2005. August 2005. Available at: http://www.asiafoundation.org/Locations/srilanka_ publications.html (accessed June 22, 2007).

27. Loganathan K. Scope and Limitations of Linking Post-Tsunami Reconstruction with Peace-Building. Colombo, Sri Lanka: Center for Policy Alternatives, February 10, 2005.

28. Rohde D. In Sri Lanka's Time of Agony, a Moment of Peace. New York Times, January 4, 2005.

29. Rohde D, Waldman A. Rival Political Factions Jockey for Power in Tsunami-Devastated Sri Lanka. New York Times, January 18, 2005.

30. Luthra D. Sri Lanka's Controversial Tsunami Deal. BBC News Online, June 24, 2005. Available at: http://news.bbc.co.uk/2/hi/south_asia/4619167.stm (accessed June 22, 2007).

31. Johnson J. Sri Lanka's Faltering Peace Process Gets Boost. Financial Times, June 24, 2005.

32. Marquand R. Crisis Lifts Sri Lankan Marxists. Christian Science Monitor, January 14, 2005.

33. Sri Lanka Suspends Tsunami Deal. BBC News Online, July 15, 2005. Available at: http://news.bbc.co.uk/2/hi/south_asia/4685291.stm (accessed June 22, 2007).

34. Sri Lanka's Supreme Court Postpones Hearing on Controversial Tsunami Aid Pact. Asia-Pacific Daily Report, Center for Excellence in Disaster Management and

Humanitarian Assistance, September 12, 2005. Available at: http://pdmin.coe-dmha.org/apdr/index.cfm?action=search (accessed June 22, 2007).

35. Luthra D. Sri Lanka—Talks or War? BBC News Online, April 19, 2006. Available at: http://news.bbc.co.uk/2/hi/south_asia/4918830.stm (accessed June 22, 2007).

36. Sri Lankan Talks End in Failure. BBC News Online, October 29, 2006. Available at: http://news.bbc.co.uk/2/hi/south_asia/6090866.stm (accessed June 22, 2007).

37. South Asia Terrorism Portal. Casualties of Terrorist Violence in Sri Lanka since March 2000. Available at: http://www.satp.org/satporgtp/countries/shrilanka/database/annual _casualties.htm (accessed July 4, 2007).

27

Educating Health Professionals on Peace and Human Rights

Neil Arya, Caecilie Böck Buhmann, and Klaus Melf

Education of health professionals over the years has been inadequate in prevention and public health, including the prevention of war and its public health consequences. Now, however, there is a growing movement to educate health professionals about mitigating the adverse consequences of war (and other forms of violence) and promoting peace and human rights.

Health professionals and students in the health professions have expressed the need for more knowledge and skills in promoting peace and human rights and in related subjects, such as global health and medical ethics.[1–3] Many medical students believe that war—and issues such as poverty, infectious disease, environmental pollution, and forced migration—will have a great impact on global health and desire education on these topics.[4–6] Major international organizations concur. For example, the United Nations General Assembly supports the teaching of peace in all types and at all levels of education.[7] And the World Medical Association supports mandatory training for physicians in medical ethics and human rights.[8] Nevertheless, teaching of these subjects has not been a high priority at medical, nursing, or public health schools.

Associations Among Violence, Social Determinants, and Ill Health

War and other forms of violence are risk factors for poor health. Poor health, however, can be a risk factor for war and other forms of violence. For example, a country that has an infant mortality rate greater than 100 per 1,000 live births is often at higher risk for war.[9] High mortality rates from infectious disease and/or malnutrition can decrease gross national product, increase rural-to-urban migration, increase competition for resources, decrease confidence in government leadership, deplete skilled administrators, and decrease capital investment—each of which may make a society more vulnerable to war.[10] At the societal level, the health consequences of war may be related to human rights violations, social injustice, and the destruction of ecosystems.

Addressing Deficits

In order to enable health professionals to promote peace and human rights—to understand complex issues and to help solve specific problems—deficits in their education in knowledge, skills, and values need to be addressed. Broader contextual issues also need to be understood. For example, medical students and physicians, with their orientation to a pathophysiological basis for disease, often cannot see linkages between the health of their immigrant, refugee, or impoverished patients and macrodeterminants of health, such as privatization of health care, criminalization of drug abuse, and promotion of the arms trade.

Knowledge deficits include concepts of peace, conflict, nonviolence, and, reconciliation; international human rights norms; and humanitarian law. Deficits in skills include the abilities to analyze conflicts, to use nonviolent communication, to act in a culturally sensitive manner, and to engage in conflict resolution, negotiation, and mediation. Deficits in values are obvious when health professionals become accomplices in inhuman acts ranging from human experimentation to torture of prisoners. Hierarchies among health workers may lead some to misuse their power and inadvertently cause violent acts against individuals or populations. Values that underlie medical ethics can help health professionals understand their responsibilities to not participate in, and to condemn, such violence.[11]

Learning from other disciplines, such as anthropology, sociology, and psychology, may help health professionals design conflict sensitive and culturally appropriate interventions to prevent violence and to foster individual and societal empowerment and resilience (the capacity to do well in difficult circumstances). These interventions can address various forms of violence, such as exploitative and repressive social structures, as well as domestic violence, child abuse, youth violence, and suicide.[12,13]

Recognizing Assets

Health professionals can be especially qualified to promote peace and human rights, but to do so, they need to apply their specific knowledge, skills, and values. In addition, health professionals must also be cautious that, in attempting to do good, they do not do harm (Box 27-1).

There is much useful knowledge in the traditional curricula of health professional schools that can be adapted to reducing the health consequences of war and promoting peace and human rights. This knowledge includes concepts of public health, especially principles of epidemiology, which can be applied to documenting the health consequences of war and economic sanctions and minimizing the adverse health effects of weapons on civilians. Such knowledge may be used to promote social change. Psychology and mental health concepts can provide an understanding of cycles of violence and the roles of depersonalization and psychic numbing in group violence and even genocide.[14] Systems analysis may enable health professionals to apply insights from health care to other sectors, such as international relations. These insights might include those derived from failures of medicine to develop ideal antibiotics; failures to understand and address social factors that contribute to causation of disease; and the tendency to focus much more on cure than on prevention.[15] Skills education of health professionals can be strengthened to enable them to assist communities to heal through health care and reconciliation activities that strengthen the social fabric. Health professionals can communicate knowledge and factual information to help counter oppressive governments, can help to personify "the enemy," and can engage in diplomacy. Values education of health professionals can also be strengthened to promote their altruism, empathy, compassion, and integrity—each of which increases their credibility and effectiveness.[16]

Health professionals can also be taught to develop superordinate goals and activities that warring parties may share. These goals transcend opposing sides in conflict. They may include, for example, goals and activities that promote the welfare of children and humanitarian ceasefires that can promote peace.

Existing Approaches to Education

There are a variety of approaches for teaching health professionals and students in the health professions about peace and human rights.

Box 27-1 Potential of Health and Development Work to Worsen Health and Safety

Neil Arya, Caecilie Böck Buhmann, and Klaus Melf

Health and development work, especially in the context of armed conflict, is often more complex than initially perceived. As a result, work that is initially perceived as beneficial to health can actually worsen the health and safety of the people it is meant to serve.[1]

Resource transfer in humanitarian and development assistance, such as after natural disasters, may distort local economic activities, lead to centralization of power and authority, and increase competition and suspicion, thereby worsening divisions among conflicting parties. Working with oppressive governments to provide medical assistance can strengthen and legitimize these regimes. By allying with groups fighting for their legitimate rights, health professionals can inadvertently support violence and prolong armed conflict. And health professionals' reliance on security personnel may imply that arms are necessary.

Bringing health professionals together in conflict zones, as in the Middle East and in the Balkans, has not always promoted peacebuilding.[2] Humanitarian ceasefires, in which health workers engage in activities to promote peace, can have the negative consequence of allowing parties to re-arm, as occurred in Sudan.[3,4] In the wake of the Rwandan genocide, Médecins Sans Frontières (MSF) withdrew from refugee camps in Goma, Zaire, when it learned that food distribution and medical aid had been commandeered by Hutu leaders who had participated in the genocide.

In weighing the pros and cons of health and development work in the context of armed conflict, health professionals must balance their responsibilities to their patients, to the institutions with which they are affiliated, and to society at large.[5]

References

1. Anderson MB. Do no harm: How aid can support peace or war. Boulder, CO: Lynne Rienner Publishers, 1999.
2. An open letter to the Palestianian and international community regarding Palestinian–Israel cooperation in health, June 2005. Available at: http://www.health-now.org/site/article.php?menuId=15&articleId=451 (accessed June 22, 2007).
3. Hendrickson D. Humanitarian action in protracted crisis: An overview of the debates and dilemmas. Disasters 1998;22:283–287.
4. Macrae J. The death of humanitarianism: Anatomy of the attack. Disasters 1998; 21:309–317.
5. Singh JA. American physicians and dual loyalty obligations in the "war on terror." BMC Medical Ethics 2003;4:4.

One approach is to teach these subjects in the context of international health. However, many schools do not teach international health. In addition, in 1993, although 61 percent of 70 medical schools in developed countries reported teaching international health, only 26 percent listed it as a separate curriculum entity.[17–19] Another approach is to use a Medicine and Human Rights framework to address subjects such as torture and other violations of civil and political rights. A broader framework of Health and Human Rights—not limited to individual patients—is used to teach about human rights violations from a public, or population-based, health perspective.[20] Subjects that can be studied in this framework include access to AIDS medications and the Health for All initiative of the World Health Organization (WHO). Medical ethics courses represent another approach to address these issues at both the macro and micro levels.

A Global Health framework focuses on socioeconomic and political factors that influence health.[21] A Social Medicine framework focuses on social determinants of health. An Ecosystem Health framework focuses on the relationship between human health and the biophysical, socioeconomic, and political environments. These three approaches are similar and complementary, but in a given context a particular approach may be more feasible or more popular.

Current Courses of Study

A broad range of courses of study based on these principles cover many of the topics mentioned. For example, the Netherlands affiliate (NVMP) of the International Physicians for the Prevention of Nuclear War (IPPNW) has organized a course at the Universities of Amsterdam and the Free University since 1992, which is now entitled, "Health and Issues of Peace and Conflict." Recently partnering with the International Federation of Medical Students' Associations (IFMSA), an umbrella group of more than 100 national medical students organizations with a deep interest in addressing medical education and global and public health issues, it plans to expand this course to all medical schools in the Netherlands. The course uses and adapts curricular materials such as those of "Medicine and Nuclear War," which was developed by IPPNW in the 1980s, and "Medicine and Peace," which was developed by the U. N. Commission on Disarmament Education, in cooperation with IPPNW and its U.S. affiliate, Physicians for Social Responsibility (PSR). At the University for the Basque region in Spain, where there has been a long history of violent conflict, a similar course is taught at a preclinical level.

The University College London has an Intercalated Bachelor of Science in International Health program. Students who are enrolled in an educational institution, such as a medical school, can earn a Bachelor of Science degree within 1 year. Many students in this program are enrolled in medical schools outside the United Kingdom. The program consists of modules inspired by the text *1x(66)Global Health Studies0x(66)* (now available free on the Internet),[21] which addresses the health effects of globalization, national debt, poverty, environmental degradation, armed conflict, and forced migration as well as concepts of human rights and humanitarian assistance. The Karolinska Institute in Sweden offers a course in International Health with components in both theory and practice, the latter of which must be taken in a low- or middle-income country.

Numerous U.S. institutions of higher education, including Harvard University, Johns Hopkins University, the University of California at Berkeley (UCB), and Emory University, use the Health and Human Rights framework, often as part of their master of public health programs or certificate courses. The first such course in the United States was developed in 1992 at Harvard. Both Harvard and Johns Hopkins offer week-long certificate courses in Health and Human Rights, the former of which has a public policy orientation. The UCB course focuses on all types of human rights—political and civil rights as well as economic, social, and cultural rights.

Students in the graduate certificate program of the Institute of Human Rights at Emory may focus on health. All students take a core course, which is cross-listed in several disciplines, including law, political science, and public health. Students may then take elective courses in such fields as "Health and Social Justice" and "Health and Human Rights." The Emory University School of Medicine offers second-year medical students a course entitled, "Human Rights, Social Medicine, and the Physician." This course, like other Social Medicine courses in the United States, focuses on individual responsibility and professional ethics.

As part of its Health as a Bridge for Peace (HBP) program, WHO organizes training sessions for health professionals and field workers that address peace-building, conflict resolution, and human rights. This training is designed to increase knowledge and to change attitudes and practice in zones of violent conflict. It is intended to encourage field workers to promote peace-building.[22]

The International Committee of the Red Cross (ICRC) has trained field workers, since 1986, in International Humanitarian Law and Human Rights as part of its Health Emergencies in Large Populations (HELP) program. Over time, these courses have been decentralized to several countries.

Médecins Sans Frontières (MSF) has begun to brief its delegates in the prevention of gender-based violence before sending them to work in refugee camps. The World Medical Association disseminates the international online course entitled "Doctors Working in Prison: Human Rights and Ethical Dilemmas," which was produced by the Norwegian Medical Association.[23]

Roles of Students

Students throughout the world continue to play a vital role in education for peace and human rights, arranging workshops, trainings, and guest lectures. They also exchange experiences and ideas for future educational programs in forums sponsored by IPPNW, IFMSA, and other organizations. In recent years, students have led IFMSA workshops on children and war, health and human rights, and refugee health and IPPNW workshops on Peace through Health, small-arms violence, and nuclear abolition. Both IFMSA and IPPNW arrange training in refugee camps on human rights combined with clinical rotations in hospitals and clinics in the same region.[24] Students have also arranged for exchange opportunities to learn about and engage in peace-related activities, through McMaster University and other educational institutions.

In 2001, a group of medical students established the IPPNW Nuclear Weapons Inheritance Project, which combines training and advocacy work on nuclear disarmament. It offers traditional training as well as role-playing exercises, practical experience, and apprenticeships. Training modules address nuclear disarmament, alternatives to nuclear weapons, dialogue technique, and health and human security[25].

Unifying the Discipline

The frameworks of Peace through Health and Medical Peace Work attempt to unify this training at the micro and macro levels, linking theory and understanding to action, advocacy, research, and field work. Peace through Health was designed to address how health workers could contribute to peace in actual or potential war zones.[26] Scholars, viewing war and other forms of violence as a social disease, have looked at a public health model of prevention for limiting the effects of violence. They attempt to incorporate all levels and types of peace work into a single framework, ranging from prevention of nuclear war to the impacts of globalization that limit human potential.[27] Thus, they see violence as being cyclical, with opportunities to reduce the risk of future violence.

Primary prevention reduces risk factors for war and strengthens factors that promote peace. Examples of primary prevention include peacekeeping, arms control, preventive diplomacy, and addressing root causes of violent conflict, such as poor governance and political corruption, human rights violations, economic and social inequalities, and community and cultural disintegration. Some people differentiate primary prevention (reducing risk factors for war) from primordial prevention (preventing these risk factors from developing).[28]

Both "top-down" and "bottom-up" approaches attempt to reduce these risk factors. The United Nations Development Program (UNDP) is responsible for coordinating global and national activities to promote the Millennium Development Goals,[29] which include reducing extreme poverty and hunger, increasing debt relief, ensuring that all children complete primary education, promoting gender equality, reducing childhood mortality, improving maternal health, reducing infectious diseases, ensuring environmental sustainability, providing safe drinking water, developing a global partnership for development, and promoting good governance. The People's Health Charter,[30] a "bottom-up" approach endorsed by many health organizations, considers health to be a fundamental human right, and inequality, poverty, exploitation, violence, and injustice to be the root causes of much morbidity and mortality among poor and marginalized people.

Secondary prevention, which can be implemented when war or violence is occurring, aims to stop further escalation of violence and to promote peaceful resolution of the conflict—termed by some as "peacemaking." Tertiary prevention, analogous to rehabilitation in medicine and ecological restoration in environmental work, consists of "peace-building," or reconciliation and reconstruction, after a war ends.

Some people envision and promote a health-based model of global security, with the primary responsibility of governments being to ensure the health and well-being of their nations' citizens. When governments fail to do this, the international community may be obliged to intervene.[31]

Courses in Peace through Health and Medical Peace Work

At McMaster University, a Peace through Health course was first offered in 2004 as an elective to third-year undergraduate students. It aims to enhance peace-building and reconciliation skills.[32] Students bring experience from various disciplines, such as Peace Studies, Health Studies, Drama, Language and Literature, and Engineering. The course involves group work and a group presentation of Peace through Health materials, some didactic teaching, and frequent guest lectures. Medical students at McMaster have developed their own problem-based elective course and an interactive online introduction to Peace through Health.[33]

The University of Tromsø in Norway first offered a graduate course on "Peace, Health, and Medical Work" in 2005, for students in medicine, other health professions, and social sciences. The course builds knowledge about human rights, global health, and disarmament as well as skills in nonviolent communication, intercultural understanding, advocacy, and media work. In addition, the Health Studies and the Peace and Conflict Studies programs at the University of Waterloo have together developed a full-credit undergraduate course in Peace through Health.[34] The course has now been made more modular and Web-based with videos, PowerPoint slides, articles, and links fully available on the Web in preparation for offering the course online and for distance education.

Course Design and Implementation

Course design and content vary for a number of reasons. Groups of students vary, from undergraduates in health sciences and humanities to students seeking a master's degree in public health, field workers, and medical specialists. Often, classes comprise students in a diverse mixture of disciplines. Some have experience with violent situations, poverty, or discrimination, and some have no such experience. Time available for courses varies, too. Some courses are elective, and others are core parts of the curriculum. Some are free, others are not. Some are for credit, others are not. Even the rigor expected of students and the requirements they must fulfill differs. And finally, the local context of courses varies. Therefore, it is impossible to develop a prototype course.

Getting these courses adopted by health professional schools, especially medical schools, requires an explanation of the health consequences of war and violence, enthusiastic support of students, dedicated faculty members, and relevant teaching materials.

Although didactic courses are popular, students seem to have greater appreciation for interactive courses and other educational experiences in which they are challenged to make decisions, learn practical skills, and participate in group activities and supervised field work. Students focus on a broad range of topics, including determinants of health, social justice, human rights norms, international law, and ethics.

It has often proved more effective to begin a course with a small group of students and allow for the subsequent evolution of demand and interest. New technologies may allow students who are geographically and culturally distant to obtain instruction in core ideas and some training more specific to their setting.

If education and training are designed to make professionals more knowledgeable, sensitive, and effective in promoting peace and human rights, courses should be evaluated in terms of both effectiveness and efficiency. Unfortunately, long-term and short-term outcomes are difficult to assess and to attribute to specific education. We are therefore left to assess such measures as students' career choices, social activism, and human rights knowledge or attitudes.

The Future

In order to continuously develop, the field of Peace through Health has a great need to build a community of researchers, academics, practitioners, and students and establish common points of reference among them.[35] Both Waterloo University and McMaster University are compiling Peace through Health resources, including course materials, case studies, evaluation tools, implementation strategies, and lists of reference materials on field work, research, and education.

Through the Medical Peace Work project,[36] several European medical peace organizations and educational institutions are strengthening the peace-health field by development and collection of teaching materials. They are producing an online multimedia course and teaching films, publishing a handbook, and developing a Web-based resource center that will include databases on courses, curricula, syllabi, presentations, film archives, educational research, and resource personnel.

In countries such as Bosnia, El Salvador, and Ecuador, there are movements within family medicine departments, medical schools, other university faculties, and communities to develop Peace through Health training, not just to study the impact of violence but also to reduce its impact and to strengthen mechanisms for social reconstruction. In Sri Lanka, the Faculty of Health Care Sciences in Batticaloa (Eastern University) has integrated a module in Peace Medicine into the mandatory training of nurses and physicians.

Education for health professionals worldwide in Peace and Human Rights is continuing to expand. We expect that mainstream medical curricula will increasingly incorporate these subjects. Use of new technology, new methods of teaching, and cross-disciplinary expertise will be important.

Acknowledgment: We thank Rob Chase, Andrew Pinto, Dabney Evans, and Joanna Santa Barbara for their review of this chapter, and Henk Groenewegen, Sonal Singh, Ed Mills, Aurora Bilbao, and Vince Iacopino for their descriptions of courses in which they have participated.

References

1. Mann JM. Medicine and Public Health, Ethics and Human Rights. Hastings Center Report 1997;27:6–13.
2. Leaning J. Human rights and medical education: Why every medical student should learn the Universal Declaration of Human Rights. BMJ 1997;315:1390–1391.
3. Rowson M. The why, where, and how of global health teaching. Student BMJ 2002; 10:215–258.

4. Melf K. Exploring Medical Peace Education and a Call for Peace Medicine. Master's Thesis. Center for Peace Studies, University of Tromsoe, Norway, 2004.
5. Bateman C, Baker T, Hoornenborg E, Ericsson U. Bringing global issues to medical teaching. Lancet 2001;358:1539–1542.
6. McMahon T, Arya N. Peace through Health. Student BMJ 2004;12:438.
7. United Nations Special Session on Disarmament, June 30, 1978. Available at: http://disarmament2.un.org/gaspecialsession/10thsesmain.htm (accessed June 22, 2007).
8. World Medical Association. Adopted by the 51st World Medical Assembly, Tel Aviv, Israel, October 1999.
9. Hotez PJ. Vaccines as instruments of foreign policy. EMBO Rep 2001;2:862–868.
10. Moodie M, Taylor WJ. Contagion and conflict: Health as a global security challenge. A report of the Chemical and Biological Arms Control Institute and the CSIS International Security Program, January 2000.
11. Miles SH. Abu Ghraib: Its legacy for military medicine. Lancet 2004;364:725–729.
12. Alpert EJ, Sege RD, Bradshaw YS. Interpersonal violence and the education of physicians. Acad Med 1997;72(1 Suppl):S41–S50.
13. Krug EG, Dahlberg LL, Mercy JA, et al. World Report on Violence and Health. Geneva: World Health Organization, 2002.
14. Lifton RJ, Markusen E. The Genocidal Mentality: Nazi Holocaust and Nuclear Threat. New York: Basic Books, 1990.
15. Arya N. The end of biomilitary realism? Time for rethinking biomedicine and international security. Med Conflict Surviv 2006;22:220–229.
16. Dyer O. Air Force doctor imprisoned for refusing third tour in Iraq. BMJ 2006; 332:931.
17. Bandaranayake DR. International health teaching: A survey of 100 medical schools in developed countries. Med Educ 1993;27:360–362.
18. Heck J, Pust R. A national consensus on the essential international-health curriculum for medical schools. Acad Med 1993;68:596–597.
19. Thomas J. Teaching ethics in schools of public health. Public Health Rep 2003; 118:279–286.
20. Mann JM, Gostin L, Gruskin S, et al. Health and human rights. Health Hum Rights 1994;1:6–23.
21. Medact. Global health studies: Proposals for medical undergraduate teaching pack, 2002. Available at: http://www.medact.org/pub_curriculum.php (accessed June 22, 2007).
22. World Health Organization. Report on the First WHO Consultative Meeting on Health as a Bridge for Peace, Les Pensières, Annecy, 1997, pp. 30–31. Available at: http://www.who.int/hac/techguidance/hbp/considering_conflict/en/print.html (accessed June 22, 2007).
23. Hoftvedt BO, Reyes H (Eds.). Doctors Working in Prison: Human Rights and Ethical Dilemmas. World Medical Association. Available at: http://lupin-nma.net (accessed June 22, 2007).
24. International Physicians for the Prevention of Nuclear War Students. Available at: http://www.ippnw-students.org/ReCap/ReCap.html (accessed June 22, 2007).
25. Buhmann C, The Nuclear Weapons Inheritance Project—Student-to-Student Dialogues and Interactive Peer Education in Disarmament Activism, Medicine, Conflict & Survival, 2007;23:92–102.
26. Arya N. Peace through Health I: Development and use of a working model. Med Conflict Surviv 2004; 20: 242–257.

27. Arya N. Globalization: The path to neo-liberal nirvana or health and environmental hell medicine. Conflict Surviv 2003;19:107–120.

28. Yusuf S, Anand S, MacQueen G. Can medicine prevent war? BMJ 1998;317:1669–1670.

29. United Nations. Millennium Goals 2000. Available at: http://www.un.org/millenniumgoals/ (accessed June 22, 2007).

30. People's Health Movement. People's Health Charter 2000. Available at: http://phmovement.org/charter/pch-english.html (accessed June 22, 2007).

31. Arya N. Do No Harm: Towards a Hippocratic Standard for International Civilization. In Re-Envisioning Sovereignty: The End of Westphalia. United Nations University and Brooking Institute, Workshop, April 2005. Canberra: Australian National University, 2006.

32. Arya N. Peace through Health II: A Framework for Medical Student Education. Med Conflict Surv 2004;3:258–262.

33. Peace Through Health, Centre for Peace Studies, McMaster University. Available at http://www.humanities.mcmaster.ca/peace-health/ (accessed July 19, 2007).

34. Peace and Conflict Studies, Conrad Grebel University College, University of Waterloo. Available at: http://www.grebel.uwaterloo.ca/pacs301 (accessed July 19, 2007).

35. Böck Buhmann C. The role of health professionals in preventing and mediating conflict. Med Conflict Surviv 2005;21:299–311.

36. Medical Peace Work. Available at: http://www.medicalpeacework.org (accessed June 22, 2007).

28

Toward a Culture of Peace

Mary-Wynne Ashford

The United Nations has declared the 2001–2010 period to be the International Decade for a Culture of Peace and Non-violence for the Children of the World. Perhaps another, equally appropriate, name for this period would be the Decade for Peace and Nonviolence for the Advancement of Public Health.

Building a culture of peace requires social policies similar to those needed for improving public health. Cultural change is difficult because we are so immersed in our own culture that we may assume that our deeply held values and attitudes are universal rather than culturally determined. As the African proverb states, "To a fish, the water is invisible." What a society values is expressed in its religion, economic system, governance, gender relations, environmental stewardship, child rearing and education, traditions of conflict resolution, popular entertainment, and health care system. Because public policies are expressions of cultural attitudes, resistance to change may be rooted in deep cultural beliefs that have not been exposed to critical discussion.

Health professionals are often reluctant to take a stand on social policies because of a concern that such advocacy is too political. But activism by health professionals has a long history. In 1848, Rudolf Virchow, then age 26, was appointed to make recommendations to address a typhus epidemic in Upper Silesia.[1] Rather than calling for more doctors or hospital beds, he urged physicians and politicians to address the social causes of disease. He outlined a revolutionary program, including full employment, higher wages, establishment of agricultural cooperatives, universal education, and the disestablishment of the Catholic Church. Virchow paired political and social reform with health care in his famous statement: "Medicine is a social science, and politics nothing but medicine on a grand scale."[1]

Prevention of war may seem to be even more political than prevention of a typhus epidemic, but the principles of effective prevention are the same. Public health interventions are usually categorized as primary, secondary, and tertiary. Primary prevention of war involves interventions for populations that are not yet in armed conflict. Primary prevention is as desirable in preventing violence as it is in preventing disease. Primary prevention of war means supporting social changes toward a culture of peace. Secondary prevention involves interventions for populations at war. It is designed to prevent further injury and death and to help resolve armed conflicts. Tertiary prevention focuses on long-term care in the wake of violence and works to mitigate the effects of trauma and prevent recurrence of war.

Societies are based on three pillars: government, the economy, and civil society.[2] *Civil society* is a term used to include all voluntary civic and social organizations that form the basis of a functioning society; it does not include commercial and government institutions. The growing influence of civil society in recent years had restrained government and the business sector by bringing conscience to bear on their decisions. Civil society supports disarmament, human rights, justice, advancement of women and minorities, and international law. Health care advocates, as part of civil society, have an important role in supporting international and national policies that promote prevention of violence and armed conflict.

The prevalence of war worldwide indicates the dominance of a culture of violence. This culture is expressed not only in armed conflict, but also in the acceptance—and often the glorification—of violence in entertainment, sports, theater, art, education, and religion (Table 28-1).

The continued proliferation of nuclear weapons indicates an unrestrained culture of violence. Mutually assured destruction is its logical outcome. A culture that would choose death for all people worldwide rather than negotiations to reconcile ideologies and national interests might best be described as a culture of death.

Many dimensions of a culture of war and violence are featured daily in mainstream media sources, but surprising new evidence suggests a global trend away from war.[3] The end of the Cold War in 1991 led to a marked decrease in the number of wars and genocides worldwide. If this change persists, it may mark a shift toward a culture of peace. Such a shift would have far-reaching effects on public health beyond the obvious reduction in battle-related morbidity and mortality.

Table 28-1. Characteristics of a Culture of Violence and a Culture of Peace and Nonviolence

A Culture of Violence	A Culture of Peace and Nonviolence
Domination by force	Cooperation and collaboration
Nuclear and other weapons of mass destruction	No nuclear weapons or weapons of mass destruction
Dictatorships tolerated	Elected, accountable governments
Huge military budgets	Small military budgets or none
Male-dominated	Gender partnership society
Competition valued	Minimal competition
Violence glorified in art, music, theater, film	Prosocial values elevated in art, music, theater, film
Win–lose philosophy	Win–win philosophy
Large income gap	Large middle class, small income gap
Racism and sexism common	Tolerance of diversity
Injustice tolerated on religious, racial, or ethnic grounds	Injustice not tolerated
Treaties and international law disregarded	Support for United Nations and international law
Social and environmental concerns trumped by military	Social and environmental concerns given high priority
Social services sacrificed for military budget	Social safety net
Punitive justice system with many in prison	Restorative justice and rehabilitation of prisoners
People committed to defeating "the enemy"	People committed to peace and justice

War is only one marker of a culture of violence, and the absence of war does not ensure a culture of peace. Furthermore, a 15-year decline in the occurrence of war may be only a temporary phenomenon. Other indicators of positive social change, however, show improvements across a wide spectrum of issues, including human rights, empowerment of women, fair trade, protection of the environment, participatory democracy, and social justice. These social changes are of great interest to health professionals because they are strongly linked to social determinants of health.

Determinants of Health

The World Health Organization (WHO) has listed determinants of health, including the following[4]:

- The socioeconomic environment (income, education, employment, working conditions, social support, and the social environment)
- Healthy child development
- The physical environment—both the natural and the built environments
- Personal health-related practices (physical activity; healthy diet and maintaining a healthy weight; use and abuse of tobacco, alcohol, and illicit drugs; use of safety equipment; gambling; sexual practices; testing for HIV and other disorders; and multiple risk behaviors)
- Health services (expenditures, delivery, access and utilization, medication expenditure and use, needs not met by existing services, and alternative health services)
- Biology and genetic endowment (birth defects, reproductive technologies, brain development, and aging).

Public Health and a Culture of Violence

Public health has been defined as what we, as a society, do collectively to ensure the conditions in which people can be healthy.[5] In times of war and other forms of armed conflict, society can do little collectively to ensure such conditions. People may not be able to meet their basic needs for food, clothing, shelter, and personal security. Even in the absence of armed conflict, a society may not ensure equitable distribution of food and material goods as well as human rights for all people. Policy decisions that deprive some individuals of the basics needed for survival and advancement are often termed "structural violence."

War is the extreme expression of a culture of violence that has dominated much of the world for 5,000 years. The United Nations recognized that preventing war and violence over the long term will require deep social change affecting complex human interactions that are often embedded in traditional practices. These practices may determine how opportunities and wealth are shared, laws are formulated, and children are raised and educated. Music, art, theater, religion, communication, and government all reflect traditions that may promote either cooperation or coercion by force. Some of the cultural changes needed have been evolving since the end of World War II, when the United Nations was founded and nations signed the Universal Declaration of Human Rights.

In order to support a state of health—defined by WHO as "complete physical, mental, and social well-being"—a society must provide conditions that not only meet survival needs but also offer a possibility of fulfilling higher needs, such as love, affection, belonging, esteem, and self-actualization. Such a society needs a complex foundation of structures and traditions that ensure security and opportunities for all of its people.

Public Health and a Culture of Peace

The United Nations defines a culture of peace as the attitudes, modes of behavior, and ways of life that reject violence and prevent conflicts by addressing their root causes in order to solve problems through dialogue and negotiation among individuals, groups, and nations.[6]

To lay the foundations for a culture of peace, the U.N. General Assembly has called for action in several areas[7]:

- Education
- Sustainable economic and social development
- Respect for all human rights
- Equality between men and women
- Democratic participation
- Understanding, tolerance, and solidarity
- Participatory communication and free flow of information and knowledge
- Promotion of international peace and security.

The Decade for a Culture of Peace offers an important opportunity for advancing public health, because each of the designated directions for action parallels work needed to foster social determinants of health.

A culture of peace promotes the positive determinants of health and supports actions to reduce the negative determinants. Armed conflict precludes positive advances in these determinants and increases the negative elements of substance abuse, high-risk sexual practices, and spread of disease. Health effects of toxic chemicals used on the battlefield may extend to the offspring of those exposed. Agent Orange, for example, is associated with birth defects including spina bifida, cleft lip, congenital neoplasms, and coloboma (an eye anomaly). Prevention of transmission of HIV to infants in war zones is almost impossible. The lack of qualified birth attendants, malnutrition, and deprivation caused by warfare all contribute to poor child development.

Etiology of War

Prevention of war, like prevention of disease, requires systematic assessment of the etiology and contributing factors that lead to its outbreak. Unless each of the causes is addressed, the conflict will not be resolved and war is likely to begin or recur.

Some of the factors that may contribute to armed conflict are:

- Competition over resources such as land, water, oil, diamonds, timber, gold, and coltan (a mineral needed in the manufacture of cell phones)
- Historical grievances heightened by nationalism, ethnocentrism, religion, or ideology exploited as a justification for violence
- Easy availability of weaponry
- Injustice and exclusion of a group from economic and social opportunities
- Characteristics of national leaders—lust for power or wealth, or a strategy to retain power (because people tend to support a national leader during wartime)
- Profits to weapons manufacturers and corporations that financially benefit from both the destruction and reconstruction of a country
- Government influenced by a military-industrial complex
- Election campaigning that promotes fear, patriotic fervor, and a candidate who advocates use of military force
- Traditions that support violent means of addressing conflicts—cultural expectations and machismo that glorify war and violence
- Media that promote hatred of specific groups
- Rapid demographic change that outstrips the capacity of a country to provide essential services and opportunities.

Transforming a Culture of Violence to a Culture of Peace

The Changing Epidemiology of War

The number of deaths in war in the 20th century is difficult to calculate, because records are often inaccurate and incomplete. Most estimates are between 110 million and 191 million deaths.[8,9] If those who died as an indirect result of war are counted, the number of deaths may be closer to 250 million.[10] This includes those who died as a result of destruction of the societal infrastructure necessary for survival, disease spread by war, and starvation resulting from battles or blockades.

Notwithstanding these numbers, the epidemiology of war seems to be changing. The *Human Security Report* of the Centre for Human Security showed a global decline in armed conflicts during the 1946–2003 period.[3] Since the end of the Cold War in 1991, the occurrence of war has decreased by 40 percent, and that of major wars and genocides by 80 percent. Battle-related deaths and international crises have also decreased. In addition, 60 dictators have been toppled nonviolently since Ferdinand Marcos was displaced in the 1986 "Velvet Revolution" in the Philippines.

The decline in armed conflict has been attributed to three factors: the successes of the United Nations in peace-building, the strengthening of international law, and the growing influence of civil society in international affairs.[3] Other major social changes have supported movement toward a culture of peace, including

- Transportation and communication systems that have made possible the global networking of civil-society organizations
- Communications systems that have enabled news reports to travel worldwide within minutes
- Government policies that have empowered women to participate in government and the economy
- Global broadcasting of nonviolent revolutions that provides lessons for activists opposing oppressive regimes.

Nonviolent revolutions began with Mohandas Gandhi, who mobilized the power of nonviolent resistance against British rule in India, eventually forcing Great Britain to give India its independence in 1947. Activists in the Philippines studied Gandhi's writings and strategies and prepared themselves to apply Gandhian principles to overturn the dictator, Ferdinand Marcos. In 1986, when a small group of dissident military leaders defied Marcos, millions of people flooded onto the streets of Manila to support them. Marcos fled, and his government was replaced by a democracy. By 1989, dissent against Soviet rule was spreading through Central and Eastern Europe. The Berlin Wall was toppled, and Germany was reunited. Poland became independent, followed by Czechoslovakia, Hungary, and Bulgaria. Since then, dictatorships have been replaced with fledgling democracies in many more countries, including Ukraine, where the "Orange Revolution" of 2004 reversed a corrupt election.

The period covered in the *Human Security Report* ended before the current wars in Iraq and Afghanistan. It is too early to determine the effect of these wars on the overall trend reported, but the end of some seemingly intractable conflicts, such as that in Northern Ireland, offers helpful insights as opposition groups choose political engagement instead of armed conflict.

The Empowerment of Women

Women usually constitute a large membership within civil-society organizations that promote peace and social justice. Increased influence of these organizations means increased prominence for the values of women, including health and social services for children, families, and the weakest members of society.

Although changes may be limited and slow, there seems to be a global shift in attitudes toward empowerment of women. An important policy to increase the number of women in government is in progress in many countries, including India, Pakistan, Bangladesh, Nepal, and Rwanda. Governments of these countries have mandated that at least one third of the seats in municipal government be reserved for women.[11] In 1992, in the state of Bihar, India, for example, 45,000 women were elected under the new law. Many were illiterate. Nongovernmental organizations throughout India began training women in literacy, human rights, and the role of local government. In addition to providing skills needed for participation in governance, this training enables women to generate income more effectively.

In France, a new parity law enacted in 2000 requires that there be equal numbers of male and female candidates standing for office at the municipal level. The percentage of women elected to municipal councils rose from 26 percent to 48 percent after the law came into force.

The Nigerian government appointed a female pharmacologist to direct the National Agency for Drug and Food Administration, with a mandate of addressing corruption in pharmaceutical and bottled-water industries.[12] With the approval of the government, she appointed only female investigators, because she believes that men are too easily tempted by bribes.

Although cultural transformation is slow and difficult, progress in ending female genital mutilation provides important insights for those who work to bring about deep cultural change. This practice, which is more than 3,000 years old, has severe health consequences. Despite being condemned by WHO more than 20 years ago, it has been very difficult to stop. Now, however, village women in Kenya, Senegal, and Sierra Leone have begun projects to end the practice.[13]

The women train together and then return to their villages to educate mothers, daughters, fathers, and sons separately, using traditional means of storytelling, singing, dancing, drumming, and art. They honor and engage the "cutters" as respected leaders who advocate abandoning the practice. They celebrate a new coming of age ceremony for girls who have not been cut: The girls spend a week in seclusion learning about women's roles and health issues. Then they join the society as adult women in a celebration with feasting and drumming. In Senegal, practice of female genital mutilation has decreased from 90 percent to 10 percent over 10 years.

By studying the experience of these African women who are accomplishing profound cultural transformation, we can deduce some lessons for developing a culture of peace:

- The entire society must be included and educated in order to transform a deeply held tradition.
- The tools for change include the arts and celebrations as well as careful, sensitive education.
- An entirely indigenous process is more successful than one led by outsiders.
- Transposing the previous practice into a new cultural tradition that fulfils the same purpose may lead to a more stable transformation.

Evolving Technologies

Information technology allows the participation of marginalized groups and has played an important role in the spread of nonviolent democracy movements. These movements share strategies of nonviolent resistance and learn how popular uprisings have removed dictators. Cell phones are revolutionizing communications in the developing world. Literacy, health, democratic decision-making, and peace are greatly facilitated by access to computers and the Internet.

The Growing Interfaith Movement

The rapid growth of interfaith groups globally supports religious moderates and increases the activities of those building peaceful relationships across religious boundaries. Interfaith choirs bring together Muslims, Christians, and Jews to sing sacred music from their different traditions. Interfaith camps in North America invite Israeli and Palestinian youth to spend a few weeks together to build understanding.[11]

A Broader Role for Health Professionals

Health professionals have unique expertise and skills to offer for the prevention of war and promotion of a culture of peace. Leaders in government and civil society look to health professionals for information about the health consequences of war and of various weapons. Research by health professionals on the impact of blockades, sanctions, and destruction of societal infrastructure exposes the disproportionate suffering of vulnerable people that is caused by these strategies.

The ethical bases of health professions offer a series of core principles that can usefully be applied to interventions in conflict resolution. Applying the principle of "Do no harm" means that aerial bombing, deployment of landmines, implementation of blockades of food and medicine, and destruction of societal infrastructure must not be permitted. Instead, the least harmful intervention should be implemented first, reducing the health consequences for all people on both sides of a conflict and ensuring the protection of the most vulnerable people. Work by health professionals in civil-society organizations has been influential in bringing about treaties to reduce nuclear weapons, ban antipersonnel landmines, and control biological and chemical weapons. Current work on small arms and light weapons involves many physicians from Africa and Latin America, where gun violence poses a serious health problem even in countries that are not at war.

Health professionals who are willing to enlarge their circle of compassion to include the world are role models who demonstrate that engagement in social issues is a responsibility of all professionals. Because competition for oil tends to fuel conflict, health professionals can advocate reducing the consumption of oil and petrochemical products. They can also reduce their individual reliance on oil and plastics. As scientists, they can promote and disseminate findings from research on the prevention of war. They can discuss proposals to prevent armed conflict that might arise from global warming or possible crises as countries compete for limited key resources, such as water, copper, and coltan. They can speak against media violence and against governments that violate or disregard national and international law. They can support interfaith dialogues and school programs to reduce racism and ethnocentrism.

Building a culture of peace means reconnecting to our sense of the sacred, to other people, and to our earth. In the process of building a culture that fosters peace and public health, we also enrich our own lives.

References

1. Taylor R, Rieger A. Rudolf Virchow on the typhus epidemic in upper Silesia: An introduction and translation. Sociol Health Illness 1984;6:201–217.
2. Perlas N. Shaping globalization: Civil society, cultural power and threefolding. Quezon City, The Philippines: Center for Alternative Development Initiatives, 2000.
3. Mack A, Nielsen Z (eds.). Human Security Report 2005: War and Peace in the 21st Century. New York: Oxford University Press, 2005.
4. Wilkinson R, Marmot M (eds.). Social Determinants of Health: The Solid Facts, 2nd ed. Denmark: World Health Organization, 2003.
5. Institute of Medicine. The Future of Public Health in the 21st Century. Washington, DC: National Academy Press, 1988.
6. U.N. Resolutions A/RES/52/13: Culture of Peace, adopted by the General Assembly January 15, 1998; and A/Res/53/243, Declaration and Programme of Action on a Culture of Peace, adopted by the General Assembly October 6, 1999.

7. U.N. Resolution A/53/25, adopted by the General Assembly, November 28, 1998.

8. Sivard R (ed.). World Military and Social Expenditures, 16th ed. Washington, DC: World Priorities, 1996.

9. World Health Organization. World Report on Violence and Health. Geneva: WHO, 2002.

10. Leitenberg M. Deaths in Wars and Conflicts in the 20th Century, 3rd ed. (Occasional paper #29.) Cornell University Peace Studies Program, 2006.

11. Ashford MW, Dauncey G. Enough Blood Shed: 101 Solutions to Violence, Terror and War. Gabriola Island, BC: New Society Publishers, 2006.

12. Frenkiel O. Bad medicine: One woman's war with fake drugs. Radio broadcast. BBC Two. July 12, 2005. Available at: http://news.bbc.co.uk/2/hi/programmes/this_world/4656627.stm (accessed June 22, 2007).

13. Spindel C. With an End in Sight: Strategies from the UNIFEM Trust Fund to Eliminate Violence against Women. New York: UNIFEM, 2000.

Appendix: A List of Some Organizations That Promote Peace

American Friends Service Committee (AFSC)
1501 Cherry Street
Philadelphia, PA 19102
Tel: 215-241-7000; Fax: 215-241-7275
Home Page: http://www.afsc.org

American Public Health Association (APHA)
800 I Street, NW
Washington, DC 20001-3710
Tel: 202-777-2742; Fax: 202-777-2533
Home Page: http://www.apha.org

American Refugee Committee (ARC)
ARC World Headquarters
430 Oak Grove Street, Suite 204
Minneapolis, MN 55403
Tel: 800-875-7060; Fax: 612-607-6499
Home Page: http://www.archq.org

Amnesty International
U.S. Office:
5 Penn Plaza, 14th Floor
New York, NY 10001
Tel: 212-807-8400; Fax: 212-463-9193
Home Page: http://www.amnesty.org

Carnegie Endowment for International Peace
1779 Massachusetts Avenue, NW
Washington, DC 20036-2103
Tel: 202-483-7600; Fax: 202-483-1840
Home Page: http://www.carnegieen
  dowment.org

The Carter Center
One Copenhill
453 Freedom Parkway
Atlanta, GA 30307
Tel: 404-420-5100 or 800-550-3560
Home Page: http://www.cartercenter.org

Center for Defense Information
1779 Massachusetts Avenue, NW
Washington, DC 20036-2109
Tel: 202-332-0600; Fax: 202-462-4559
Home Page: http://www.cdi.org

Centers for Disease Control and
    Prevention (CDC)
1600 Clifton Road
Atlanta, GA 30333
Tel: 404-639-3311
Home Page: http://www.cdc.gov

Centre for Conflict Resolution
UCT Hiddingh Campus
31-37 Orange Street
Cape Town 8000
South Africa
Tel: 27 21 422 2512; Fax: 27 21 422
    2622
Home Page: http://www.ccrweb.ccr
    .uct.ac.za

Centre for Peace Studies
McMaster University
1280 Main Street West
Hamilton, Ontario L8S 4K1
Canada
Tel: 905-525-9140 ext. 24265; Fax: 905-
    570-1167
Home Page: http://www.humanities
    .mcmaster.ca/~peace

Center for Strategic and Budgetary
    Assessments
1667 K Street, NW, Suite 900
Washington, DC 20006
Tel: 202-331-7990; Fax: 202-331-8019
Home Page: http://www.csbaonline
    .org

Collaborative Learning Projects and the
    Collaborative for Development Action,
    Inc. (CDA)
17 Dunster Street, Suite #202
Cambridge, MA 02138
Tel: 617-661-6310; Fax: 617-661-3805
Home Page: http://www.cdainc
    .com

Council for a Livable World
322 4th Street, NE
Washington, DC 20002
Tel: 202-543-4100
Home Page: http://www.clw.org

Council for Responsible Genetics
5 Upland Road, Suite 3
Cambridge, MA 02140
Tel: 617-868-0870; Fax: 617-491-5344
Home Page: http://www.gene-watch.org

Doctors of the World (Médecins du Monde)
U.S. Office:
80 Maiden Lane, Suite 607
New York, NY 10038
Tel; 212-226-9890 or 888-817-4357
Home Page: http://www.doctorsoftheworld
    .org
Main Office:
14 Heron Quays
London E14 4JB
United Kingdom
Tel: 44 20 7515 7534; Fax: 44 20 7515 7560
Home Page: http://www.medecinsdumon
    de.org.uk

Doctors Without Borders (Médecins Sans
    Frontières)
U.S. Office:
333 7th Avenue, 2nd Floor
New York, NY 10001-5004
Tel: 212-679-6800; Fax: 212-679-7016
Home Page: http://www.doctorswithout
    borders.org
Main Office:
Rue de Lausanne 78
1211 Geneva
Switzerland
Tel: 41 22 849 8400; Fax: 41 22 849 8404
Home Page: http://www.msf.org

Educators for Social Responsibility (ESR)
ESR National Center:
23 Garden Street
Cambridge, MA 02138
Tel: 617-492-1764; Fax: 617-864-5164
Home Page: http://www.esrnational.org

Federation of American Scientists
1717 K Street, NW, Suite 209
Washington, DC 20036
Tel: 202-546-3300; Fax: 202-675-1010
Home Page: http://www.fas.org

Francois Xavier Bagnoud Center for
  Health and Human Rights
Harvard University School of Public
  Health
651 Huntington Avenue, 7th Floor
Boston, MA 02115
Tel: 617-432-0656; Fax: 617-432-4310
Home Page: http://www.hsph.harvard.edu/
  fxbcenter

Friends Committee on National
  Legislation
245 Second Street, NE
Washington, DC 20002
Tel: 202-547-6000; Fax: 202-547-6019
Home Page: http://www.fcnl.org

Global Health Council
1111 19th Street, NW—Suite 1120
Washington, DC 20036
Tel: 202-833-5900; Fax: 202-833-0075
Home Page: http://www.globalhealth
  .org

Greenpeace
U.S. Office:
702 H Street, NW, Suite 300
Washington, DC 20001
Tel: 800-326-0959
Home Page: http://www.greenpeace.org

Human Rights Watch
350 Fifth Avenue, 34th Floor
New York, NY 10118-3299
Tel: 212-290-4700; Fax: 212-736-1300
Home Page: http://www.hrw.org

Institute for Defense and Disarmament
  Studies
675 Massachusetts Avenue
Cambridge, MA 02139
Tel: 617-354-4337; Fax: 617-354-1450
Home Page: http://www.idds.org

Institute for Energy and Environmental
  Research
6935 Laurel Avenue
Takoma Park, MD 20912
Tel: 301-270-5500; Fax: 301-270-3029
Home Page: http://www.ieer.org

Institute for Multi-track Diplomacy
1901 North Fort Myer Drive, Suite 405
Arlington, VA 22209
Tel: 703-528-3863; Fax: 703-528-5776
Home Page: http://www.imtd.org

International Association of Lawyers
  Against Nuclear Arms (IALANA)
U.S. Office:
Lawyers Committee on Nuclear Policy
675 Third Avenue, Suite 315
New York, NY 10017-5704
Tel: 212-818-1861; Fax: 212-818-1857
Home Page: http://www.ialana.net

International Campaign to Ban
  Landmines
Chemin Balexert 7
1219 Geneva
Switzerland
Tel: 41 22 920 0325; Fax: 41 22 920
  0115
Home Page: http://www.icbl.org

International Center for Technology
  Assessment
660 Pennsylvania Avenue, SE, Suite 302
Washington, DC 20003
Tel: 202-547-9359; Fax: 202-547-9429
Home Page: http://www.icta.org

International Committee of the Red Cross
  (ICRC)
Avenue de la Paix 19
CH-1202 Geneva
Switzerland
Tel: 41 22 734 6001; Fax: 41 22 733
  2057
Home Page: http://www.icrc.org

International Federation of Red Cross and
Red Crescent Societies
P.O. Box 372
CH-1211 Geneva 19
Switzerland
Telephone: 41 22 730 42 22
Fax: 41 22 733 03 95
Home Page: http://www.ifrc.org

International Peace Bureau
41, rue de Zurich
CH-1201 Geneva
Switzerland
Tel: 41 22 731 6429; Fax: 41 22 738 9419
Home Page: http://www.ipb.org

International Physicians for the Prevention
of Nuclear War (IPPNW)
727 Massachusetts Avenue
Cambridge, MA 02139
Tel: 617-868-5050; Fax: 617-868-2560
Home Page: http://www.ippnw.org

International Rescue Committee (IRC)
122 East 42nd Street
New York, NY 10168-1289
Tel: 212-551-3000; Fax: 212-551-3180
Home Page: http://www.theirc.org

The Joan B. Kroc Institute for International
Peace Studies
University of Notre Dame
P.O. Box 639
Notre Dame, IN 46556
Tel: 219-631-6970; Fax: 219-631-6973
Home Page: http://www.nd.edu/~krocinst

Lawyer's Alliance for World Security
1779 Massachusetts Avenue, NW, Suite 615
Washington, DC 20036
Tel: 202-332-0600; Fax: 202-462-4559
Home Page: http://www.cdi.org/laws

MEDACT (UK affiliate of IPPNW)
The Grayston Centre
28 Charles Square
London N1 6HT
United Kingdom
Tel: 44 20 7324 4739; Fax: 44 20 7324 4734
Home Page: http://www.medact.org

National Priorities Project
17 New South Street
Northampton, MA 01060
Tel: 413-584-9556; Fax: 413-584-9647
Home Page: http://www.nationalpriorites
.org

Oxfam America
226 Causeway Street, 5th Floor
Boston, MA 02114
Tel: 617-482-1211; Fax: 617-728-2594
Home Page: http://www.oxfamamerica
.org

Peace Action
1100 Wayne Avenue. Suite 1020
Silver Spring, MD 20910
Tel: 301-565-4050; Fax: 301-565-0850
Home Page: http://www.peace-action.org

Physicians for Global Survival (Canadian
affiliate of IPPNW)
#208-145 Spruce Street
Ottawa, Ontario K1R 6P1
Canada
Tel: 613-233-1982; Fax: 613-233-9028
Home Page: http://www.pgs.ca

Physicians for Human Rights (PHR)
2 Arrow Street, Suite 301
Cambridge, MA 02138
Tel: 617-301-4200; Fax: 617-301-4250
Home Page: http://www.physiciansforhu
manrights.org

Physicians for Social Responsibility (U.S.
affiliate of IPPNW)
1875 Connecticut Avenue, NW, Suite
1012
Washington, DC, 20009
Tel: 202-667-4260; Fax: 202-667-4201
Home Page: http://www.psr.org

Project on Defense Alternatives
The Commonwealth Institute
P.O. Box 398105
Cambridge, MA 02139
Tel: 617-547-4474; Fax: 617-868-1267
Home Page: http://www.comw.org/pda

Stockholm International Peace Research
   Institute (SIPRI)
Signalistgatan 9
SE-169 70 Solna
Sweden
Tel: 46 8 655 97 00; Fax: 46 8 655
   97 33
Home Page: http://www.sipri.org

20/20 Vision
8403 Colesville Road, Suite 860
Silver Spring, MD 20910
Tel: 301-587-1782
Home Page: http://www.2020vision.org

Union of Concerned Scientists
2 Brattle Square
Cambridge, MA 02238-9105
Tel: 617-547-5552; Fax: 617-864-9405
Home Page: http://www.ucsusa.org

United Nations Children's Fund
   (UNICEF)
3 United Nations Plaza
New York, NY 10017
Tel: 212-326-7000; Fax: 212-887-7465
Home Page: http://www.unicef.org

United Nations Development Program
   (UNDP)
One United Nations Plaza
New York, NY 10017
Tel: 212-906-5000; Fax: 212-906-5364
Home Page: http://www.undp.org

United Nations High Commissioner for
   Human Rights (UNHCHR)
1211 Geneva 10
Switzerland
Tel: 41 22 917 9000; Fax: 41 22 917 9022
Home Page: http://www.ohchr.org

United Nations High Commissioner for
   Refugees (UNHCR)
Case Postale 2500
1211 Geneva
Switzerland
Tel: 41 22 739 8111
Home Page: http://www.unhcr.org

Women's Action for New Directions
   (WAND)
691 Massachusetts Avenue
Arlington, MA 02476
Tel: 781-643-6740; Fax: 781-643-6744
Home Page: http://www.wand.org

World Health Organization (WHO)
Avenue Appia 20
1211 Geneva 27
Switzerland
Tel: 41 22 791 21 11; Fax: 41 22 791 31 11
Home Page: http://www.who.int

Worldwatch Institute
1776 Massachusetts Avenue, NW
Washington, DC 20036
Tel: 202-452-1999; Fax: 202-296-7365
Home Page: http://www.worldwatch.org

Index

Page numbers followed by "f" denote figures; those followed by "t" denote tables

Aaland Islands Convention, 81
Abu Ghraib, 199–200, 229f, 234–236, 259
Aceh, 428–433
Acetylcholinesterase, 122
Activism, 452–453, 458
Advocacy, 16–17
Afghanistan, 12, 64, 108, 228, 352
Africa. *See also specific country*
   arms expenditures by, 94
   landmines in, 108
   posttraumatic stress disorder in, 63–64
Agent Orange, 320–322
Aiming For Prevention campaign, 390
Air pollution, 69–70
Alfred P. Murrah Federal Building, 13, 63
Al-Qaeda, 248
American Public Health Association, 16,
      329–330, 383f
Amputations, 103, 109
Andean Strategy, 289, 299
Angola, 34, 108, 218

Annan, Kofi, 367
Antarctic Treaty, 81
Anthrax, 135, 142, 143t, 145
Antiadrenergic agents, 61
Anti-Ballistic Missile (ABM) Treaty, 167
Antipersonnel landmines, 74–75. *See*
      Landmines
Anxiety, 182–183
Argentina, 305, 419
Arias, Oscar, 294
Armed conflict. *See also* War
   in Central America, 289
   changing patterns of, 32–34
   civilian deaths from, 218
   in Cold War period, 32
   contributing factors, 457
   deaths from, 24–25, 218. *See also*
      Conflict-related deaths
   in developing countries, 414
   dissemination of information, 349
   human development and, 30–31

Armed conflict (*continued*)
impact of, 339–340
inequalities in, 32–33
internal, 28
interventions to prevent, 348
multinational forces in, 28
public health prevention of health
consequences of. *See* Public health
prevention of health consequences
risk factors for, 348t, 348–349, 446–447
secondary effects of, 91
temporal phases of, 342
types of, 346
Armored combat vehicle, 88
Arms. *See also* Guns; Small arms and light
weapons
expenditures on, 10–11, 94
exporting countries, 89
governmental purchases of, 94
small, 33, 87–88
Arms brokers, 96
Army of the Republic of South Vietnam,
315
Asphyxiants, 119, 120t–121t
Aum Shinrikyo cult, 117, 127–128

Bachelet, Dr. Michelle, 305
Bangladesh, 207
Battle tank, 88
Behavioral science consultation teams,
236
Biodefense research laboratory, 139–140
Biological Defense Research Program,
138
Biological warfare, 83, 137t
Biological weapons
anthrax, 135, 142, 143t, 145
botulism, 146–147
brucellosis, 143t
categorization of, 140t, 140–141
description of, 135
Ebola virus, 144t, 149
environmental effects of, 80
glanders, 143t
hemorrhagic fevers, 144t, 149
history of, 136–141
Marburg virus, 144t, 149
plague, 143t, 145–146
Q fever, 143t

research on, 139–140
smallpox, 144t, 147–148, 148f
Soviet Union production and testing of,
138, 158t, 161
tularemia, 143t, 146
U.S. production and testing of, 136, 138
Biological Weapons Convention (BWC),
138, 366
Blast injuries, 91
Blister agents. *See* Vesicants
Blunt trauma, 91
Bomb craters, 70, 71f
Bombay, India, 157t
Bosnia, 9, 70, 218, 373
Botulism, 146–147
"Brain drain," 414
Brussels Declaration of 1874, 130
Brutality, 5–9
Bubonic plague, 146
Bureau for Crisis Prevention and
Recovery, 416
Burundi, 198
Bybee, J.S., 230

Cambodia, 62, 103–105, 323, 331, 369
Cambodia Mine Action Centre, 113
Carbamate pesticides, 122
CARE, 385–386
Caroline Incident, 361
Center for Research on the Epidemiology
of Disasters, 424
Centers for Disease Control and
Prevention, 14
Central African Republic, 385–386
Central American Free Trade Agreement
(CAFTA), 297, 308–309
Centre for Human Security, 457
Chad, 385
Chamorro, Violetta, 294
Charter of the United Nations, 47–48
Chechnya, 39, 264–278
Chelyabinsk, Russia, 12, 77
Chemical agents and weapons
aerosol form, 118
asphyxiants, 119, 120t–121t
children exposed to, 125
cholinesterase inhibitors, 120t–121t,
122–123
on civilian populations, 125–126

classification of, 118–124
contingency planning for, 125–126
delayed effects of, 125
delivery of, 117–118
destruction of, 132–133
detection of, 125
environmental effects of, 80
Geneva Protocol of 1925 prohibitions,
    130–131
history of, 127–130, 130t
international law regarding, 130–132
latency period of, 118
long-term effects of, 125
proliferation control, 132–133
properties of, 118–119
public health preparedness, 124–125
respiratory tract irritants, 120t–121t,
    123–124
terrorist use of, 127–128
vapor form, 118
vesicants, 120t–121t, 124
Chemical warfare, 83, 117, 128–130
Chemical Weapons Convention (CWC),
    131, 366
Chernobyl, 78
Chiapas, Mexico, 301–302
Child soldiers, 185–187, 189–190
Children
    anxiety in, 182–183
    chemical agent exposure, 125
    Darfur genocide of, 211
    death of, 180
    depression in, 183
    disability of, 181
    ethnic cleansing targeting of, 180
    growth retardation of, 181–182
    illness of, 181
    immunization programs, 182
    injuries to
        description of, 181
        landmine, 102–103, 107, 181
    international humanitarian law
        protections for, 189
    in Iraq War, 255, 257
    loss of family relationships, 185
    malnutrition in, 181–182, 220f, 257
    measures to help, 188–191
    moral impact, 184
    peace education for, 189

posttraumatic stress disorder in, 62,
    183, 187
prostitution of, 188
psychological injuries to, 182–184
radioactive fallout-related malignancies
    in, 78
rape of, 188, 190
in reconstruction of war-torn societies,
    191
refugees, 216, 219, 220f
rehabilitation of, 190–191
resilience of, 185
sociocultural impact, 184–185
spiritual impact, 184
starvation of, 181–182
torture of, 188
trafficking of, 201
vulnerability of, 9, 179–180
war effects on, 179–191
Chile, 289, 303–305
China, 158t, 169t
Chinese Rebellion of 1850–1864, 71
Cholinesterase inhibitors, 120t–121t,
    122–123
Chronic pain, 55
Civil society, 453
Civil wars
    in El Salvador, 291–292
    in Sri Lanka, 433–436
    in United States, 8
Civilians
    assaults on, 39
    chemical attacks on, 125–126
    "conventional" means used to kill, 39
    ethnic cleansing, 39–40
    explosives that injure, 89–91
    extrajudicial killing of, 39–40
    failing to provide care to, 398
    Geneva Convention Protocol I
        protections for, 90
    gun ownership by, 98–99
    high-risk conflicts for injury, 33
    indirect assaults on, 42–43
    indiscriminate attacks on, 90–91
    indiscriminate weapons used to assault, 41
    Iraq War, 251–252, 256f
    landmine injuries to, 102–104
    mental health impact of war on, 61–63
    vulnerability of, 34

Clausewitz, Carl von, 308
Clostridium botulinum, 146
Cluster-bomb submunitions, 75
"Coercive interrogation," 231
Cognitive-behavioral therapies, 60
Cold War
    description of, 31, 39
    nuclear weapon proliferation after,
        168
Collective violence, 26–27
Colombia, 298–301
Combat aircraft, 88
"Combat neurosis," 52
Combat trauma
    in Iraq War, 57–58
    posttraumatic stress disorder secondary
        to, 57
"Comfort women," 197
Commission for the Historical
    Clarification of Human Rights
    Violations and Acts of Violence,
    295–296
Commission on Weapons of Mass
    Destruction, 367
Communal conflict, 8
Communicable diseases, 351, 376–377
Complex humanitarian emergency,
    208–209
Complex political emergency, 209
Comprehensive Nuclear Test Ban Treaty
    (CTBT), 167–168
Condor Cordillera war, 306
Confidentiality breaches, 395
Conflict phase, of armed conflict, 342,
    343t–344t, 350–352
Conflict resolution, 17–18
Conflict-related deaths
    causes of, 23
    criteria for, 29
    historical data, 25–32
    inaccuracies in, 27
    information sources, 24–25, 27
    in 20th century, 25–26, 29f
Congo, 24, 279–287, 383. *See also*
    Democratic Republic of Congo
Contras, 292
Convention against Torture and other
    Cruel, Inhuman or Degrading
    Treatment, 365

Convention on Conventional Weapons
    amendments to, 105–106
    description of, 93
    ineffectiveness of, 106
    mine bans, 105–107
Convention on the Prohibition of the Use,
    Stockpiling, Production and
    Transfer of Anti-Personnel Mines
    and on Their Destruction, 104–107
Convention on the Rights of the Child, 189
"Convention with Respect to the Laws and
    Customs of War on Land," 364
Conventional weapons
    definition of, 70, 87
    disarmament efforts, 92–95
    heavy systems, 88–89
    improvised explosive devices, 87, 89
    manufactured explosives, 89
    nuclear weapons vs., 366
    prohibition efforts, 92–95
    small arms and light weapons, 87–88
Costa Rica, 302–303
Covenant of the League of Nations, 358
Criminal justice, 417
Crude mortality rate (CMR)
    Democratic Republic of Congo war,
        281–283, 285
    description of, 214–215, 216f
    in health zones reporting violence, 378
    in refugee camps, 371f
Cyanide poisoning, 119

Darfur, 5, 210–212, 219, 384
Deaths
    conflict-related. *See* Conflict-related
        deaths
    direct, 24, 29–30
    indirect, 24–25, 30
    statistics regarding, 23
    in 20th century, 25–26
Debayle, Anastasio Somoza, 425
Decade for a Culture of Peace and
    Nonviolence for the Children of the
    World, 452, 456
Defense Threat Reduction Agency, 125
Dehumanization, 237
Democide deaths, 26
Democratic Republic of Congo, 279–287,
    383

Department of Veterans Affairs, 59
Depleted uranium, 12, 70, 260
Depression, 52, 54, 62, 64, 183, 352
Dianisidine chlorosulfate, 128
Diarrheal diseases, 217, 222, 350
2,4-Dichlorophenoxyacetic acid, 73
Dioxin, 320–322
Direct deaths
    definition of, 24
    statistics regarding, 29–30
Disarmament, Demobilization, and
        Reintegration, 415
Disasters
    in Aceh, 428–433
    aftermath of, 425–428
    economic effects of, 426
    global distribution of, 31
    humanitarian assistance for, 427,
        436–437
    natural, 424–428
    secondary effects of, 426–427
    in Sri Lanka, 433–436
Displaced persons
    in Colombia, 300
    health consequences, 214–220
    internally, 220–221
    Iraq War, 257–258
    mortality rates in, 214–215
    public health program for, 222–224
    raping of, 221
    refugees. See Refugees
    relief programs for, 221–225
    return of, 411, 414
    statistics regarding, 212, 214t
Doctors Without Borders. See Médecins
        Sans Frontières
Documentation, 16
Domestic violence, 200
Dominguez, Jorge, 306–307
Drone aircraft, 12
"Dum-dum bullets," 363
Dunant, Henri, 362

East Timor, 34, 215, 414
Ebola virus, 144t, 149
Economic sanctions
    advocacy for ban on, 17
    description of, 10
    populations affected by, 190

Education
    courses of study, 444–445, 448
    existing approaches to, 442, 444
    future of, 449
    knowledge deficits, 441
    Medical Peace Work courses,
        447–448
    Peace through Health courses,
        447–448
    skills, 442
El Salvador, 43, 290–292, 306, 390
Embargoes, 323–325. See also Economic
        sanctions
Emergency contingency planning,
        125–127
Emergency derogation, 49
Emergency response teams, 416
Endemic disease control, 223
Energy Employees Occupational Illness
        Compensation Program, 162
Environment
    biological weapons effect on, 80
    chemical weapons effect on, 80
    in Colombia, 300
    hazardous waste effects on, 80
    health professionals advocacy for,
        18
    Iraq War effects on, 260
    landmine effects on, 103–104
    nuclear weapons dismantling and
        destruction effects on, 77, 161
    peacetime impacts on, 76–80
    Vietnam War destruction of, 70
    wartime impacts on
        description of, 11–12
        forest clearing, 71–73
        intentional, 70–75
        intentional release of dangerous
            forces, 75–76
        oil releases, 74
        unintentional, 69–70
Environmental warfare, 75–76, 83
Epidemic preparedness, 223–224
Epidemiology, 23, 457–458
Eritrea, 5, 28
Ethiopia, 4–5, 28, 39, 62, 358, 370
Ethnic cleansing, 39–40, 180, 194,
        196
Ethyl bromoacetate, 128

Explosives
    improvised explosive devices (IEDs),
        87, 89
    injuries inflicted by, 91–92
    landmines. *See* Landmines
    plastic, 91
    terrorist use of, 91
    in Vietnam War, 316
    volatile, 91
Exposure therapies, 61
Extrajudicial killings, 39–40
Eye movement desensitization and
    reprocessing, 61

Farabundo Marti Front for National
    Liberation, 290
Fay, George, 235
Figueres, Jose "Pepe," 302–303
Firearms
    civilian ownership of, 98–99
    diversion of, 96–97
    global supply of, 96–98
    governmental efforts to control, 98
    nongovernmental organizations' efforts
        to control, 98
    secondary effects of, 95
    supply and demand for, 97–99
    violence caused by, 94–95
First Indochina War, 313
Forest clearing, 71–73
Fossil fuels, 75
Fourth World Conference on Women, 203
France, 11, 158t, 169t
Francisella tularensis, 146
Free Trade Agreement of the Americas,
    308
Fresh water impoundments, 75–76
Freud, Sigmund, 357

Gandhi, Mohandas, 458
Gangs, 11
Garcia, Anastasio Somoza, 292
Gender-based violence, 378
Geneva Conventions
    conventional weapons prohibition
        efforts, 93
    general discussions of, 12, 33, 38, 44
    prisoners of war, 364
    Protocol I, 47, 81, 83, 90, 365

    Protocol II, 81, 83, 365
    rules of conduct of armies, 362
Geneva International Centre for
    Humanitarian Demining, 110
Geneva Protocol of 1925, 130–131
Genital mutilation, 194, 204, 459
Genocide
    in Cambodia, 369
    in Darfur, 210
    deaths from, 26
    in Rwanda, 212, 279–280, 373
Gerakan Aceh Merdeka, 429, 431–432
Germany, 8
Glanders, 143t
Goma, Zaire, 373–374
Great Britain, 136
"Greek Fire," 92
Group therapy, 61
Growth retardation, 181–182
Gruinard Island, 80
Guantánamo Bay, 228, 236
Guatemala, 295–298
Guernica, 4f
Guerrillas, 299
Gulf War. *See* Persian Gulf War
Guns. *See also* Firearms; Small arms and
    light weapons
    civilian ownership of, 98–99
    diversion of, 96–97
    global supply of, 96–98
    supply and demand for, 97–99
    violence caused by, 94–95

Hague Conventions
    description of, 12, 46
    1899, 363
    ignoring of, 46
    II, 82
    IV, 82
    1907, 363
    1914, 364
    VIII, 82
Hague Peace Conference of 1899, 130
Harsh interrogations, 228, 231, 234–235
Hayden, Michael V., 230
Hazardous wastes
    environmental effects of, 80
    from nuclear weapons production, 161
Health as a Bridge for Peace program, 445

Health professionals and workers
    activism by, 452–453
    burnout by, 412
    in conflict zones, 443
    education of, 440–449
    organizational support for, 413
    peace promotion by, 460–461
    postconflict situation effects on, 412–413
    psychological symptoms by, 412
Hemorrhagic fevers, 144t, 149
Hepatitis E, 217, 219
Herbicides
    description of, 72f, 73
    in Vietnam War, 320–323
Herzegovina, 9, 70, 218
Heymann, Philip, 231
High-altitude bombers, 12
"Highly coercive interrogation," 231
Hiroshima, 41, 46, 153f, 153–154
HIV, 194, 217–218, 414
Holocaust, 6
Honduran–Salvadoran war, 306
Honduras, 293, 306
Horn of Africa, 370
Hospitals
    destruction of, 43
    in North Vietnam, 319
    in South Vietnam, 318
Human Development Index (HDI), 30–31
Human rights
    education in, 445
    health professionals advocacy for, 18
    international protections, 37–38,
        44–49
    Iraq War effects on, 258–259
    medical neutrality, 43
    types of, 37
Human rights violations
    in Colombia, 299–300
    description of, 37–49
Human Security Report, 457–458
Human trafficking, 201
Humanitarian assistance organizations
    communicable disease control, 376–377
    data collection and use by, 371, 376
    delivery of health services, 376
    description of, 369–370
    emergency response teams, 416
    environmental settings for, 372

gender considerations in programs,
    378
in Goma, Zaire, 373–374
health standards for, 375–376
mortality rates affected by, 371–372
natural disaster responses by, 427,
    436–437
physical protection by, 377
resource transfer, 443
roles and responsibilities of, 375
Rwandan genocide, 373
Sphere Project, 374–376
witnessing and documenting of conflict
    by, 378–379
women protected by, 377–378
Humanitarian Charter, 374–375
Humanitarian law, 45–47
Hussein, Saddam, 258
Hydrogen bombs, 154–155, 156f

Immunizations, 182, 222–223, 397
Improvised explosive devices (IEDs)
    description of, 87, 89
    prohibition efforts, 93
Incendiary weapons
    description of, 12
    history of, 92
India, 5, 158t, 169t, 207, 459
Indiscriminate attacks, 90–91
Indiscriminate weapons, 41
Indonesia, 429, 432
Industrialized mass murder, 40
Infant mortality rates, 441
Infectious diseases
    in Democratic Republic of Congo war,
        283–286
    description of, 218–219
    diarrhea, 217, 222, 350
    violence and, 284–285
Information technology, 460
Infrastructure destruction
    description of, 10
    Iraq War, 42, 257
    Persian Gulf War, 42
    women affected by, 197
Infrastructure reconstruction, 353
Injury deaths
    causes of, 23
    information sources, 24–25

"Instructions for the Government of
Armies of the United States in the
Field," 362
Intellectual corruption, 44
Interfaith groups, 460
Internal conflicts, 32
Internally displaced persons, 220–221,
257–258
International Action Network on Small
Arms (IANSA), 386
International Agency for Research on
Cancer (IARC), 80
International Association of Lawyers
Against Nuclear Arms (IALANA),
366–367, 388
International Atomic Energy Agency
(IAEA), 166
International Campaign for the Abolition
of Nuclear Weapons, 388–389
International Campaign to Ban
Landmines, 104–106, 110
International Committee of the Red Cross
(ICRC), 104, 235, 420
International Convention Against Torture,
230
International Covenant on Civil and
Political Rights, 44, 48
International Covenant on Economic,
Social and Cultural Rights, 44
International Criminal Court, 47, 417
International Criminal Tribunal, 305
International law
"Convention with Respect to the Laws
and Customs of War on Land," 364
history of, 362–363
Lieber Code, 362–363
war fought according to, 361–365
International Medical Corps, 385
International Physicians for the Prevention
of Nuclear War (IPPNW), 171,
330, 366, 382f, 387–388, 444, 446
Interrogations, 228, 231, 234–235
Iodine-131, 17, 162
Iran, 28, 156, 157t
Iran–Iraq War, 243
Iraq, 5, 28
"brain drain" in, 414
chemical agents used by, 130
environmental contamination in, 70

ethnic cleansing in, 40
Oil-for-Food Program, 245
posttraumatic stress disorder in, 64
refugees from, 64
torture techniques, 228
Iraq War
child mortality rates, 255, 257
civilian injuries and casualties, 251–252,
256f
combat trauma in, 57–58
deaths from, 250, 251f
diversion of resources for, 259–260
economic environment affected by,
261
health consequences of, 243, 250–257
health services in Iraq affected by,
257
human rights effects, 258–259
infrastructure destruction caused by,
257
justification for, 245, 248
mental health problems secondary to,
250–251
physical environment affected by, 260
refugees of, 257–258
sociocultural environment affected by,
260–261
soldier's view of, 253–254
status of Iraq, 249t
timeline of, 245–250, 246t–248t
U.S. casualties in, 250, 252f
U.S. spending for, 10, 260–261
Vietnam War vs., 261
views on, 253–255
women's rights affected by, 259
Irish Republican Army, 97
Israel, 169t, 232–233

Janajweed militia, 221
Jathika Hela Urumaya, 435
Jordan, 258
"Just war" doctrine, 45

Kellogg-Briand Pact, 358–359
Khmer Rouge, 62, 228, 324
Korean War, 76
Kosovo, 62, 215, 373
Kurds, 40, 216, 219
Kuwait, 5, 11–12, 73f

"La Violencia," 298
Landmines
  in Africa, 108
  banning of, 104
  in Cambodia, 103–105
  causalities caused by, 107–108
  children injured by, 102–103, 107, 181
  civilian injuries caused by, 102–104
  countries with highest number of, 102
  description of, 5, 74–75
  environmental effects of, 103–104
  future of, 111, 114
  history of, 104–105
  injuries caused by
    amputations for, 103, 109
    medical treatment for, 107–108
    psychosocial consequences of, 109
    public health systems affected by,
      108–109
    rehabilitation for, 109–110
  Physicians for Human Rights efforts
    to ban, 384
  prevalence of, 102
  production of, 105
  public awareness of, 111–112
  reasons for using, 104–105
  risk education about, 112–113
  unexploded, 113
  in Vietnam, 316–317, 324
Laos, 331
Large-caliber artillery system, 88
Latin America wars
  Chiapas, Mexico, 301–302
  Chile, 303–305
  Colombia, 298–301
  Costa Rica, 302–303
  description of, 288–290
  El Salvador, 290–292
  Guatemala, 295–298
  internal conflicts as cause of, 307–308
  interstate conflicts as cause of, 306–307
  Nicaragua, 292–295, 309
  politics and, 308–309
  prevention of, 306–308
Latin American arms expenditures, 94
Latin American Nuclear Weapon Treaty,
  82–83
League of Nations, 363
Leahy, Patrick, 111

Letter bombs, 92
Leukemia, 78
Lewisite, 124
Liberation Tigers of Tamil Eelam, 386,
  434
Lieber, Francis, 362
Lieber Code, 362–363
Life integrity rights, 37, 42
Lung fibrosis, 164

M-19, 298
Machel Report, 189
Malaria, 217, 294–295, 352
Malignancies, from radioactive fallout,
  78–79
Malnutrition
  in children, 181–182, 220f, 257
  definition of, 219
  description of, 9
  in El Salvador, 291
  public health prevention of, 350–351
  in refugees, 218–219
  risk factors for, 350
  in Vietnam, 326–327
Marburg virus, 144t, 149
Marcos, Ferdinand, 458
Marginalized populations, 307–308
Martens Clause, 363–364
Mass murder, 40, 45
Mass rape, 61, 197
Measles, 217
Medact, 389
Médecins Sans Frontières (MSF), 297,
  382–384, 404, 443, 445
Medical care workers
  best interests of patient served by, 393
  in combatant roles, 399
  ethical behavior by, 393
  ethical dilemmas for
    battlefield triage, 396–397
    failing to provide care to civilians,
      398
    failing to provide optimal care to
      U.S. military personnel, 399
    failure to keep adequate records, 395
    immunizations, 397
    medical care used as a weapon, 400
    medical priorities for military
      purposes, 394–395

Medical care workers (*continued*)
  medical research on military
    personnel without informed
    consent, 395
  militarily useful research and
    development, 400
  moral actions, 401
  overriding of patients' wishes, 396
  patient confidentiality breaches, 395
  torture, 401
  treating of enemy military personnel,
    398
  Geneva Convention obligations of,
    397–399
  military service alternatives for,
    404–405
  mixed-agency conflicts, 393–394
  as moral agents, 403–405
  moral protest actions, 401–403
  opposition to war by, 405
  right to refuse military service, 402–403
  self-censorship by, 402
  societal education about war by, 405
Medical neutrality, 43
Mental health
  of civilians, 61–63
  in Iraq, 64, 250–251
  posttraumatic stress disorder. *See*
    Posttraumatic stress disorder
  societal effects, 54
Mental health treatment
  by Department of Veterans Affairs, 59
  economic effects of, 58–59
"Mercy euthanasia," 396
Metropolitan Medical Response System,
    125, 127
Mexico City, 291
Militarism, 244–245
Military dictatorships, 409
Military expenditures, 10, 11t
Military personnel
  confidentiality breaches, 395
  medical research on, 395
  overriding of wishes of, 396
  protest actions by, 401–402
Military service, 245, 402–403
Military sexual assault trauma, 59–60
Mines. *See* Landmines
Mine Ban Treaty, 104–107, 110

Mine Protocol II, 82
Mine risk education, 112–113
MINUGUA, 295
Missile systems, 89
Missing persons, 420–421
Mixed agency, 393–394
Model Nuclear Weapons Convention, 172
Mortality
  crude mortality rate. *See* Crude mortality
    rate
  humanitarian assistance organizations'
    effect on, 371–372
  infant mortality rates, 441
  refugee, 214–215
  statistics regarding, 23
Mosquito-borne diseases, 70
Mozambique, 108, 185, 415, 419
Munitions industry workers, 163
Mustard, 124–125
Myanmar, 384

Nagasaki, 41, 46, 153–154, 154f
Napalm, 93
Natural disasters
  in Aceh, 428–433
  aftermath of, 425–428
  economic effects of, 426
  global distribution of, 31
  humanitarian assistance for, 427,
    436–437
  natural, 424–428
  secondary effects of, 426–427
  in Sri Lanka, 433–436
Naval war, 82
Nazi, 304
Neutrality, 81
Nguyen Minh Triet, 330
Nicaragua, 292–295, 309
Nicholas II, 358
Nigeria, 459
"Night commuters," 188
Nixon, Richard, 325
Nongovernmental organizations
  CARE, 385–386
  consequences of war documented by,
    389
  conventional weapons efforts, 92
  firearms control efforts by, 98
  functions of, 381

history of, 381–382
HIV prevention programs by, 218
International Medical Corps, 385
International Physicians for the
    Prevention of Nuclear War
    (IPPNW), 171, 330, 366, 382f,
    387–388
Médecins Sans Frontières (MSF),
    382–384
mitigating the effects of war by, 382
nuclear weapon disarmament campaigns
    by, 387–389
Oxfam, 386
Physicians for Human Rights (PHR),
    384–385
Red Cross, 381–382
Save the Children, 386–387
small arms violence reduced by, 98,
    389–390
surveillance systems by, 347
Vietnam assistance from, 329
workers of, 34
Nonrenewable fuels, 75
Non-state actors, 12
Nonviolent conflict resolution, 17–18
North America Free Trade Agreement
    (NAFTA), 309
North Korea, 156, 158t, 169t
North Vietnam, 319–320, 327–328
Nuclear facilities, 76
Nuclear Nonproliferation Treaty (NPT),
    166–167, 170, 366, 388
Nuclear Posture Review, 168
Nuclear power, 170–171
Nuclear war, 82–83
Nuclear weapons
    abolition of, 171
    acute radiation sickness caused by,
        155t
    casualty predictions, 156, 157t
    Comprehensive Nuclear Test Ban Treaty
        (CTBT), 167–168
    conventional weapons vs., 366
    countries with, 367
    deterrent uses of, 367
    development of, 366
    dismantling and destruction of, 77, 169
    environmental effects, 161
    explosive force of, 152

global stockpile of, 169t
health impacts of, 153–165, 155t
    on Hiroshima, 153–154
    hydrogen bombs, 154–155, 156f
    inspections for, 166
    international control of, 165–168
    mechanism of action, 152
    military spending on, 165
    on Nagasaki, 153–154
    nongovernmental organizations' efforts
        to eliminate, 387–389
    Nuclear Nonproliferation Treaty (NPT),
        166–167, 170, 366, 388
    Partial Test Ban Treaty (PTBT),
        165–166
    plutonium stockpile caused by, 168
    post–Cold War proliferation of, 168
    present-day scenarios for, 156–158,
        157t
    production of
        description of, 160–162
        health effects to workers involved in,
            163–164
        resource diversion for, 165
    public health threats from, 161–162
    radiation from, 154
    radioactive fallout from, 78–79,
        159–160
    recommended future restrictions on,
        169–172
    research of, 168
    "rogue nation" acquisition of, 367
    secrecy associated with, 162, 165
    test ban treaties, 165–168
    testing of, 158t, 158–160
    U.S. production of, 77, 160–161, 165,
        169t
    weapons of mass destruction, 365
Nuclear Weapons Convention (NWC),
    172
Nuclear-weapons-free zones, 167
Nuremberg Code, 395
Nuremberg Principles, 44, 304
Nuremberg Trials, 46, 304

Oil-for-Food Program, 245
Oklahoma City bombing, 13, 63
Operation Desert Storm, 244
Organophosphorus pesticides, 122

Organization for the Prohibition of
  Chemical Weapons, 131, 132f
Organization of American States, 306
Organophosphorus compounds, 122–123
Ottawa Convention, 106–107
Over-evacuation, 396
Oxfam, 386

Pacifism, 402
Pakistan, 5, 158t, 169t, 207, 425
Palestinians, 233
Pan American Health Organization
  (PAHO), 289
Pappas, Thomas, 234
Partial Test Ban Treaty (PTBT), 165–166
Paternalism, 396
Peace
  culture of, 453, 454t, 456–460
  education about, 189
  health professionals' role in promoting,
    460–461
  organizations that promote, 463–467
Peace agreements, 190
Peacetime forces
  environmental impact of, 76–80
  reasons for maintaining, 76–77
Pellagra, 219
Penetrating trauma, 91
Pentagon, 12
People's Army of Vietnam, 315
Permanent Court of Arbitration, 358
Persian Gulf War
  description of, 12, 42
  health consequences of, 243, 245
  oil releases during, 73f, 74
  Oil-for-Food Program, 245
  posttraumatic stress disorder in veterans
    of, 55
  refugees of, 257–258
Peruvian Truth Commission, 418
Pharmacotherapy, 61
Phosgene, 123
Physicians for Human Rights (PHR), 302,
  384–385, 416
Physicians for Social Responsibility
  (PSR), 444
Pinochet, Augusto, 304–305
Plague, 143t, 145–146
Plan Colombia, 289–290

Plastic explosives, 91
Plutonium, 164, 168
Pol Pot, 369
Political marginalization, 307
Postconflict phase. *See also* Postwar period
  balance of power, 418
  criminal justice in, 417–418
  definition of, 409–411
  health care restoration, 414
  health workers affected by, 412–413
  lack of financial resources, 415
  missing persons, 420–421
  prosecution for crimes, 419
  psychological healing, 420
  public health prevention of health
    consequences in, 342, 344t–345t,
    352–354
  reconciliation commissions, 418
  rehabilitation programs, 415–416
  transition process, 415
  truth commissions, 418
Posttraumatic stress disorder (PTSD)
  in Afghanistan populations, 64, 352
  in African populations, 63–64
  barriers for mental health care for, 58
  in children, 62, 183, 187
  in civilians, 62
  comorbidities, 53–55
  coping with, 63–64
  cultural considerations, 63
  description of, 5
  developmental childhood trauma and, 57
  diagnosis of, 52–53
  epidemiology of, 55–58
  evolution of, 51–52
  from explosive attacks, 91–92
  features associated with, 53
  gender and, 57
  in Iraq War soldiers, 251
  medical comorbidities, 55
  military sexual assault trauma as cause
    of, 59–60
  multiple deployments and, 58
  neurobiology of, 60
  neuroimaging studies of, 60
  pharmacotherapy for, 61
  posttraumatic environment and, 57
  prevalence of, 55–56
  psychosocial interventions for, 65

in refugees, 62–63, 411
risk factors, 56–57, 351
substance-use disorders associated with, 53–54
symptoms of, 52–53, 64–65, 183
treatment of, 60–61
underdiagnosis of, 56
in Vietnam veterans, 54–56, 331
violent behavior and, 54
Post-Tsunami Operational Management Structure, 435
Postwar period. *See also* Postconflict phase
victimization of women in, 200–201
violence in, 94
Poverty, 328
Pralidoxime, 123
Prazosin, 61
Preconflict phase, of armed conflict, 342, 343t, 347–349
Preemptive war, 361
Prevention
primary, 15, 446, 453
public health. *See* Public health prevention
secondary, 15, 18, 45, 447, 453
tertiary, 15, 19
Prisoners of war
description of, 325
Geneva Conventions regarding, 364
provisions for, 46
Proportionality, 49
Prosecution for crimes, 419
Prostitution, 188
Protocol on Prohibitions or Restrictions on the Use of Incendiary Weapons, 92
Psychological injuries
to children, 182–184
posttraumatic stress disorder. *See* Posttraumatic stress disorder
in refugees, 411
risk factors for, 351
from torture, 229
Psychotropic medications, 377
PTSD. *See* Posttraumatic stress disorder
Public health
culture of peace and, 456
culture of violence and, 455–456
definition of, 3, 455

nuclear weapons threats to, 161–162
war effects on, 3–4, 19
Public health prevention of health consequences
communicable diseases, 351
in conflict phase, 342, 343t–344t
diarrheal diseases, 350
framework for, 340–342
malnutrition, 350–351
in postconflict phase, 342, 344t–345t
in preconflict phase, 342, 343t
strategies for improving, 346–347
unified model for. *See* Unified model
Public health professionals, 15–19

Q fever, 80

Radiation Exposure Compensation Program, 162
Radiation sickness, 155t
Radiation-induced thyroid cancer, 160
Radioactive fallout, 78–79, 159–160
Radioactive materials, 77
Rape
of children, 188, 190
ethnic cleansing, 194, 196
HIV transmission through, 194
mass, 61, 197
measures to reduce, 190
posttraumatic stress disorder secondary to, 57, 59–60
war-related, 6, 9
of women, 9, 194, 221
"Rape of Nanking," 6
Rations, 222
Reagan administration, 292–293
Reconciliation commissions, 418–419
Red Cross, 381–382
Refugee camps
crude mortality rates in, 371f
description of, 221–222
Refugees
children, 216, 219
countries with highest number of, 208, 209t
from Darfur, 5, 210–212, 219
death of, 216–218
description of, 31
diarrheal diseases in, 217

Refugees (*continued*)
global distribution of, 208, 209t
high-risk groups, 216, 219
from Iraq, 64
Kosovar, 215
Kurdish, 216, 219
malaria in, 217
malnutrition in, 219
measles epidemics in, 217
mortality rates in, 214–215
nutritional deficiencies in, 218–220
Persian Gulf War, 257–258
posttraumatic stress disorder in, 62–63, 411
psychological trauma in, 411
rations for, 222
relief programs for, 221–225
return of, 411, 414
from Rwanda, 212, 373
statistics regarding, 207–208
United Nations High Commissioner for Refugees (UNHCR), 208, 370, 418
Vietnam, 324
vulnerability of, 10
women, 197, 200
Rehabilitation
of children, 190–191
from landmine injuries, 109–110
postconflict, 415–416
Relief programs, for refugees and displaced persons, 221–225
REMHI Commission, 296
Renunciation of War Pact, 81
Resources diversion
description of, 10
for Iraq War, 259–260
for Vietnam War, 330–331
Respiratory tract irritants, 120t–121t, 123–124
Responsibility to Protect, 203
Rotblat, Józef, 171
Routinization, 236–237
Russell–Einstein Manifesto, 387
Russia, 169t
Rwanda
conflicts in, 6, 34
diarrheal diseases in, 350
ethnic cleansing in, 40
genocide in, 212, 279–280, 373

health workers affected by, 412
mass raping of women in, 199
mortality rates, 373–374
posttraumatic stress disorder, 63–64
refugees from, 212, 373

Sanctions, 10, 17, 190
Sandinistas, 294
Sarin attacks in Japan, 117, 127–128
Save the Children, 386–387
Scurvy, 220
Seabed Treaty, 83
Secondary prevention, 15, 18, 45, 447, 453
Selective serotonin reuptake inhibitors, 61
Self-defense, 45
SEMTEX, 91
September 11, 2001, 12, 14, 91, 233, 244
Septicemic plague, 146
Sexual assaults, 5, 221. *See also* Rape
Sexual violence, 9, 11
"Shell shock," 51
Sierra Leone, 197–198, 417, 419
Siracusa Principles, 49
Skills education, 442
Sleep deprivation, 235
Small arms, 33
Small arms and light weapons. *See also* Arms; Firearms; Guns
Aiming For Prevention campaign, 390
"culture of violence" created by, 97
deaths from, 94, 95t
definition of, 87–88
diversion of, 96–97
global supply of, 96–98
governmental efforts to control, 98
national stockpiles of, 97
nongovernmental organizations' efforts to control, 98, 389–390
secondary effects of, 95
violence caused by, 94–95
Small Arms Survey, 94
Smallpox, 144t, 147–148, 148f
Soldiers
children as, 185–187
women as, 197–198
Somalia, 220–221, 370

Somatization, 55
Somoza, Anastasio, 292
South Africa, 97
South America, 289–290
South Pacific Nuclear Free
    Zone Treaty, 82
South Vietnam, 314, 317–319, 323–324
Southeast Asia Nuclear Weapon Free
    Treaty, 82–83
Southeast Asian Treaty Organization
    (SEATO), 314
Soviet Union, 138, 158t, 161, 169t
Specter, Arlen, 111
Sphere Project, 374–376
Spitsbergen Treaty, 81
Spousal abuse, 200
Sri Lanka, 433–436
Starvation, 181–182
Strategic Arms Limitation Talks, 167
Stream manipulation, 74
Sudan, 24, 210, 385
Suicide, 55
Surplus weapons, 99
Surveillance, 16

Tai Ping Movement, 71
Tamils, 433–434
Tear gas, 123
Teenage gangs, 11
Terrorism
    chemical agents used in, 127–128
    description of, 13–14
    explosives used in, 91
    torture methods and, 229–230
Tertiary prevention, 15, 19
2,3,7,8-Tetrachlorodibenzo-*p*-dioxin,
    320–322
Thailand, 327, 369
Third Reich, 8
Thirty Years War, 45
Thyroid cancer, 160
Thyroid tablets, 17
Tokyo War Crimes Trial, 9
Torture
    at Abu Ghraib, 199–200, 229f,
        234–236
    of children, 188
    condemnation of, 228–229
    definition of, 227, 230

    dehumanization and, 237
    description of, 6
    factors necessary for, 236–237
    harsh interrogations, 228, 231,
        234–236
    interrogation methods, 228
    justifications for, 231–232
    mechanisms of, 227
    medical care worker's ethical dilemmas
        regarding, 401
    political repression uses of, 228
    posttraumatic stress disorder secondary
        to, 57
    prevalence of, 227
    psychological effects of, 229,
        236–237
    safeguards against, 234–235
    studies of, 236–237
    terrorism and, 229–230
    by United States, 233–234
    waterboarding, 228
Toxic metals, 163–164
Triage, 396–397
Trial of the Major War Criminals, 304
2,4,5-Trichlorophenoxyacetic acid, 73,
    320
Trinitrotoluene, 163
Truth commissions, 418–419
Tsunamis, 424, 428, 433–435
Tularemia, 143t, 146

Unexploded ordnance, 316–317, 350,
    352
Unified model
    applications of, 345–347
    conflict phase application of,
        350–352
    description of, 342
    postconflict phase application of,
        352–354
    preconflict phase application of,
        347–349
United Kingdom, 11, 136, 158t, 169t
United Nations
    Charter of, 359–361
    Children's Fund, 10, 245
    Conference on the Illicit Trafficking in
        Small Arms and Light Weapons
        in All Its Aspects, 98

United Nations (*continued*)
Crime Prevention and Criminal Justice
Commission, 98
Development Program, 416, 447
employees of, 34
Environment Program, 70
High Commissioner for Refugees, 208,
370, 418
history of, 359
Registry of Conventional Arms, 93
Security Council Resolution 1325,
202–203
United Nations-African Union mission in
Darfur, 211
United States
biological weapons production and
testing by, 136, 138
firearm exports by, 97
militarism in, 244–245
military service in, 245
in Nicaragua wars, 292–293
nuclear weapon production by, 77,
160–161, 165, 169t
Vietnam War effects on, 330–332
Weapons of Mass Destruction
Commission, 170–171
United States Agency for International
Development (USAID),
308–309
United States Campaign to Ban
Landmines, 111
Universal Declaration of Human Rights,
44, 48, 308
Uppsala Conflict Data Project, 24,
30–31
Uranium, depleted, 12, 70, 260
Uranium miners, 160, 162

Vaccinations
anthrax, 145
smallpox, 148
Venezuelan equine encephalitis, 80
Vesicants, 120t–121t, 124
Vessey Initiative, 329
Victim-activated Landmine
Abolition Act of 2006, 111
Viet Cong, 315
Vietnam
assistance for, 329–330

demographics of, 315
description of, 11
economic reform effects, 328–329
embargo of, 323–325
exports by, 329
food shortages in, 326–327
geography of, 315–316
health care services in, 327–329
history of, 314–315
infant mortality rate in, 326
infrastructure in, 328
malnutrition in, 326–327
population of, 326
poverty in, 328
refugees from, 324
South, 314
U.S. promises to rebuild, 325
Vietnam Association of Victims of Agent
Orange, 321–322
Vietnam Memorial, 332
Vietnam War
Agent Orange use in, 320–322
background, 314–317
civilians in
deaths of, 316
health services for, 317–320
deaths in, 313, 314t, 331
dioxin exposure, 320–321
environmental destruction during, 70,
316, 320, 322–323
explosives used in, 316
health facilities destroyed during,
320
health services during, 317–320
herbicides used in, 320–323
immediate effects of, 316–317
injuries sustained in, 331–332
Iraq War vs., 261
landmine injuries in, 108, 324
long-term effects of, 323–325
missing in action soldiers from, 325
North Vietnam, 319–320
postwar effects of, 323–325
prisoners of war, 325
South Vietnamese, 317–319
unexploded bombs and landmines after,
316–317
United States effects of, 330–332
veterans of, 54–56, 331–332

Violence
  collective, 26–27
  culture of, 453, 454t, 455–456
  cycle of, 11
  description of, 3, 373
  firearms-related, 94–95
  gender-based, 378
  health affected by, 441
  infectious diseases and, 284–285
  postwar, 94
  sexual, 9, 11
Violent behavior, 54
Viral hemorrhagic fevers, 144t, 149
Vitamin A deficiency, 219

War. *See also* Armed conflict;
    specific war
  brutality of, 5–9, 361–362
  cognitive effects of, 65
  conventional, 81–82
  definition of, 3, 38
  epidemiology of, 457–458
  etiology of, 456–457
  inevitability of, 357
  legal constraints, 80–83
  opposition to, 405
  preemptive, 361
  prevention of, 453, 456–457
  psychiatric effects of, 65
  risk factors for, 348t, 348–349,
    446–447
  writings about, 357–358
"War on drugs," 299
"War on terror," 14, 228
Warship, 89
Water pollution, 69–70
Waterboarding, 228. *See also* Torture
Weapons
  advances in, 12
  biological. *See* Biological weapons
  chemical. *See* Chemical agents and
    weapons
  conventional. *See* Conventional
    weapons
  expenditures on, 10–11
  health effects of production of,
    163–164
  incendiary. *See* Incendiary weapons
  indiscriminate, 41

  nuclear. *See* Nuclear weapons
  surplus, 99
Weapons of mass destruction (WMDs),
    365–367
Weapons of Mass Destruction
    Commission, 170–171
Widows, 200
Wildfires, 76
Women
  at-risk populations, 193–194
  civil infrastructure destruction effects
    on, 197
  in combatant role, 197–198
  cultural factors that affect, 195–197
  Darfur genocide of, 211
  in decision-making bodies, 203–204
  domestic violence against, 200
  empowerment of, 458–460
  gender training for troops, 203
  genital mutilation of, 194, 204, 459
  HIV transmission to, 194
  humanitarian assistance organizations'
    protection of, 377–378
  humiliation of male enemies by
    exploitation of, 196–197
  inferior social status of, 195
  Iraq War effects on, 259
  in labor force, 202
  lack of protection for, 199
  opportunities for, 204
  in postwar period, 200–201
  in prewar period, 198
  raping of, 9, 194, 221
  refugees, 197, 200
  rights of, 195, 201–202
  roles and responsibilities of, 195–196
  spousal abuse, 200
  trafficking of, 201
  U.N. Security Council Resolution
    1325 for, 202–203
  vulnerability of
    description of, 9
    measures to end, 201–204
    predisposing factors for, 194–198
  in war period, 198–200
  widows, 200
Wood, Leonard, 399
World Health Organization (WHO),
    23–24, 366, 413, 454

World Medical Association (WMA), 440
World Trade Center (WTC), 12, 13, 91
World War I
  chemical agents used in, 128
  description of, 26, 44
World War II
  biological agent testing, 136
  civilian deaths in, 47
  efforts to prevent, 358–359
  environmental warfare in, 76
  exploitation of women in, 197

general discussions of, 11, 26–28,
  44, 46
mental health issues, 56

Yersinia pestis, 145–146
Yudhoyono, Susilo Bambang, 430
Yugoslavia, 40, 65

Zaire, 280, 373
Zapatista Army for the National
  Liberation, 301

CPSIA information can be obtained
at www.ICGtesting.com
Printed in the USA
LVHW02s1959291117
557996LV00003B/6/P

9 780195 311273